SEXUAL HEALTH

Selected Titles in ABC-CLIO's
**CONTEMPORARY
WORLD ISSUES**
Series

American Families in Crisis, Jeffrey S. Turner
Animal Rights, Clifford J. Sherry
Campaign and Election Reform, Glenn H. Utter and
        Ruth Ann Strickland
Climate Change, David L. Downie, Kate Brash, and
        Catherine Vaughan
Corporate Crime, Richard D. Hartley
DNA Technology, David E. Newton
Domestic Violence, Margi Laird McCue
Education in Crisis, Judith A. Gouwens
Emergency Management, Jeffrey B. Bumgarner
Environmental Justice, David E. Newton
Gangs, Karen L. Kinnear
Gay and Lesbian Rights, David E. Newton
Globalization, Justin Ervin and Zachary A. Smith
Identity Theft, Sandra K. Hoffman and Tracy G. McGinley
Lobbying in America, Ronald J. Hrebenar and Bryson B. Morgan
Modern Sports Ethics, Angela Lumpkin
Nuclear Weapons and Nonproliferation, Sarah J. Diehl and
        James Clay Moltz
Obesity, Judith Stern and Alexandra Kazaks
Policing in America, Leonard A. Steverson
Renewable and Alternative Energy Resources, Zachary A. Smith and
        Katrina D. Taylor
Rich and Poor in America, Geoffrey Gilbert
Sentencing, Dean John Champion
Sexual Crime, Caryn E. Neumann
U.S. National Security, Cynthia A. Watson
U.S. Social Security, Steven G. Livingston
U.S. Trade Issues, Alfred E. Eckes, Jr.
Waste Management, Jacqueline Vaughn

For a complete list of titles in this series, please visit
www.abc-clio.com.

Books in the Contemporary World Issues series address vital issues in today's society, such as genetic engineering, pollution, and biodiversity. Written by professional writers, scholars, and nonacademic experts, these books are authoritative, clearly written, up-to-date, and objective. They provide a good starting point for research by high school and college students, scholars, and general readers as well as by legislators, businesspeople, activists, and others.

Each book, carefully organized and easy to use, contains an overview of the subject, a detailed chronology, biographical sketches, facts and data and/or documents and other primary-source material, a directory of organizations and agencies, annotated lists of print and nonprint resources, and an index.

Readers of books in the Contemporary World Issues series will find the information they need to have a better understanding of the social, political, environmental, and economic issues facing the world today.

SEXUAL HEALTH

A Reference Handbook

David E. Newton

**CONTEMPORARY
WORLD ISSUES**

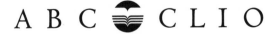

A B C CLIO

Santa Barbara, California
Denver, Colorado
Oxford, England

Library of Congress Cataloging-in-Publication Data

Newton, David E.
  Sexual health : a reference handbook / David E. Newton.
    p. cm. — (Contemporary world issues)
  Includes bibliographical references and index.
  ISBN 978-1-59884-366-8 (alk. paper) — ISBN 978-1-59884-367-5 (ebook)
  1. Hygiene, Sexual. 2. Sex—Handbooks, manuals, etc. I. Title.
  RA788.N49 2010
  613.9'5—dc22   2009037221

14 13 12 11 10   1 2 3 4 5

This book is also available on the World Wide Web as an eBook.
Visit www.abc-clio.com for details.

ABC-CLIO, LLC
130 Cremona Drive, P.O. Box 1911
Santa Barbara, California 93116-1911

For Gary Sikkema, worthy student, fellow traveler on the road of life, good friend!

Contents

List of Tables, xv
Preface, xvii

1   **Background and History, 1**
    Introduction, 1
    Sexually Transmitted Infections, 2
        An Ancient Issue, 2
        Types of Infections, 3
        Symptoms, Prognosis, and Treatment, 5
        Chlamydia, 5
        Syphilis, 6
        Gonorrhea, 8
        Herpes, 9
        Hepatitis, 10
        HIV/AIDS, 12
    Pregnancy and Contraception, 14
        Barrier Methods, 15
        Hormonal Methods, 17
        Intrauterine Devices, 19
        Fertility Awareness and Abstinence, 19
        Sterilization, 20
        A Concluding Observation, 21
    Sexual Orientation and Gender Identity, 21
        Terminology, 22
        Gay, Lesbian, Bisexual, Transgender, and Questioning
            Youth Issues, 24
        Options for GLBTQ Youth, 26
        Progress: A Mixed Blessing?, 28
    References, 28

2 **Problems, Controversies, and Solutions, 31**
Introduction, 31
Sex Education: Yes or No?, 33
Public Opinion on Sex Education, 34
The Content of Sex Education Courses, 36
  Abstinence-Only Education, 36
  Condom Instruction, 42
  Homosexuality, 44
  Abortion, 50
  What Should Schools Teach about Sex?, 52
Issues That Transcend School Programs, 53
  Access to Contraceptive Devices, 53
  Access to Contraceptives outside of Schools, 57
  The Controversy over Plan B, 58
  Pharmacist Choice in Filling Contraceptive Prescriptions, 59
  Human Papillomavirus (HPV), 62
In Conclusion, 65
References, 66

3 **Worldwide Perspective, 75**
Sex Education, 76
  Europe, 76
  Asia and Australasia, 81
  The Muslim World, 84
  Latin America, 85
  Africa, 87
New Issues of Concern in Human Sexuality, 87
  The HIV/AIDS Pandemic, 88
  Other Sexually Transmitted Infections, 94
  Contraception and Family Planning, 96
  Sexual Orientation and Gender Identity, 98
References, 101

4 **Chronology, 107**

5 **Biographical Sketches, 127**
Mary Steichen Calderone, 127
Min-Chueh Chang, 129
Anthony Comstock, 130
Paul Ehrlich, 131
Kevin Jennings, 132
Alfred Kinsey, 133

Charles Knowlton, 135
Beverly LaHaye, 136
Hideyo Noguchi, 137
Elise Ottesen-Jensen, 138
Robert Parlin, 139
Paul VI, 140
Gregory Goodwin Pincus, 141
John Rock, 142
John D. Rockefeller III, 143
Margaret Sanger, 145
Matthew Shepard, 146
Marie Stopes, 148
Brandon Teena, 149
Karolina Olivia Widerström, 150
Harald zur Hausen, 151
References, 152

6   **Data and Documents, 153**
Documents, 153
    Texas Sex Education Law (1995), 153
    Separate Program for Abstinence Education (1996), 154
    Memorandum for the Administrator of the United
        States Agency for International Development (2001),
        156
    South Dakota House Bill 1215 (2006), 157
    Responsible Education About Life Act (2007), 159
    Mandatory HPV Vaccination (2007), 161
    Access to Birth Control Act (2007), 163
    Mexico City Policy (2009), 167
Court Cases, 168
    Griswold v. Connecticut (1965), 168
    Roe v. Wade (1973), 170
    Curtis v. School Committee of Falmouth (1995), 171
    Parker v. Hurley, 474 F. Supp. 2d 261 (2007), 174
    Gonzalez v. School Board of Okeechobee County (2008), 177
Reports, 180
    The Surgeon General's Call to Action to Promote
        Sexual Health and Responsible Sexual Behavior
        (2001), 180
    The Content of Federally Funded Abstinence-only
        Education Programs (2004), 182
Data, 184

Cases of Sexually Transmitted Diseases Reported by
State Health Departments and Rates per 100,000
Population: United States, 1941–2007, 184
Estimated Number of Cases of Other Sexually
Transmitted Infections in the
United States, 1966–2007, 184
Characteristics of Women Who Obtained Legal
Abortions—United States, 1973–2005, 188
Pregnancy and Live Birthrates for Females
15–19 Years of Age, by Age, Race,
and Hispanic Origin: United States,
Selected Years, 1980–2000, 192
Percentage of High School Students Who Were
Currently Sexually Active, Who Used a Condom
during or Birth Control Pills before Last Sexual
Intercourse, by Sex, Race/Ethnicity, and
Grade, 2003, 193
Worldwide Data on HIV/AIDS, 2008, 194
Estimated Number of Orphans Due to AIDS, 2008, 194

7 **Directory of Organizations, Associations,
and Agencies, 197**
Governmental Agencies, 197
Agency for Healthcare Research and Quality (AHRQ), 197
Division of STD Prevention (DSTDP) Centers for
Disease Control and Prevention, 198
The Kinsey Institute for Research in Sex, Gender, and
Reproduction, 198
National Institute of Allergy and Infectious Diseases
(NIAID), 199
Office of Population Affairs (OPA), Office of
Public Health and Science, U.S. Department
of Health and Human Services, 200
United Nations Population Fund (UNPF), 200
World Health Organization (WHO), 201
Nongovernmental Agencies, 202
Abortion Access Project (AAP), 202
Abstinence the Better Choice (ABC), 202
Advocates for Youth, 203
American Association of Sex Educators,
Counselors and Therapists (AASECT), 203

American Sexually Transmitted Diseases
    Association (ASTDA), 204
American Social Health Association (ASHA), 204
Association of Reproductive Health
    Professionals (ARHP), 205
AVERT, 205
Bixby Center for Global Reproductive Health, 206
BOMA-USA, 206
Catholics for Choice (CFC), 207
Center for Reproductive Rights (CRC), 207
Centre for Development and Population
    Activities (CEDPA), 208
Concerned Women for America (CWA), 209
Contraceptive Research and Development
    Program (CONRAD), 209
Couple to Couple League (CCL), 210
EngenderHealth, 211
Family Health International (FHI), 211
Family Research Council (FRC), 212
Focus on the Family, 212
Guttmacher Institute (GI), 213
International Consortium on Emergency Contraception
    (ICEC), 213
International Society for Sexually Transmitted
    Diseases Research (ISSTDR), 214
International Union against Sexually Transmitted
    Infections (IUSTI), 214
Ipas, 215
Kaiser Family Foundation, 215
NARAL—Pro-Choice America, 216
National Campaign to Prevent Teen and Unplanned
    Pregnancy, 216
National Right to Life (NRL), 217
National Women's Health Resource Center (NWHRC), 218
Pharmacy Access Partnership, 218
Planned Parenthood Federation of America (PPFA), 219
Population Action International (PAI), 219
Population Council (PC), 220
Pro-Choice Public Education Project (PEP), 221
Religious Coalition for Reproductive Choice (RCRC), 221
Reproductive Health Technologies Project (RHTP), 222

Sexuality Information and Education Council of the
    United States (SIECUS), 223
United States Conference of Bishops, 223
Young People's Sexual Health (YPSH), 224
Gay and Lesbian Youth Group, 224
    Gay and Lesbian Community Center of the Ozarks
        (GLCCO), 225
    Gay, Lesbian and Straight Education Network (GLSEN), 225
    Human Rights Campaign (HRC), 225
    Matthew Shepard Foundation (MSF), 226
    Parents, Families & Friends of Lesbians & Gays (PFLAG),
        226
    Sexual Minority Youth Assistance League (SMYAL), 227
    Utah Pride Center, 227
    Youth Guardian Services (YGS), 228
    Youth Pride, 228

8   **Selected Print and Nonprint Resources, 231**
    General, 231
        Books, 231
        Articles, 233
        Reports, 236
        Web Sites, 239
    Sexually Transmitted Infections, 241
        Books, 241
        Articles, 243
        Reports, 245
        Web Sites, 248
    Contraception and Abortion, 250
        Books, 250
        Articles, 252
        Reports, 254
        Web Sites, 256
    Sexual Identity and Sexual Orientation, 260
        Books, 260
        Articles, 262
        Reports, 264
        Web Sites, 267

Glossary, 269
Index, 277
About the Author, 291

List of Tables

1.1   Cases of Certain STIs in the United States, 2007, 5
1.2   Effectiveness of Various Contraceptive Methods, 16
3.1   Youth Education on Sexual Orientation in 16 European
      Countries, 100
6.1   Cases of Sexually Transmitted Diseases Reported by State
      Health Departments and Rates Per 100,000 Population:
      United States, 1941–2007, 185
6.2   Estimated Number of Cases of Other Sexually Transmitted
      Infections in the United States, 1966–2007, 189
6.3   Characteristics of Women Who Obtained Legal Abortions—
      United States, 1973–2005, 190
6.4   Pregnancy and Live Birthrates for Females 15–19 Years
      of Age, by Age, Race, and Hispanic Origin: United States,
      Selected Years, 1980–2000, 193
6.5   Percentage of High School Students Who Were Currently
      Sexually Active, Who Used a Condom During or Birth
      Control Pills before Last Sexual Intercourse, by Sex, Race/
      Ethnicity, and Grade, 2003, 194
6.6   Worldwide Data on HIV/AIDS, 2008, 195
6.7   Estimated Number of Orphans due to AIDS, 2008, 196

Preface

Adolescence is a period of great turmoil in a person's life. A flood of hormones changes the body of a girl into that of a woman, the body of a boy into that of a man, often at a rapid pace. The relative calm and peacefulness of childhood is replaced by a rush of new biological sensations, emotional feelings, social challenges and interpersonal questions with which one has never had to deal before. For the first time, a person has to think about relating with other individuals of the same and opposite sex in new ways, ways that involve the possibility of sexual contact and intercourse.

But sexuality, for all the joys and physical pleasures it brings, is a risky human behavior. When two bodies come into contact, a host of possibilities arise. Some of these possibilities are glorious, the chance of bringing new life into the world. But some possibilities are less than wonderful. In the first place, the chance of bringing new life into the world may not be the best possible outcome for two 16-year-olds who have just been introduced to the experience of sexual activity. They may have too much of their adolescence left before them to contemplate starting a family of their own. How do teenagers feeling the power of hormonal drives develop control over their emotional feelings and physical desires to make sure they do not find themselves in an impossible family situation? It is thus that family planning can become an issue of serious consequence for young people who are barely beyond the stage of childhood themselves. Society must find a way to provide information and guidance for teenagers faced with such problems. Some people argue that the family is the best or only place for such discussions to occur. Other people see that education in human sexuality is a reasonable and desirable function of the school also. Still other people look to other agencies—

religious groups, health centers, nongovernmental organizations, and the like—to provide these services.

Sexual contact between two people can also have profound health consequences. Sometimes, diseases can be spread that are irritating and inconvenient, but hardly life threatening. Still, they are conditions with which a person has to deal. In other cases, sexually transmitted infections can, indeed, be among the most serious diseases a person can contract, even resulting in death. The HIV/AIDS pandemic has made the modern world more aware of that fact than any disease in modern history. Teenagers need information as to how they can avoid such infections. Again, adults differ as to the best way to achieve this objective, with some arguing for sexual abstinence until marriage as the only way to avoid the risk of pregnancy as well as that of sexually transmitted infections. Others say that the human sex drive is so strong that expecting adolescents to be abstinent is unrealistic, and society must find ways to teach teenagers about the ways of avoiding not only pregnancy, but also diseases that can be spread through sexual contact.

Finally, adolescence is also a period when many boys and girls begin to question their own sexual orientation and gender identity, questions that they almost certainly have never thought about before. Almost-men find themselves physically and emotionally attracted to other males, and almost-women find themselves drawn to other females. And on another level entirely, some males may begin to question the concordance (or lack of it) between their biological gender (male or female) and how they feel in the depths of their hearts about their own gender.

The sex drive so deeply ingrained in human beings is, thus, the source of countless issues and controversies as one grows through adolescence. And given the depth of feeling that most people have about sexual issues, it is hardly surprising that some of these issues and controversies are at the center of the greatest social and political debates in progress in the United States and around the world. This books attempts to provide an introduction to those issues and to resources available for analyzing them further. The first chapter of the book provides some broad general background about the process of conception and the methods by which it can be controlled; an introduction to the subject of sexually transmitted infections; and a discussion of the development of sexual orientation and gender identity. Chapter 2 of the book discusses some of the issues surrounding pregnancy and contraception, sexually transmitted infections, and sexual orientation and gender identity. It attempts to present an unbiased review of arguments for and against a number of specific issues with which society is now dealing, questions such as the type of sex education children and adolescents should have, the role of educational institutions in providing contraceptive information and materials, and the extent to which schools should become involved in discussions of same-sex relationships.

Chapter 3 looks to the status of many of these same issues in countries around the world. Given varying cultural, social, and religious attitudes toward human sexuality, it is hardly surprising that almost every philosophy and set of practices about the education of young people about sexuality can be found somewhere in the world. This chapter reviews some of those philosophies and practices. Chapters 4 through 8 provide resource materials intended for those readers who would like to learn more about these topics. Chapter 4 provides a chronology of important events related to the issues discussed in this book, while Chapter 5 provides biographical sketches of some important individuals in the history of human sexuality.

Chapter 6 contains excerpts from some important documents dealing with issues related to human sexuality: laws, regulations, policy statements, court decisions, and statistics and data. Chapter 7 lists a number of print and electronic resources to which the reader can turn for more detailed information on any of the topics discussed in the book, while Chapter 8 lists organizations interested in issues of sexual health to whom one can turn for further information. Finally, a glossary provides definitions of some basic terms used in the book.

1

Background and History

Introduction

Aaron was stunned. He had never expected to get a telephone call like this one. The public health nurse wanted him to come in . . . to be tested for syphilis! His friend, Dale, had just been to the clinic and tested positive for syphilis. Dale had named Aaron as a sexual contact. Now Aaron had to be tested too.

Aaron knew that syphilis was a dangerous disease. He had heard that people went blind and even died from the disease. What had he done wrong? Should he have been more careful? Dale was a good friend. Why had Dale not told him about the possible risks of their having sex together? Could the infection be cured? Maybe he could find something in the drug store to take against the disease. Aaron was so embarrassed! How could he ever face Dale again? Or any of his friends? Or his family?

Many people experience medical problems associated with their reproductive systems at least once in their lives. Such problems are usually—but not always—the result of contact with another person, as with Aaron and Dale. They may be a question of disease, as in cases involving syphilis, gonorrhea, chlamydia, HIV/AIDS, or a number of other conditions. Or they may involve issues of contraception, in the case of a sexual contact that may have resulted in pregnancy. Or they may involve emotional rather than physical issues, centering on questions about a person's sexual identity or sexual orientation. This chapter provides background on these three large areas of sexual health: sexually transmitted infections, contraception and pregnancy, and sexual identity and sexual orientation.

1

Sexually Transmitted Infections

The issue with which Aaron has to deal involves a group of diseases known collectively as sexually transmitted infections (STIs). At one time (and still among many individuals), the diseases were known as sexually transmitted diseases (STDs) or venereal diseases (VDs). Diseases that fall into this category include amebiasis, bacterial vaginosis, campylobacter fetus, candidiasis, chancroid, chlamydia, condyloma acuminata, cytomegalovirus, enteric infections, genital mycoplasmas, genital warts, giardiasis, gonorrhea, granuloma inguinale, hepatitis, herpes, HIV disease, lymphogranuloma venereum, molluscum contagiosum, pediculosis pubis, salmonella, scabies, shingellosis, syphilis, trichomoniasis, yeast infections, and vaginitis.

Some of these diseases are rare and unfamiliar to most people; others are very common and a problem for many people. Some diseases are mild and pose little threat to a person who develops the condition; others are life-threatening. In any case, all STIs are medical problems, that is, they are caused by specific microorganisms, such as bacteria or viruses; they can be recognized by certain characteristic signs and symptoms; they may have both short- and long-term consequences for one's overall health; and they usually can be treated and, in many cases, cured.

But, like many medical issues, sexually transmitted infections have nonmedical consequences in one's life: social, moral, ethical, legal, and emotional, for example. Even the possibility of having syphilis for Aaron means more than simply having to go to the hospital, being tested, and being treated. It also means the possibility of assessing one's own sexual practices, talking with close friends and family, and reconsidering what one knows and believes about himself or herself as a person. These issues come wrapped not only in the experience of dealing with STIs, but in dealing with any issue related to one's sexual health, including pregnancy and contraception, and one's sexual identity and sexual orientation. Medical issues that almost anyone can deal with in a relatively emotion-free state become especially troubling when they have to do with one's reproductive system.

An Ancient Issue

Venereal diseases have been a major medical problem in the world for at least five centuries, and probably much longer than that.

Part of the problem in unraveling the history of these diseases in history is that ancient records do not offer unambiguous clinical symptoms that allow a modern reader to determine precisely what disease a person has. Thus, some scholars find passages in the Bible itself that appear to refer to syphilis, such as references that might indicate that Abraham's wife, Sarah, may have had the disease (Cohen 1991, 166). Considerable debate among experts has developed over attempts to decide the sexually transmitted diseases to which ancient writers from the time of ancient China and the Egyptians may have alluded (see, for example, Goldman 1971; Heymann 2006; Rothschild 2005; Willcox 1949).

What seems to be clear is that the first mention of sexually transmitted infections in Western Europe dates to about 1495, when a disease called the great pox (to distinguish it from small-pox) broke out among French troops besieging Naples (McAllister 2000). As was to become a common pattern, the French blamed the disease on their enemies and called it the Italian disease. Later, the Italians themselves called the disease the French disease; the Dutch called it the Spanish disease; the Russians called it the Polish disease; the Turks called it the Christian disease; and much later, the Tahitians called it the British disease. These names reflected the fact that the disease commonly showed up in port cities, where it was presumably introduced by sailors arriving from another country.

In any case, the epidemiology and symptomology of syphilis were poorly known until at least the end of the 18th century. It was not until 1767 that syphilis and gonorrhea were even recognized as separate diseases. In that year, Scottish physician John Hunter infected himself with pus from a patient with gonorrhea, only to discover that he later developed symptoms not only of that disease, but also of syphilis. He was able to track the development of the latter disease, describing in careful detail for the first time the stages through which the disease developed until, in 1793, it caused an aneurysm responsible for his death (Androutsos, Magiorkinis, and Diamantis 2008).

Types of Infections

As noted previously, sexually transmitted infections can range from harmless, but annoying diseases to serious and potentially fatal conditions. An example of the former is the condition known as *Pediculosis pubis*. The term *pediculosis* refers to a group of infections caused by a group of insects that belong to the order Phthiraptera. These are tiny insects that live off blood and typically attach themselves to the base of a hair, from which they feed off their host. Perhaps the best-known example of the pest is *Pediculosis capitis*, the common head louse. Its close cousin, *Pediculosis pubis*, occurs most commonly in the pubic region, although it may also be found in other hairy areas, such as the eyelashes or in underarm hair. The most common symptom of an infection by this insect is itchiness, which becomes more severe over time. The only long-term problem is that scratching of infected areas may produce sores, which themselves may lead to more serious infections. The disease is readily treated with a variety of over-the-counter medications which, although not necessarily 100 percent effective, will eventually cure the problem.

Most STIs are of considerably more concern than *Pediculosis pubis*. The American Social Health Association has assembled a number of important statistics about these diseases. First, more than half of all Americans will contract a sexually transmitted infection at some point during their lifetime. Second, about 65 million Americans are currently living with some type of STI, and about 19 million new cases are reported every year. Third, about half of all new cases of STI occur among men and women age 15 to 24. Fourth, each year in the United States, about one in four teenagers contract one type of STI. Fifth, fewer than a third of all U.S. physicians routinely screen for STIs. Sixth, about one half of all sexually active men and women will contract at least one STI before the age of 25 (American Social Health Association 2009).

The most common sexually transmitted infection in the United States is chlamydia. In 2007, 1,108,374 cases of chlamydia were reported to the U.S. Centers for Disease Control and Prevention (CDC) in the 50 states and the District of Columbia. Experts believe that the true number of cases is probably much larger, perhaps as many as 2,291,000, because many women do not realize that they have the infection. Such is the case with other STIs, which always raises questions about the accuracy of STI statistics. Not only are people sometime unaware or unwilling to report an STI, but also figures for various diseases are difficult to compare because some public health departments may be required by law to report the number of cases for some diseases, but not for others. In any case, the number of cases of the most important sexually transmitted diseases for 2007 (the last year for which data are available) is shown in Table 1.1.

TABLE 1.1
Cases of Certain STIs in the United States, 2007

Disease	Number of Cases
Chlamydia	1,108,374
Gonorrhea	355,991
Genital herpes	317,000
Genital warts	312,000
Vaginal trichomoniasis	205,000
Pelvic inflammatory disease	146,000
Syphilis	40,920
HIV/AIDS	35,962
Hepatitis[1]	8,347
Chancroid	23

Sources: Division of STD Prevention, *Sexually Transmitted Disease Surveillance 2007* (Washington, D.C.: Department of Health And Human Services. Centers for Disease Control and Prevention. National Center for HIV/AIDS, Viral Hepatitis, STD, and TB Prevention. Division of STD Prevention, December 2008), table 1, p. 100; Centers for Disease Control and Prevention, "Basic Statistics," http://www.cdc.gov/hiv/topics/surveillance/basic.htm#aidscases; "Surveillance for Acute Viral Hepatitis—United States, 2007," *Morbidity and Mortality Weekly Report* 58 (SS-3; May 22, 2009), table 2, p. 11.
[1] Hepatitis A: 2,979; hepatitis B: 4,519; hepatitis C: 849

Symptoms, Prognosis, and Treatment

For each specific sexually transmitted infection, a set of basic information is useful. The first is the signs and symptoms of the disease, the physical conditions associated with the disease, conditions such as fever, nausea, blurred vision, and achy muscles. The second set of information concerns prognosis, the likely course of the disease. The third set of information relates to treatments that are available, both for relief of symptoms and possible cure, as well as for prevention of the disease in the first place. This outline serves as the basis for the discussion of the following sexually transmitted infections.

Chlamydia

Chlamydia is the most common sexually transmitted infection in the United States. It is caused by the bacterium *Chlamydia trachomatis,* which is transmitted most commonly by any type of sexual activity in which body parts come into contact with each other. The disease can also be transmitted from a woman to a newborn baby during childbirth. The disease occurs most commonly among women, causing abnormal vaginal discharge, discomfort during urination, and some itchiness. Men who have chlamydia may experience an unusual discharge from the penis and some pain and burning during urination. Perhaps the most important point about chlamydia, however, is that no symptoms may appear, and a person may be unaware that he or she has the infection. This fact is troublesome because in women the infection may spread from its initial site in the vagina into the urethra and cervix, where it can cause long-term reproductive problems, such as sterility. The most serious consequence of untreated chlamydial infection is pelvic inflammatory disease (PID), which can cause permanent damage to the fallopian tubes and other parts of the reproductive system. Experts estimate that 40 percent of all untreated chlamydial infections eventually result in a PID infection. The most serious health consequence of PID is an ectopic pregnancy (a pregnancy that occurs outside the uterus), which can result in death.

As with many STIs, the more serious consequences of chlamydia can be avoided by early detection and treatment. The *Chlamydia trachomatis* bacterium is easily killed with antibiotics, azithromycin or doxycycline being the drugs of choice. The best way to avoid a chlamydial infection is abstinence, not having sexual contact with another person, but that option is difficult or impossible for most people. Alternatively, one should be open with a sexual partner about her or his health status in order to avoid contact with someone who is or may be infected. The CDC also recommends annual tests for chlamydia for all sexually active women under the age of 25 and for older women who have risk factors for the disease, such as a number of sexual partners or many new partners.

Syphilis

Historically the most feared of all STIs, syphilis has gradually come under control in the United States and most other parts of the world. In the United States, the number of syphilis cases has fallen from more than 485,000 in 1941 to a low of less than 32,000 in 2000. It has since increased moderately to just over 40,000 in 2007 (Division of STD Prevention 2008, 100).

Syphilis is caused by the microorganism *Treponema pallidum*, belonging to the Spirochaetaceae family, which gets its name from the spiral-shaped appearance of its members. The microorganism survives reasonably well in the warm, moist environment of the mucous membranes that line the mouth, vagina, rectum, and other parts of the human body, but it dies quickly in almost any other environment. It is transmitted from one person to another during any act in which two individuals come into close contact, such as during oral, anal, or vaginal sexual contact. Because the organism is fragile, however, contact between an infected and uninfected person does not guarantee that the second individual will develop the disease.

If transmission does occur, symptoms do not appear until the organism has become established and started to multiply. This period of incubation may range anywhere from about 9 to 90 days, with an average of about three weeks, during which time a person is asymptomatic (does not shown signs of infection). At this point, an ugly sore, or chancre, may appear at the site of contact. The chancre is a symptom of the *primary stage* of syphilis. The chancre may develop on the penis, vagina, rectum, or mouth and, in some cases, may appear to be no more than a simple pimple that is easy to ignore. In other cases, it is larger and may break open, forming an ugly, hard-to-ignore open sore. In any case, if left untreated, the chancre or sore heals within two to four weeks. An individual may easily conclude that the disease has disappeared and requires no further attention.

Such is not the case, however, as the spirochetes that cause the disease remain in the body, growing and multiplying within the bloodstream. At some point—at any time between one and six months, with an average of six to eight weeks—a new set of symptoms will appear. These symptoms include a skin rash that covers all or part of the body, most characteristically on the palms of the hands or soles of the feet, where rashes normally do not occur. In about a quarter of all cases, an individual will also experience flu-like symptoms, including headache, sore throat, runny nose, nausea, and constipation. Other symptoms include fever and weight loss and, in some cases, loss of hair. A person is most contagious during this stage of the disease.

If untreated, these symptoms may also disappear, again prompting a person to conclude that the disease has disappeared. Again, this conclusion is erroneous because the spirochete remains in the body, although it has now stopped growing and multiplying. No further symptoms may appear for a very long time—known as the latent period—before reappearing months or years after the initial infection. At that point, the most serious stage of syphilis—known as late or tertiary syphilis—develops.

This stage of the disease is characterized by a number of very serious disorders affecting the muscular, cardiovascular, and nervous systems that disable and damage a person's body. The disease may eventually end in death.

Shortly after the first cases of syphilis had been reported on the Italian peninsula in about 1495, a method for treating the disease had been developed—the use of mercury salts which had previously been used to treat leprosy and other diseases of the skin. In fact, for more than 500 years, mercury compounds remained the drugs of choice for dealing with the disease, in spite of the fact that such compounds are themselves poisonous. Thus, in many cases, the cure was worse than the disease, prompting the famous saying, "Spend one night with Venus [the goddess of love]; spend the rest of your life with Mercury (Candida Martinelli's Italophile Site 2009). That situation finally changed in 1910, when German bacteriologist Paul Ehrlich (1854–1915) discovered a chemical called arsphenamine that was effective in killing the syphilis spirochete. Arsphenamine was marketed under the name of Salvarsan, or 606, the latter name reflecting the fact that it was the 606th drug that Ehrlich had tried in his effort to find a treatment for syphilis.

Today, syphilis is easily treated in its early stages. A single dose of penicillin given during the primary stage will kill the spirochetes that cause the disease. For individuals who are in more advanced stages of the disease, a series of inoculations are necessary, and for anyone allergic to penicillin, alternative antibiotics are available. Thus, the disease that once was the scourge of most of the world can be cured more easily than the common cold.

Gonorrhea

Gonorrhea is caused by the bacterium *Neisseria gonorrhoeae*, which like the causative agent of all STIs, grows in any moist, warm region of the body, ranging from the reproductive tract to the anus to the mouth and eyes. Women are often asymptomatic for gonorrhea, or symptoms may be so mild as to be mistaken for a simple bladder or vaginal infection. Men may also be asymptomatic, although they more commonly experience a burning sensation or pain during urination and/or a discharge from the penis. These symptoms appear anywhere from 1 to 30 days after exposure, with an average of 3 to 5 days. As with syphilis, untreated cases of gonorrhea eventually go into remission and symptoms disappear. But also as with syphilis, disease organisms have not disappeared from the body and may cause more serious problems at a later date. For men, these problems may include urethritis, prostatitis, and epididymitis, which can result in sterility. For women, the most serious complication from untreated gonorrheal infection is pelvic inflammatory disease (PID), which can range from mild to severe. About a million American women develop PID each year, with gonorrheal infections being an important cause. In the most serious cases, PID can be very painful, causing damage to the fallopian tubes and increasing the chance of an ectopic pregnancy.

Although the *Neisseria gonorrhoeae* bacterium is killed by a number of antibiotics, treatment of the disease has become more difficult in recent years because of the evolution of drug-resistant strains of the microorganism. In 2007, the CDC issued new recommendations for the treatment of these drug-resistant forms of the disease which make use of the antibiotics ceftriaxone, cefixime, or spectinomycin (Centers for Disease Control and Prevention 2009b).

Herpes

The term *herpes* refers to a large number of diseases in humans and other animals caused by one of more than a dozen different viruses. Eight of those diseases affecting humans are caused by viruses classified as human herpesvirus 1 through 8, which are responsible for diseases such as chicken pox and shingles (human herpesvirus 4), infectious mononucleosis (human herpesvirus 5), and Kaposi's sarcoma (human herpesvirus 8). The two sexually transmitted forms of the disease are caused by human herpesvirus 1 and 2, better known as herpes simplex virus type 1 and type 2 (HSV-1 and HSV-2). HSV-1 and HSV-2 are very similar to each other, sharing about 50 percent of their DNA. The most important difference between the two types is their preferred sites in the body. HSV-1 most commonly resides in nerve cells near the ear, while HSV-2 tends to become established in nerve tissue at the base of the spine. When HSV-1 becomes active, it most commonly causes the painful but relatively harmless condition known as cold sores or fever blisters. When HSV-2 becomes active, it is responsible for the development of the condition known as genital herpes, a painful infection of the genital area. Either form of the virus can cause an infection in either part of the body, although the distribution described here tends to be most common.

As with all STIs, herpes infections are spread by intimate contact between an infected person and an uninfected person. The first signs of the disease include blister-like sores that may be very painful and may be accompanied by fever and flu-like symptoms. In many cases, symptoms do not appear, and a person may not be aware that she or he has been infected with the virus. According to some estimates, more than one in five American adults have been infected with HSV-2 at some time in their lives, most of whom are not aware of that fact (Herpes.com 2009). The incubation period for the disease is about two weeks, and any sores that appear tend to disappear another two to four weeks later. As with other STIs, the disappearance of symptoms is not an indication that the disease has been cured, however. Instead, the viruses responsible for the disease remain embedded in nerve tissue and may become activated again at a future date. The number and severity of additional outbreaks vary significantly from person to person and appear to be dependent on three major factors: (1) the severity of the first outbreak (that is, the ability of a person's immune system to combat the first appearance of the virus); (2) the length of time a person has been infected (the number and severity of infections tend to decrease over time); and (3) the variety of virus causing the infection (HSV-1–caused genital herpes tends to be less severe than HSV-2–caused genital herpes).

Genital herpes tends to receive bad press from the general public, largely because people are embarrassed to have sexual partners or others find out about their condition. From a medical standpoint, however, the disease is usually no more serious (although just as uncomfortable and inconvenient) as a cold sore (Herpes.com 2009). Somewhat uncommonly, genital herpes may progress to more serious conditions, and, perhaps, may be associated with increased risk for other viral infections, especially HIV/AIDS. The most serious consequence of genital herpes is potential infection of a newborn child during birth to a woman with the infection, a condition that is potentially fatal for the child.

There is currently no cure for genital herpes, although medications are available to relieve its symptoms. Three commonly recommended drugs are the antivirals famciclovir, acyclovir, and valacyclovir.

Hepatitis

Hepatitis is an inflammation of tissues in the liver. The disease can be caused by a number of factors, including alcohol abuse. Hepatitis can be either acute, in which case the disease lasts less than about six months, or chronic, in which case it continues for an extended period of time. Most cases of acute hepatitis are caused by a group of viruses designated as hepatitis virus A, hepatitis virus B, hepatitis virus C, hepatitis virus D, and hepatitis virus E. Other possible hepatitis viruses have been hypothesized, but not yet confirmed. The diseases caused by these viruses have the same names as the viruses themselves: hepatitis A, hepatitis B, hepatitis C (originally called non-A, non-B), hepatitis D, and hepatitis E. The first two of these forms are the most common sexually transmitted forms of hepatitis.

Hepatitis A was formerly called infectious hepatitis. It is transmitted through contaminated food or water and by means of oral-anal sex. In oral sex, one person places his or her mouth on the anus of a second person, often coming into contact with contaminated fecal matter in the process. That fecal matter, as well as contaminated food or water, may contain the hepatitis virus A responsible for the disease. Symptoms of the disease normally appear about two to six weeks after exposure and mimic flu symptoms: fever, nausea, diarrhea, abdominal pain, fatigue, and loss of appetite. One of the clearest symptoms, as it is for all forms of hepatitis, is jaundice, a yellowing of the skin and the whites of the eyes. The disease usually runs its course in about two to six months, after which most people recover completely. The disease does not recur because the immune system has developed antibodies to the virus, and long-term serious effects are rare, and generally due to other infections that may be present at the same time. No treatment is available for a hepatitis A infection, although a vaccine is available. The CDC recommends that travelers expecting to visit countries with less than optimal food and water supplies be vaccinated for hepatitis A. People who plan to engage in oral-anal sex should also be aware of the possible health issues involved in this activity.

Hepatitis B was formerly called serum hepatitis because it can be transmitted through contaminated blood and blood products. It is one of the most common diseases in the world, with an estimated two billion individuals having been exposed to the hepatitis B virus. The most important means of transmission are blood transfusions that involve contaminated blood, unprotected sexual activities, sharing of contaminated needles, and transmission from a woman to her child during childbirth. The symptoms associated with hepatitis B are similar to those for hepatitis A but include the appearance of clay-colored bowel movements, a very distinctive symptom of the infection. Symptoms may appear anywhere from six weeks to six months, but most commonly about 90 days, after exposure. In the vast majority of cases, symptoms clear (disappear) after a few weeks or months, and reoccurrence of the disease is unlikely. In a small number of cases, the disease becomes chronic, with the virus remaining in a person's bloodstream for many years. In the most serious cases, the infection may eventually lead to cirrhosis of the liver (in which normal liver tissue is replaced by scar tissue), liver cancer, and even death. Seven drugs are currently approved by the U.S. Food and Drug Administration (FDA) for the treatment of hepatitis B infections: lamivudine, adefovir, tenofovir, telbivudine, entecavir, interferon alpha-2a, and pegylated interferon alfa-2a. The decision as to whether to begin treatment for a hepatitis B infection and which drug to use should be made on a case-by-case basis discussion between a patient and her or his physician. A vaccine for hepatitis B is also available and is recommended for travelers who plan to visit areas in which the risk for infection is high and for other individuals at risk for infection in their daily lives, including those who are sexually active with a number of different partners.

HIV/AIDS

The acronym HIV stands for *human immunodeficiency virus*, the agent responsible for acquired immune deficiency syndrome (AIDS). The first cases of HIV/AIDS were seen in the United States in the early 1980s. HIV spread rapidly through the gay community, among intravenous drug users and Haitians, among hemophiliacs, and finally to the heterosexual community, both in the United States and throughout the world. Today the disease is regarded as a worldwide pandemic, meaning an epidemic that has spread over a wide geographical area. In its latest report, the CDC estimated that there were 1,056,400–1,156,400 people in the United States living with AIDS, of whom 21 percent were undiagnosed. An additional 56,300 new cases of the disease were reported in 2006, the last year for which data are available. The CDC also estimated that 583,298 people had died of AIDS since it was first reported in the 1980s, 14,561 of those deaths having occurred in 2006 (Department of Health And Human Services. Public Health Service. Centers for Disease Control and Prevention 2008, 14, 20; Centers for Disease Control and Prevention 2009b).

The term *HIV/AIDS* is often used to describe an infection that has a very long incubation period. A person who has become infected may not show symptoms of the disease for many months or years. The average time between infection and so-called full-blown AIDS has been estimated at about 10 years. During this period, an individual is usually not aware that he or she has been infected. Only a blood test can detect the presence of the AIDS virus, and that test may not show results for at least six months after infection.

During the incubation period, the AIDS virus slowly attacks and disables the immune system, exposing an infected individual to ever greater risk from a number of diseases against which the body is usually able to protect itself. HIV/AIDS is, thus, a progressive disease in which a person's health gradually worsens. The CDC now defines the transition of an HIV infection to full-blown AIDS as the point at which a person has a CD4 T-cell count of less than 200 or has had one or more opportunistic infections. CD4 cells are a critical component of the immune system. When they decrease sufficiently in number, the body is no longer able to combat diseases very effectively. The term *opportunistic infection* refers to a number of conditions that are usually relatively harmless because the immune system is able to combat them effectively. Some typical opportunistic infections are a form of pneumonia called *Pneumocystis jirovecii* (formerly *Pneumocystis carinii*); a rare type of cancer, Kaposi's sarcoma; a type of streptococcus caused by the bacterium *Streptococcus pyogenes*; and a yeast infection caused by the fungus *Candida albicans*.

For the first decade of the HIV/AIDS epidemic, no treatment was available for the disease and death rates were very high, generally over 95 percent. Today, a number of medications have been developed for treating the infection. The most effective therapy involves the use of a combination of at least three drugs to destroy or inactivate the virus. The availability of this cocktail has dramatically reduced the death rate from HIV/AIDS. Efforts have been made to develop a vaccine against the virus, but without success thus far. One problem is that the virus tends to evolve rapidly so that a vaccine developed against one strain of the virus may not be effective very long. By far the most important approach to dealing with the HIV/AIDS epidemic is education. The more individuals know about the disease and the better they understand the value of and methods for practicing safer sex, the better their chances of avoiding becoming infected with HIV. The term *safer sex* refers to all those practices that one can employ during sexual acts that are likely to reduce the risk of contracting HIV/AIDS or, for that matter, any other sexual infection.

Pregnancy and Contraception

Pregnancy has long been considered one of the preeminent events in a woman's life, the opportunity to bring new life into the world. At the same time, pregnancy has been the source of anxiety and fear for many women throughout history. One reason for such concern has been the challenge of raising larger and larger families. While children have been an economic asset to families throughout much of human history (since they provide additional labor), they can also be a burden because of the cost of rearing and caring for them. Of equal concern to women has been the medical risk they face during childbirth. Until recently, bringing a new life into the world could be a medically dangerous venture. While no valid and reliable statistics are available for most of history, most specialists believe that women have always faced a relatively high risk of death as a result of childbirth. According to a recent study by the World Health Organization (WHO), the primary causes of maternal death during childbirth are severe bleeding and hemorrhaging, infections, unsafe abortions, eclampsia (convulsions associated with the birth process), obstructed labor, and the presence of infections and other diseases, such as malaria, anemia, and cardiovascular disorders (Department of Reproductive Health and Research 2004, 45).

It should hardly be surprising, then, that women have been searching for ways to avoid becoming pregnant or to abort a pregnancy as far back as records exist. For thousands of years, of course, humans had no understanding of the process by which a woman becomes pregnant, so nothing resembling scientific methodology was available for the design of contraceptive methods. One approach was to use a variety of substances, applied to the vaginal region, to avoid pregnancy. Those substances included olive oil, tobacco juice, ginger, beeswax, honey, crocodile dung, and lemon juice. Vaginal suppositories made of these materials—called pessaries—were often used during or just following intercourse. Oral contraceptives were also employed. They included foam from a camel's mouth, concoctions made of metallic ores, alcoholic drinks, and a variety of herbal teas. Physical acts were also thought to be helpful. One of the most commonly cited of these acts was one recommended by the Greek physician Soranus of Ephesus (fl. first–second centuries CE), who suggested that women jump backward seven times in order to dislodge sperm in their uterus ("A Brief History of Contraceptives" 2009; Herodotus Wept 2009).

As an understanding of the mechanisms by which conception occurs developed over the centuries, so did the sophistication of technologies designed to prevent conception. Today, a number of options are available to a woman who chooses to be sexually active, while avoiding pregnancy. Most of those options can be classified under one of five categories: barrier methods, such as condoms and diaphragms; hormonal methods, such as "The Pill" and "The Patch"; emergency methods, such as Plan B; behavioral techniques, such as coitus interruptus and abstinence; and abortion. Only the last of these options is not discussed in this book. The topic of abortion is so complex and so controversial that it cannot be discussed in a general overview like the one presented here. The bibliography in Chapter 8, however, lists a number of references dealing with the topic.

Barrier Methods

Any contraceptive technology designed to prevent sperm from reaching a woman's uterus or the eggs it contains is called a barrier method. Many of the oldest methods of contraception, including the whole range of pessaries, were barrier methods. The most common barrier methods used today are condoms, diaphragms, cervical caps, and spermicides.

Condoms are made for either male or female use. A male condom is a thin sheath of latex rubber or polyurethane plastic worn over a man's erect penis. It captures semen produced during ejaculation that occurs during an orgasm, along with the sperm contained with the semen. The effectiveness of the male condom is 85–98 percent (see Table 1.2), which can be increased if combined with some other conceptive method, such as a spermicide. The female condom is used when a man chooses not to use a male condom. It is a plastic pouch inserted into the vagina that captures semen produced during ejaculation. Like the male condom, it is available without prescription in most pharmacies and is more effective when combined with another contraceptive, such as a spermicide.

Spermicides are chemicals that kill sperm or make them sufficiently inactive that they are unable to reach and fertilize an egg

TABLE 1.2
Effectiveness of Various Contraceptive Methods

Method	Effectiveness (%)
Barrier methods	
Cervical cap[1]	
Has experienced childbirth	70
Has not experienced childbirth	85
Condom[2]	
Male	85–98
Female	79–95
Diaphragm[2]	84–94
Spermicides[2]	71–82
Hormonal methods[2]	
Oral contraceptives	
The Pill	92–99
The mini-pill	92–99
Vaginal ring	92–99
Injection	97–99
Implant	99
Skin patch	92–99
Emergency contraception	at least 75
Fertility awareness and abstinence[2]	
Abstinence	100
Fertility awareness	75–99
Sterilization[2]	
Male/female	99

Sources: [1] American College of Obstetricians and Gynecologists, "Contraception," http://www.acog.org/publications/ patient_education/bp022.cfm. Accessed on June 8, 2009.
[2] Centers for Disease Control and Prevention, "Unintended Pregnancy Prevention: Contraception," http://www.cdc. gov/ReproductiveHealth/UnintendedPregnancy/Contraception.htm. Accessed on June 8, 2009.

in a woman's uterus. The active ingredient in most spermicides is an organic chemical by the name of nonoxynol-9. Spermicides are available without prescription in most pharmacies and come in a variety of forms, including jellies, foams, creams, suppositories, tablets, and vaginal films. Vaginal films and tablets must be inserted into the vagina at least 10 minutes, and no more than an hour, before intercourse, and they must be left in place for six to eight hours after intercourse. They must be reapplied prior to each act of sexual intercourse, and they work most efficiently in combination with some other type of contraception, such as a condom or diaphragm.

Diaphragms and cervical caps are thin rubber or plastic cups that fit inside the vagina and cover the cervix, preventing sperm from reaching the uterus and egg. They come in various sizes and are available only by prescription. Cervical caps come in four sizes, while diaphragms are sized according to the diameter of the device, as determined by a medical professional. The prescription for a diaphragm or cervical cap may change depending on a number of factors, including weight changes, urinary tract infections, births or abortions, pelvic surgery, or discomfort for a woman or her partner during intercourse. Both devices should be used only with spermicides, which are applied on the surface of the diaphragm or cervical cap prior to intercourse. A woman should consult with her health professional about the proper method for inserting a diaphragm or cervical cap.

Hormonal Methods

Another category of contraceptive methods involves the introduction of hormones into a woman's body to reduce the probability of pregnancy occurring. The hormones involved are estrogen or progestin or a combination of the two. These hormones have three major effects on the reproductive system: they prevent ovulation, reduce the probability of implantation of a fertilized egg in the uterine wall, and/or increase the viscosity of cervical mucus, making it more difficult for a sperm to reach an egg.

Today, at least 30 different products based on the use of hormones are commercially available in the United States. They can be classified as oral contraceptives, injections, implants, patches, or vaginal rings.

Oral contraceptives are among the best known of all methods of contraception currently available. The first such product, Enovid, was approved for use in the United States by the U.S. Food and Drug Administration in June 1957. It and later versions became widely known simply as The Pill. The more than 30 versions of The Pill are all alike in that they contain two different hormones, one derived from estrogen and one from progestin (related to progesterone found naturally in the human body). For this reason, they are sometimes referred to as *combination oral contraceptives*. Combination oral contraceptives differ from one another in two ways. First they may contain different versions of the two hormones. The most common estrogen derivative is ethinyl estradiol, while the progestin component may be any one of a number of compounds, including norethindrone, norgestrel, norgestimate, or desogestrol. Second, the concentration of components within pills may be constant throughout a complete cycle of the product (a monophasic design), or it may vary for pills taken at various times throughout the cycle (biphasic or triphasic designs). Oral contraceptives are available only by prescription, and the proper product and regime should be determined in consultation between a woman and her physician. A different form of The Pill, sometimes known as The Mini Pill, contains a progestin derivative only. It is recommended for women who are breast-feeding or are allergic to estrogen derivatives.

The hormones needed to prevent pregnancy can also be administered by other methods:

> *Injections* are used to deliver a single progestin-derivative hormone called depot medroxyprogesterone acetate (DMPA, or Depo-Provera) once every three months (four times a year). The primary advantage of injections is that they are more convenient (four times a year) than oral contraceptives (365 times a year), and they may provide protection against some medical problems, such as uterine cancer, pelvic inflammatory disease, and ectopic pregnancies.

> *Patches* are small Band-Aid-like devices worn on the buttocks or back. They contain a combination of an estrogen derivative and a progestin derivative that is released slowly over time from the patch and that is absorbed by the skin into the bloodstream. A new patch is worn once a week for three weeks, and then no patch is worn on the fourth week. It addition to the benefit of convenience, patches may also provide protection against some forms of cancer, reduce risk of pelvic inflammatory disease, and reduce cramping.

> *Vaginal rings* are flexible plastic rings inserted into the upper vagina at the opening to the cervix. They contain a combination of estrogen and progestin derivatives that is released slowly into the bloodstream during the three weeks they are in place. They are removed during the fourth week, and then reinserted to begin another cycle of use. Vaginal rings have essentially the same advantages and benefits as do patches.

> *Implants* are thin, rodlike devices made of flexible plastic inserted under the skin in a woman's upper arm. They contain a progestin derivative that prevents ovulation for

up to three years. Insertion and removal of the rods are simple procedures that are performed in a physician's office. A number of side effects, most of them mild, are related to use of implants, including headaches, increased bleeding, vaginitis, and weight gain.

Emergency contraception is another form of hormonal birth control that is similar to oral contraception because it is taken by mouth, but different because it is not taken on a regular basis to prevent fertilization. Emergency contraception is sometimes referred to as the "morning-after" pill because it is taken after sexual intercourse has occurred, in an attempt to prevent a pregnancy from developing. The only emergency contraception currently licensed for use in the United States is known as Plan B, which contains the hormone levonorgestrel, a derivative of progestin. The precise mechanism by which Plan B and other emergency contraceptives prevent pregnancies is somewhat complicated, depending in large part on the point in a woman's cycle during which she takes the drug.

Intrauterine Devices

As their name suggests, intrauterine devices (IUDs) are devices that are inserted into a woman's uterus and then act to prevent fertilization of an egg by sperm. Two devices are currently available, one that contains hormones and one made of copper. Both devices are T-shaped and inserted into the uterus by a trained medical professional. The Mirena intrauterine system (IUS) contains a small amount of a progestin derivative that, when released into the uterus, prevents ovulation and implantation and thickens cervical mucus, thus reducing the ability of sperm to reach an egg. The copper T IUD has a shape similar to the IUS, but is made of copper, which deteriorates slowly releasing particles of the element to the uterus, with a similar effect. Both forms of the IUD come with short strings attached that allow access to the device after it is implanted. The IUS can remain in the uterus for up to 5 years, and the copper T IUD, for up to 10 years.

Fertility Awareness and Abstinence

The preceding contraceptive methods all make use of some material or object to reduce the risk of pregnancy. Two other popular approaches to birth control use neither. Abstinence is one. The term refers to a person's decision to refrain entirely from sexual intercourse that could result in a woman's becoming pregnant. This method is the only contraceptive technique for which effectiveness is 100 percent. If one does not have intercourse, pregnancy cannot result. The issue (discussed in more detail in Chapter 2) is the extent to which most people can remain abstinent for extended periods of time in order to achieve this objective.

Another approach to contraception relies on a woman's becoming familiar with her own reproductive cycle and determining the times at which she is more or less likely to become pregnant. This approach is sometimes called natural family planning (NFP) because it does not depend on any artificial devices such as pills, patches, injections, or barriers. One form of NFP is called the cervical mucus method, in which a woman regularly examines the mucal discharge from her cervix. Prior to ovulation, this mucus tends to become thinner and more watery, making it easier for sperm to travel through the uterus to an egg. With practice, a woman can recognize changes in the consistency of her cervical mucus and refrain from sexual intercourse until it has returned to its more normal state. A second NFP method is called the sympto-thermal method because it relies on a woman's becoming familiar with changes in body temperature that take place throughout her menstrual cycle. As ovulation begins, body temperature also starts to rise by small amounts. By taking her temperature on a daily basis, a woman can estimate the point where she is in her cycle and refrain from intercourse during ovulation. In most cases, both cervical mucus properties and body temperature are taken as an indication of the times at which to avoid sexual intercourse.

Sterilization

The contraceptive methods discussed thus far are all reversible. That is, a man or woman can choose to stop using a particular method at almost any time, and conception can occur (almost) the next time there is intercourse. More drastic methods of contraception involve surgical techniques to prevent ovulation or release of sperm. In men, such procedures are called vasectomies, and in women, tubal ligation or, colloquially, "having one's tubes tied." In a vasectomy, the tube leading from the testes to the penis (the vas deferens) is blocked, preventing release of sperm into the semen. The procedure does not inhibit a man from having an erection and ejaculation, but it does prevent sperm from being released during ejaculation. Tubal ligation involves the cutting, tying, banding, or otherwise blocking of a woman's fallopian tubes, preventing the release of an egg into the uterus. The procedure does not affect a woman's menstrual cycle or her ability to engage in sexual intercourse.

Both vasectomies and tubal ligations are sometimes thought of as permanent forms of contraception. In fact, both procedures are reversible, although the success rate for pregnancies after a reversible procedure tend to be low to moderate. In both cases, the success rate depends on a number of factors, especially the patient's age. For both procedures, the rate of conception after reversal surgery has been estimated at between 30 and 75 percent (University of Florida Health System 2009; VasectomyMedical. com 2009).

A Concluding Observation

The information provided in this section should be regarded only as a general overview to the topic of contraception. The decision as to whether or not to use a contraceptive, the method to use, and the specific procedures to follow vary significantly from person to person. They depend on a person's age, gender, personal values, philosophy of life, religious beliefs, and a host of other factors. In any case, the decision made by a young woman or young man almost always benefits from a discussion of the options available with a parent, adult trusted counselor, and/or medical professional.

Sexual Orientation and Gender Identity

Childhood is usually a pretty simple time in a person's life. Boys are boys, and girls are girls. Adults sometimes help kids keep the distinctions clear by dressing boys and girls differently, by treating them in different ways, and by making sure they know that they are expected to act in different ways. Also, boys tend to hang out with boys, and to regard girls as "icky" or unappealing in other ways. Girls prefer to hang out with other girls, regarding boys as "gross" or not people one wants to spend time with.

But, at about age 10 or so, things change. Hormones become active in both male and female bodies and childhood standards and norms no longer hold true. Boys, at least most of them, begin to feel that maybe girls are not so bad after all. It may be all right to spend some time with them . . . actually, to spend a lot of time with them in more intimate ways than they had ever imagined before. And most girls are willing to give boys a second chance . . . and even a third and fourth chance, to see if there might not be more to the male sex than they had ever imagined.

But some boys continue to like hanging out with other boys, and even begin to feel that they would like to do more than just play baseball and smoke cigarettes behind the barn with them. Even though they have received the message thousands of times that it's time to start going out with girls, somehow a date with a boy seems more appealing and more natural. And some girls feel the same way about other girls. And yet other boys and girls just are not sure to whom they are most strongly attracted, boys or girls . . . or both!

Finally, some boys and girls are no longer entirely sure they are really male or female at all. The hormones that begin to flow in a male's body may suddenly carry a strange and terrifying message: "Did you know that you are really a girl, and not a boy?" Or, on the other hand, "You have been brought up as a girl, but now is the time to admit that you feel more like a boy."

It is no wonder that adolescence has often been called the period of Sturm und Drang, "storm and stress," as almost-men and almost-women for the first time in their lives begin to assess their own sexual nature.

Terminology

No discussion of sexual orientation and gender identity can proceed without a clear understanding of the meaning of a number of essential terms. To begin with these two terms themselves, *sexual orientation* means the sex to which a person is primarily attracted physically, emotionally, and sexually. To say that one is *heterosexually oriented* means that one is attracted primarily to someone of the opposite sex; someone who is *homosexually orientated* is attracted primarily to someone of the same sex. The terms *homosexual* and *heterosexual* are not very good as nouns, because they tend to define a person exclusively or primarily in terms of her or his sexual orientation. "That woman is a homosexual" suggests that her sexual orientation is the most important defining characteristic one can assign to her, which typically is not the case. Some people are attracted to both sexes, perhaps equally, but usually to some extent or another. They are said to have a bisexual orientation.

The issue of one's sexual orientation has long been a matter of considerable controversy in the United States and many other (but not all) parts of the world. As a result, a very large vocabulary of pejorative terms have grown up to talk about anyone whose sexual orientation is outside the usual heterosexual norm recognized by society. Gay, lesbian, faggot, fairy, queer, and dyke are only a few of those terms, none of which is especially helpful in discussing the issues of sexual orientation in this book.

The term *gender identity* means something very different from sexual orientation. Gender identity refers to the perception that one has of his or her own sexual status. A man may have been born with male genitalia and still feel deep down in his heart and soul that he is somehow a woman. Someone born with the reproductive system of a woman might still feel that she is a man in a woman's body. Although these feelings are not typical of most men and women, they are not uncommon, and they are the basis of profound psychological and emotional struggles for people who experience them. Such individuals sometimes decide that they can no longer live a lie, and commit to a series of medical procedures through which they change their physical gender, from male to female or male to female. Such individuals are known as transgendered individuals.

Gay men, lesbians, bisexuals, and transgendered individuals all experience a common reaction from general society, often a feeling of not belonging. It is small wonder, then, that a number of social and political organizations have grown up to deal with issues common to those who belong to one of these categories. These groups often define themselves as gay, lesbian, bisexual, and transgendered (GLBT) groups and, in some cases, throw in the word *queer* (as in gay, lesbian, bisexual, queer, and transgendered) as an in-your-face political statement to the general community. Groups interested in issues of sexual orientation and gender identity may also add yet another term to their name: *questioning*, resulting in organizations that call themselves gay, lesbian, bisexual, transgendered, and questioning (GLBTQ). The term *questioning* refers to and emphasizes the fact that many adolescents are at a stage in their lives when they really do not know the category to which they belong, that is, whether they are more attracted to someone of the same sex, of the opposite sex, or to both sexes, or even how they feel about their own sexual identity.

A final category of individuals to be mentioned includes transvestites, sometimes the least understood of all nontypical groups. Transvestites are individuals who take pleasure in dressing and acting as members of the opposite sex: men dress as women, and women dress as men. Such individuals are almost without exception heterosexual. The term almost always applies to the former case—men who dress as women—because that condition is regarded as somehow abnormal or unnatural. On the contrary, many women dress and act in a manner not unlike that of men in everyday society, so the practice is generally not regarded as abnormal or unnatural. Instead, it is more likely to be regarded as a statement of status in (at least) American society. That is, it is permissible for a woman to want to move up in the world by dressing like her superior, a man, while it is largely unthinkable that a man would want to move down in the world by dressing like a woman. But that analysis is for another time.

Gay, Lesbian, Bisexual, Transgender, and Questioning Youth Issues

One reason that adolescence is such a difficult time in a person's life is that so many questions have to be answered in the transition from being a child to being an adult. Does one want to simply adopt and accept the attitudes, beliefs, and lifestyle of one's parents, or should one break away and form a new and independent life? Should one be a Democrat, Orthodox Jew, and attorney because those are the choices one's parents made or want their children to make? Or does one's conscience push one toward the Republican party, atheism, and a career as a concert pianist?

The matters of sexual orientation and gender identity are not so much matters of choice—evidence now suggests that both characteristics have strong genetic roots—but deciding how to act on one's innermost convictions about these issues *is* a decision one has to make. In a society in which homosexual behavior and transgenderism are still the subject of considerable disapproval, acknowledging to oneself and one's family and friends that one may be lesbian, gay, or a potentially transgendered individual can be far more difficult than announcing that one is no longer a Democrat or an Orthodox Jew.

Public opinion polls suggest that attitudes about homosexual behavior in the United States have undergone significant changes in the past few decades. In its most recent poll on the question (June 2008), the Gallup Poll organization found that the nation was evenly split on the question of whether or not homosexual relations are "morally acceptable" or "morally wrong," with 48 percent of respondents agreeing with each position. But that result represents a significant shift in less than a decade. When the same question was asked in 2001, the majority of respondents—53 percent—agreed that homosexual relations were "morally wrong," while only 40 percent thought they were "morally acceptable" (Gallup 2009). This trend is more apparent when viewed over a longer time span. In 1983, Gallup asked respondents whether they thought homosexuality was "an acceptable alternative lifestyle or not": 51 percent of respondents said no, while 34 percent said yes. Twenty-five years later, when Gallup asked the same question, these positions had been reversed: 57 percent of respondents agreed that homosexuality "was acceptable," while 40 percent said that it was not (Gallup 2009).

These data send mixed messages to adolescents in the United States who are questioning their sexual orientation and gender identity. For one thing, they indicate that at least 4 out of 10 Americans still regard homosexual behavior as morally unacceptable. That means that something like 4 out of 10 parents, school teachers and counselors, religious leaders, neighbors, family friends, and others with whom one comes into contact on a daily basis regards "you," the questioning teenager, as morally repugnant. Many of the resources on which adolescents depend for support and guidance in dealing with difficult personal questions—such as one's religious beliefs, political commitments, sexual orientation, and gender identity—may not, therefore, be available in dealing with this issue.

The problems faced by adolescents dealing with issues of sexual orientation and gender identity have been documented in a number of surveys and studies. In 2001, for example, the Massachusetts Department of Public Health reported on a study it conducted of suicides and suicide attempts among high school students in the state. It found that about 40 gay, lesbian, and bisexual students had attempted suicide at least once, compared to a rate of 10 percent among heterosexual students (Healy 2001). Similar results have been reported in a number of other studies on suicide rates among teenagers (2005 Youth Risk Behavior Survey 2007, 50; Trevor Project 2009).

In one of the most comprehensive (if somewhat dated) studies of the issues faced by GLBTQ students, more than 40 percent of respondents reported not feeling safe in school because of their sexual orientation or gender identity; more than 90 percent heard homophobic remarks from fellow students; 30 percent heard similar remarks from faculty and administrators; and 69 percent reported having experienced some form of verbal or physical harassment. Even among those respondents who said they felt safe at their schools, 46 percent reported verbal harassment, 36 percent reported sexual harassment, 12 percent reported physical harassment, and 6 percent reported some type of physical assault (The Body 2001).

One consequence of the problems GLBTQ students face is their tendency to turn to alcohol and illegal drugs as a form of relief and compensation. A study by researchers at the University of Pittsburgh in 2008 found that the rate of alcohol and substance abuse among gay, lesbian, and bisexual students is about 190 percent that of heterosexual students and, among some subgroups of GLB students, the rate may reach 400 percent that of their heterosexual counterparts. Lead researcher Michael P. Marshal explained that

> homophobia, discrimination and victimization are largely what are responsible for these substance use disparities in young gay people. . . . History shows that when marginalized groups are oppressed and do not have equal opportunities and equal rights, they suffer. Our results show that gay youth are clearly no exception. (Addiction 2008)

Options for GLBTQ Youth

Some adolescents are fortunate in that they can turn to trusted resources—parents, teachers, religious leaders, friends, neighbors, and relatives—when they have questions about their sexual orientation or gender identity. Somewhat strangely enough, the one group of individuals whom they may not be able to turn are older gay men, lesbians, bisexuals, and transgendered individuals. The problem has traditionally been that older GLBT individuals are hesitant to offer their help to younger men and women and boys and girls for fear of being labeled as predators. The connection between child molestation and homosexual behavior has been emphasized for so long that concerns about one's legal safety may prompt many older GLBT individuals from associating with younger questioning youth under almost any circumstances. The abundance of evidence that refutes this connection has made this problem only slightly less of an issue (see, for example, Newton 1978).

In any case, a number of resources have been developed over the past two decades to which GLBTQ youth can turn for assistance in dealing with their own questions about sexual orientation and gender identity. Without much doubt, the availability of the Internet has been a key factor in increasing the number of these resources to which young people can turn. For example, Youth Resource is a project of Advocates for Youth that provides information on a range of topics of interest and concern to GLBTQ youth. It provides a link to dozens of local organizations, such as school and campus groups, to which one can turn for direct advice and assistance. A search for the state of Alabama, for example, returns the names of 4 youth groups that deal with sexual orientation and gender identity issues among teenagers, 1 campus organization, and 13 peer- education groups. Another online resource is the National Youth Advocacy Coalition, whose primary objective is to "strengthen the role of young people in the LGBTQ rights movement" (National Youth Advocacy Coalition).

A number of nonelectronic resources are also available for GLBTQ youth. Perhaps the best known of these resources is the Gay, Lesbian, and Straight Education Network (GLSEN), founded in 1990 to work to "to assure that each member of every school community is valued and respected regardless of sexual orientation or gender identity/expression" and "to develop school climates where difference is valued for the positive contribution it makes in creating a more vibrant and diverse community" (GLSEN 2009).

Resources are also available for adults who want to learn more about ways in which they can act as a resource for GLBTQ youth. Probably the oldest and most widely respected of these organizations is Parents and Friends of Lesbians and Gays (PFLAG). PFLAG was founded in 1972 by Jeanne Manford after her son was beaten in a gay pride parade in New York City. Manford's goal was to provide a safe haven for parents of gays and lesbians and to provide information and support for mothers and fathers who were unsure how to deal with news that a son or daughter was gay or lesbian. Today PFLAG has more than 200,000 members in over 500 chapters in all 50 states and the District of Columbia. In addition to working with individual parents, the organization works on a local and national basis for equal rights for all individuals regardless of sexual orientation or gender identity.

Progress: A Mixed Blessing?

In some ways, dealing with issues of sexual orientation and gender identity are easier for young men and women today than it was a half century ago. In the 1950s, many GLBTQ youth probably knew little or nothing about homosexuality. One of the most common themes in the biographies of gay men and lesbians of the times was that "I thought I was the only person in the world like me." Today, stories of gay men, lesbians, bisexuals, and transgendered individuals appear everywhere in the public media. One consequence of this change has been that the age at which young men and women acknowledge being gay, lesbian, or bisexual has become younger and younger (Elias 2007). In that context, perhaps "coming out of the closet" (acknowledging one's sexual orientation) may be easier for teenagers in the 21st century than it ever was in the United States.

On the other hand, "being out" means that young men and women often have to deal with difficult issues at an earlier age than ever before. As with issues of sexually transmitted infections and contraception, questions about sexual orientation and gender identity are increasingly problems about which adolescents need more accurate information and guidance from adults.

References

Addiction. 2008. "Gay Youth Report Higher Rates of Drug and Alcohol Use." http://www.addictionjournal.org/viewpressrelease.asp?pr=74. Accessed on June 10, 2009.

American Social Health Association. 2009. "STD/STI Statistics > Fast Facts." http://www.ashastd.org/learn/learn_statistics.cfm. Accessed on June 5, 2009.

Androutsos G., E. Magiorkinis, and A. Diamantis. 2008. "John Hunter (1728–1793): Father of Modern Urology." *Balkan Military Medical Review* 11: 52–55.

The Body. 2001. "Fact Sheet: Lesbian, Gay, Bisexual and Transgender Youth Issues." http://www.thebody.com/content/whatis/art2449.html. Accessed on June 10, 2009.

"A Brief History of Contraceptives." 2009. http://home.snu. edu/~dwilliam/f97projects/contraception/history.htm. Accessed on June 8, 2009.

"Candida Martinelli's Italophile Site." 2009. http://italophiles.com/ carnevale.htm. Accessed on June 7, 2009.

Centers for Disease Control and Prevention. 2009a. *MMWR Weekly*. http://www.cdc.gov/mmwr/preview/mmwrhtml/mm5739a2.htm. Accessed on June 8, 2009.

Centers for Disease Control and Prevention. 2009b. "Updated Recommended Treatment Regimens for Gonococcal Infections and Associated Conditions—United States, April 2007." http://www.cdc. gov/std/treatment/2006/updated-regimens.htm. Accessed on June 7, 2009.

Cohen, Mark Nathan. 1991. *Health and the Rise of Civilization*. New Haven, CT: Yale University Press, 1991.

Department of Health and Human Services. Public Health Service. Centers for Disease Control and Prevention. December 2008. *HIV/ AIDS Surveillance Report*. Atlanta, GA: Centers for Disease Control and Prevention.

Department of Reproductive Health and Research. World Health Organization. 2004. *Maternal Mortality in 2000*. Geneva: World Health Organization.

Division of STD Prevention. December 2008. *Sexually Transmitted Disease Surveillance 2007*. Washington, D.C.: Department of Health And Human Services. Centers for Disease Control and Prevention. National Center for HIV/AIDS, Viral Hepatitis, STD, and TB Prevention. Division of STD Prevention.

Elias, Marilyn. 2007. "Gay Teens Coming Out Earlier to Peers and Family." *USA Today*, February 7. http://www.usatoday.com/news/ nation/2007-02-07-gay-teens-cover_x.htm. Accessed on June 10, 2009.

Gallup. 2009. "Americans Evenly Divided on Morality of Homosexuality." http://www.gallup.com/poll/108115/americans- evenly-divided-morality-homosexuality.aspx. Accessed on June 10, 2009.

GLSEN. 2009. "Our Mission." http://www.glsen.org/cgi-bin/iowa/all/ about/history/index.html. Accessed on June 10, 2009.

Goldman, Leon. 1971. "Syphilis in the Bible." *Archives of Dermatology* 103 (5; May): 535–36.

Healy, Patrick. 2001. "Massachusetts Study Shows High Suicide Rate for Gay Students." http://www.glsen.org/cgi-bin/iowa/all/news/ record/399.html. Accessed on June 10, 2009.

Herodotus Wept. 2009. "Early Contraceptives." http://herodotuswept. wordpress.com/2007/11/14/early-contraceptives/. Accessed on June 8, 2009.

Herpes.com. 2009. "The Truth about HSV-1 and HSV-2." http://www. herpes.com/hsv1-2.html. Accessed on June 7, 2009.

Heymann, Warren R. 2006. "The History of Syphilis." *Journal of the American Academy of Dermatology* 54 (2; February): 322–23.

Marshal, Michael P. et al. 2008. "Sexual Orientation and Adolescent Substance Use: A Meta-analysis and Methodological Review." *Addiction* 103 (4; April): 546–56.

McAllister, Marie E. 2000. "Stories of the Origin of Syphilis in Eighteenth-Century England: Science, Myth, and Prejudice." *Eighteenth-Century Life* 24 (1; Winter): 22–44.

National Youth Advocacy Program. 2009. http://www.nyacyouth.org/about/index.php. Accessed on June 10, 2009.

Newton, David E. 1978. "Homosexual Behavior and Child Molestation: A Review of the Evidence." *Adolescence* 13 (49; Spring): 29–43.

Rothschild, Bruce M. 2005. "History of Syphilis." *Clinical Infectious Diseases* 40 (10; May): 1454–63.

The Trevor Project. 2009. "Suicidal Signs." http://www.thetrevorproject. org/info.aspx. Accessed on June 10, 2009.

2005 Youth Risk Behavior Survey. December 2007. Boston: Massachusetts Department of Elementary and Secondary Education.

University of Florida Health System. 2009. "Tubal Reversal." http://www.obgyn.ufl.edu/ENDO/PatientHandouts/Tubal%20Reversal.pdf. Accessed on June 9, 2009.

VasectomyMedical.com. 2009. "Vasectomy Reversal." http://www. vasectomymedical.com/vasectomy-reversal-success-rates.html. Accessed on June 9, 2009.

Willcox, R. R. 1949. "Venereal Disease in the Bible." *British Journal of Venereal Diseases* 25: 28–33.

2

Problems, Controversies, and Solutions

Introduction

The factual information that young men and women need in order to understand and deal with issues of sexual health is available from a number of sources: parents, medical professionals, teachers and counselors, and (sometimes) church leaders, neighbors, other adults, and friends. For more than a century in the United States, some people have been advocating sex education classes in schools as the best means for providing this information. The age at which sex education should begin, the topics to be included, the composition of sex education classes, and a number of other issues are still being debated.

School-based sex education in the United States is usually said to have begun in 1913, when Ella Flagg Young, then superintendent of schools in Chicago, initiated the so-called Chicago Experiment, a series of lectures on sexual hygiene for separate groups of boys and girls in the city's high schools. Young's decision reflected a growing concern that was sweeping the country at the time about the appalling increase in the rate of sexually transmitted infections. Many observers thought that this medical problem was caused by a deteriorating moral atmosphere, caused in part by the urbanization of American society and the flood of immigrants reaching the nation's shores. Proponents of an expanded program of sex education, for both adults and adolescents, saw their effort as having both a medical and a moral component. Solving the problem of increased rates of sexually transmitted infections required not only better information about the human

31

reproductive system, but also stronger moral training for young people experiencing sexual urges for the first time. Indeed, some proponents of sex education for the young specifically argued that instruction of this kind would encourage young people to avoid sexual activities entirely until marriage. As one historian has observed, "Many of the proponents of sex purity saw sex education as a way to desexualize society, except in the marriage bed" (Tyack and Hansot 1990, 222; see also Fass 2004; Jensen 2007).

After a vigorous debate within the school board and the community at large, Flagg received approval for her program, which was eventually to reach more than 20,000 students in three lectures on the topics: "personal sexual hygiene," "problems of sex instincts," and "a few of the hygienic and social facts regarding venereal disease" (Moran 1996, 501). The Chicago Experiment survived only one year, however. Objections from within the school system itself and the community in general continued throughout the year. The most common objection was that a delicate matter such as human sexuality had no place in public schools. This view was reflected in a letter to the *Chicago Tribune* that appeared on page 1 of the December 11, 1913, issue of the newspaper. "I honestly fear," the governor wrote, "that if sex hygiene be taught in the schools and young boys and girls in the open class room are made aware of things which may be taught in the line of sex hygiene, it may create, and probably will create, in their young minds a prurient curiosity which will induce, rather than suppress, immorality and unchastity" (as cited in Jensen 2007, 230). A parent who objected to the program was perhaps somewhat more blunt in her feelings:

> If any person attempted to "instruct" my innocent children in subjects that modesty tells us to ignore, I would horsewhip the "educator," and thus give him or her a needed lesson in respecting the rights of parents to bring up their little ones in innocence of the terrible evils of life. (as cited in Jensen 2007, 230–31)

Criticisms such as these carried the day in Chicago, and Flagg's program was not renewed for 1914. In fact, Flagg herself lasted only another two years as superintendent, resigning in 1915 over an issue unrelated to the sex education controversy.

Perhaps the most significant point about the Chicago Experiment is that it raised fundamental questions about the role (if any) that the education of young men and women in topics related to human sexuality should have in public schools. That debate continues today within the context of a number of specific issues, such as whether sex education even belongs in the public schools, the age at which children should be taught about sexuality, the topics that should be included in a class on sexuality, and the role of parents and other adults outside the school system. The rest of this chapter is devoted to a review of some of these issues, their current status in the United States, public attitudes about the issues, and laws and regulations related to the issues.

Sex Education: Yes or No?

Probably the most fundamental question related to the issue of sex education for adolescents in the United States is simply whether or not such instruction should be available to students in public schools, a question first posed with regard to Ella Flagg Young's Chicago Experiment. The debate over this question continues in the first decade of the 21st century, with many of the same arguments offered as were presented in 1913. On the pro side of the debate, the case is made that adolescents need instruction in issues of sexually transmitted infections, pregnancy and contraception, sexual orientation and gender identity, and other issues in order to make better and more informed decisions about their own sexual behaviors. Opponents of sex education in the public schools agree that this goal is desirable, but argue that such instruction should take place in the home, not in schools. This disagreement is not one that can be resolved by turning to research for answers. The choice is fundamentally one of a person's personal philosophy and outlook on life.

A second issue is, however, more amenable to scientific analysis: are school-based sex education programs effective? That is, do such programs actually change the behavior of young men and women who sit through sex education classes in schools? During the 1980s and 1990s, a number of studies were conducted on this question. Most of these studies produced little or no support for the hypothesis that sex education classes change the sexual behavior of adolescents. As an example, a study reported in 1986 that "data reveal no significant relationship between exposure to sex education and the risk of premarital pregnancy among sexually active adolescents" (Dawson 1986, 162). Another study showed that young women who have had a sex education course are neither more nor less likely to use contraception than are those who had no such instruction (Zelnick and Kim 1982, 117; also see Marsiglio and Mott 1986 and Furstenberg, Moore, and Peterson 1986).

Since the turn of the century, very few or no national studies have been conducted to assess the effectiveness of sex education programs (Mueller, Gavin, and Kulkarni 2008). That situation changed in 2008, however, with the release of a comprehensive study on the association between sex education classes and patterns of sexual behavior among adolescents. That study was based on data collected from a sample of 2,019 males and females between the ages of 15 and 19 who had never been married, as reported in the 2002 National Survey of Family Growth, conducted by the Centers for Disease Control and Prevention. The authors of the study pointed out that two important changes had taken place since the last national studies at the end of the 20th century. First, a significantly larger number of teenagers have been exposed to sex education programs in elementary and secondary schools. Second, the age at which students first receive sex education instruction has decreased significantly. These factors, the authors suggest, may help explain the quite different results they obtained, in comparison with earlier studies.

The most significant of those findings was that 71 percent of teenage boys and 59 percent of teenage girls who had attended sex education classes in school were less likely to have sexual intercourse before the age of 15 that those who had not had such instruction. In addition, males who had been in sex education classes were almost three times (2.77 times) as likely to use some form of contraception as those who had not attended such classes. For some subgroups, these results were even more striking. Among African American females, the likelihood of engaging in sexual intercourse before the age of 15 was reduced by 91 percent among those who had attended sex education courses in school (Mueller, Gavin, and Kulkarni 2008, 89; Science Daily 2007).

Public Opinion on Sex Education

In some respects, the battle over the teaching of sexuality in American schools is over. A number of public opinion polls indicate that the vast majority of Americans now support some form of sex education in schools. In 2004, for example, National Public Radio, the Henry J. Kaiser Family Foundation, and the John F. Kennedy School of Government at Harvard University (NPR/KFF/JFK) sponsored a poll of the general public and of public school principals about the role of sex education in American schools. The results of that poll were conclusive, with only 7 percent of respondents in the general poll expressing the view that sex education should not be taught in schools. Almost three quarters of principals (74%) said that sex education was simply not an issue in their schools, with there being no complaints, discussions, or comments from parent groups, religious and community leaders, or elected officials about the teaching of sexuality in schools (NPR/Kaiser/Kennedy School Poll 2004a; NPR 2004). Indeed, the issue is no longer *whether* sex education should be taught in schools, but *what topics* should be included.

One of the interesting findings of the NPR/KFF/JFK poll was that the general public appears to be relatively satisfied with the topics that most experts believe should be included in sex education courses. Of a list of 18 topics read to respondents, 11 received more than a 90 percent approval rating from respondents, including topics such as sexually transmitted infections (99%), HIV/AIDS (98%), and contraception (94%). Three additional topics received more than 80 percent approval, including abortion, how to use and where to get contraceptives, and how to use a condom. Only four topics received a lower rating, but still more than 70 percent approval: masturbation, homosexuality, oral sex, and oral contraceptives without parental knowledge and/or approval (NPR/Kaiser/Kennedy School Poll 2004a; NPR 2004).

The NPR/KFF/JFK poll also pursued the question of how the views of evangelical Christians differ from nonevangelicals on issues of sex education. Not surprisingly, the survey discovered that the former group tends to be somewhat more leery about the role of sex education in the school curriculum. Twelve percent of evangelicals said that sex education should not be provided in schools under any circumstances, three times the rate for nonevangelicals. Evangelicals were also significantly more likely to disapprove of certain specific topics in sex education than were nonevangelicals: twice as many disapproved of mentioning oral sex in classes (41% to 20%), discussions about homosexuality (37% to 18%), information about obtaining contraceptives without parental approval (42% to 20%), and discussions about masturbation (27% to 13%); and three times as many objected to instructions about the use of a condom (26% to 9%) and the use of contraceptives (21% to 7%) (NPR/Kaiser/Kennedy School Poll 2004; NPR 2004a). Overall, the most significant conclusion to be drawn from this poll appears to be that a large majority of Americans appear to favor the inclusion of sex education in schools and approve of the topics most commonly recommended by professional sex educators.

The Content of Sex Education Courses

A large majority of Americans appear to favor the inclusion of sex education in schools and approve of at least some of the topics most commonly recommended by professional sex educators. Americans still differ significantly as to whether topics such as the use of condoms, the availability of contraceptives, and sexual orientation and gender identity should be included in sex education courses, whether all students should be required to attend classes on such topics, and how they should be presented. The sections that follow review some of the specific issues about sex education in schools that are still the subject of debate among Americans.

Abstinence-Only Education

Perhaps the single most controversial issue concerning sex education in American schools today relates to so-called abstinence-only programs. Abstinence-only sex education programs focus on the principle that refraining from sexual intercourse is the only certain way to avoid conception and sexually transmitted infections. Such programs teach about abstinence exclusively, with (usually) no mention of other methods of contraception or avoiding STIs. By contrast, sex education programs that teach a wider array of subjects are generally known as comprehensive sex education programs.

History

Abstinence-only sex education programs first became popular in the late 1990s as the result of an amendment to a welfare-reform bill sponsored by Senator Rick Santorum (R-PA) and Senator Lauch Faircloth (R-NC) in 1996. That amendment established a program for special grants to states for abstinence-only-until-marriage programs in schools. The bill was approved by the U.S. Congress, signed by President George W. Bush, and became part of the Social Security Act (chapter 42 of the United States Code).

The program is now commonly known as Title VI. In order to qualify for grant money, a program has to meet a number of conditions. It must have "as its exclusive purpose, teaching the social, psychological, and health gains to be realized by abstaining from sexual activity." In addition, the program must teach

- [that] abstinence from sexual activity outside marriage [is] the expected standard for all school age children;
- that abstinence from sexual activity is the only certain way to avoid out-of-wedlock pregnancy, sexually transmitted diseases, and other associated health problems;
- that a mutually faithful monogamous relationship in [the] context of marriage is the expected standard of human sexual activity;
- that sexual activity outside of the context of marriage is likely to have harmful psychological and physical effects;
- that bearing children out-of-wedlock is likely to have harmful consequences for the child, the child's parents, and society.

It also must teach

- young people how to reject sexual advances and how alcohol and drug use increases vulnerability to sexual advances and
- the importance of attaining self-sufficiency before engaging in sexual activity (United States Code Title 42. Chapter 7. Subchapter V §710).

Abstinence-only sex education programs are also funded in two other ways by the federal government. The Adolescent Family Life Act (AFLA) is the older of these two programs. It was included as Title XX of the Public Health Service Act of 1981 "to promote abstinence from sexual activity among adolescents and to provide comprehensive health care, education and social services to pregnant and parenting adolescents" (U.S. Department of Health and Human Services. Office of Public Health and Science. Office of Population Affairs 2009). More recently, the U.S. Congress established a program known as Special Projects of Regional and National Significance–Community-Based Abstinence Education (SPRANS–CBAE) (U.S. Department of Health and Human

Services. Health Resources and Services Administration 2000). As of mid-2009, the U.S. government had provided more than $1.5 billion dollars for abstinence-only education through these three programs (Sexuality Information and Education Council of the United States 2008).

Arguments in Favor of Abstinence-Only Sex Education

The argument for abstinence-only programs is implicit in the legislation on which their funding is based, especially the Title VI legislation of Senators Santorum and Faircloth. That argument was restated most recently in a number of letters written by pro-abstinence-education organizations and individuals as the U.S. Congress and President Barack Obama have considered the possibility of cutting back on federal funding of such programs. For example, the National Abstinence Education Association wrote to Senators Tom Harkin and Arlen Specter, chair and ranking member of the Senate Subcommittee on Labor, Health, and Human Services that

> the recent statistics by the CDC, which revealed that 1 in 4 adolescent girls have at least one STD, certainly underscores the need for a strong commitment to the risk elimination message of abstinence-centered programs.
>
> Two of the four STDs tracked in the recent CDC study can easily be spread by skin to skin contact which means that transmission can take place without intercourse and in spite of the use of a condom. Only abstinence will adequately stem this epidemic among teens.
>
> Abstinence education is taught to some 2.5 million youth across the country. Preserving intact funding for this approach is the only way we assure that teens receive the information and skills needed to prevent the physical and emotional consequences of sexual activity. Parents overwhelmingly support the currently funded approach. Teens are also increasingly choosing to be abstinent, so this is a message that resonates with both teens and their parents.
>
> There is also a growing body of research that shows that abstinence education is a good investment and is showing empirical success. A number of studies show that students who participate in abstinence programs delay sexual onset, reduce partners when sexually active and

even discontinue sexual activity if previously sexually experienced. They are also no less likely to use a condom than their peers, if they do become sexually active. (National Abstinence Education Association 2008)

Research on Abstinence-Only Sex Education

Opponents of abstinence-only have a somewhat different view of these programs than those expressed in this letter. They point to a number of research studies which suggest that abstinence-only programs have little or no effect on attitudes or behaviors of students who have completed abstinence-only courses. In April 2007, for example, Mathematica Policy Research, Inc., reported on a study of four federally funded Title V programs in Miami, Florida; Milwaukee, Wisconsin; Powhatan, Virginia; and Clarksdale, Mississippi. Researchers found that "youth in the program group were no more likely than control group youth to have abstained from sex and, among those who reported having had sex, they had similar numbers of sexual partners and had initiated sex at the same mean age" (Trenholm et al. 2007, xvii). Researchers concluded that these programs had "no overall impact on teen sexual activity, no differences in rates of unprotected sex, and some impacts on knowledge of STDs and perceived effectiveness of condoms and birth control pills (Trenholm et al. 2007, 59).

Researchers have also examined some specific aspects of abstinence-only education programs. For example, Janet E. Rosenbaum at the Johns Hopkins University School of Public Health reported in January 2009 on a study of the so-called virginity pledge, sometimes taken as a measure of the success of abstinence-only programs. In this pledge, men and women promise to remain virgins until they are married. In her longitudinal study of 3,440 students who had taken a virginity pledge in 1995, Rosenbaum found that, five years later, 82 percent of the sample denied ever having taken the pledge. More significantly, she found that students who had attended an abstinence-only program did not differ significantly from a matched cohort of students who did not attend such a program on issues related to premarital sex, sexually transmitted infections, and anal and oral sex variables. The only differences found between experimental and control groups were that those who attended abstinence-only programs were less likely to use condoms or other birth control devices either during their first sexual experience or their last (prior to the survey) experience (Rosenbaum 2009, 110).

In a 2007 study, researchers explored the effect of abstinence-only programs on a single topic in sex education: HIV/AIDS infections. They found that among the 15,940 participants in their study

> overall, the trials did not indicate that abstinence-only programs can reduce HIV risk as indicated by behavioral outcomes (e.g., unprotected vaginal sex) or biological outcomes (e.g., sexually transmitted infection). Instead, the programs consistently had no effect on participants' incidence of unprotected vaginal sex, frequency of vaginal sex, number of sex partners, sexual initiation, or condom use. (Underhill, Operario , and Montgomery 2007)

One of the troublesome objections sometimes made about abstinence-only programs is that they not only omit discussions of any topic on sexuality other than abstinence, but also that the information they provide is sometimes inaccurate. In order to examine this issue, the Special Investigations Division of the Minority Staff of the Committee on Government Reform conducted a study in 2004 of a number of abstinence-only programs funded under the Special Programs of Regional and National Significance Community-Based Abstinence Education. Researchers concluded that "over 80% of the abstinence-only curricula, used by over two-thirds of SPRANS grantees in 2003, contain false, misleading, or distorted information about reproductive health" (Special Investigations Division. Minority Staff of the Committee on Government Reform 2004, i). The types of errors found in these programs included incorrect information about the effectiveness of contraceptives and the risks of abortion, a blurring of the line between scientific information and religious doctrine, a presentation of stereotypes about boys and girls as factual information, and a number of straightforward scientific errors (Special Investigations Division. Minority Staff of the Committee on Government Reform 2004, i–ii).

Another issue that concerns opponents of abstinence-only programs is the emphasis given such programs by the federal government, which annually gives about $170 million for the support of abstinence-only sex education. Critics claim that this emphasis puts the federal government "out of step not only with research, but also with public opinion" ("Few Americans Favor Abstinence-only Sex Ed" 2006). Public opinion surveys appear to confirm the latter half of this complaint. For example, a study of

1,096 adult Americans in late 2005 and early 2006 asked whether respondents favored abstinence-only sex education programs or comprehensive programs (that included both abstinence and other approaches to sex education), as well as their attitudes about various aspects of sex education programs. Researchers found that 82 percent of respondents favored a comprehensive approach to the teaching of sexuality, and 68 percent approved instruction on the proper use of condoms. Thirty-six percent of respondents favored an abstinence-only approach to sex education (Bleakley, Hennessy, and Fishbein 2006, 1151).

The Future of Abstinence-Only Sex Education

A significant change in federal policy about abstinence-only programs was announced by White House domestic policy coordinator Melody Barnes in May 2009. The 2010 federal budget would drastically reduce funding for such programs, she said, with most of the money saved being earmarked for teen pregnancy prevention programs. The shift in policy came, Barnes said, in response to research findings that abstinence-only programs simply do not achieve the goals for which they are designed. "In any area where Americans want to confront a problem, they want solutions they know will work," Barnes said, "as opposed to programming they know hasn't proven to be successful" (Jayson 2009).

Proponents of abstinence-only education strongly disagreed with President Obama's decision to withdraw funding from such programs. In a press release on the topic, the National Abstinence Education Association said that

> the president's budget ignores research that documents a 50% decrease in sexual onset among teens that are enrolled in abstinence programs. . . .
>
> At a time when teens are subjected to an increasingly sexualized culture, it is essential that common-sense legislators from both sides of the aisle reject this extreme attempt to defund the only approach that removes all risk. Members of Congress would be well advised to listen to youth and parents in their districts who overwhelmingly support these valuable programs. (National Abstinence Education Association 2009)

This statement suggests that a number of individuals still strongly support the principle of abstinence-only sex education in American schools and that the debate over the content of sex education is likely to continue for the foreseeable future.

Condom Instruction

One of the most controversial topics in school sex education programs involves instruction in the use of condoms. Most sex educators believe that condom use is an important component in conducting a safe sexual life since condoms are an effective method of preventing many sexually transmitted infections and pregnancy. No one argues that condoms are a perfect solution for these problems, although they are among the most effective anti-infective and contraceptive devices readily available to teenagers and adults. In fact, evidence suggests that a large majority of adults favor the inclusion of instruction about condom use in any effective school program of sex education (NPR/Kaiser/Kennedy School Poll 2004b, 11). The point at which condoms often become an issue in schools is the decision by some schools and some school systems to provide free condoms for students who request them. According to the most recent data available (from 1996), 2.2 percent of all schools in the United States and 0.3 percent of all school systems made condoms available to students at no cost (Kirby and Brown 1996). A somewhat more recent survey for the state of Massachusetts found somewhat larger numbers: 15 percent of all high schools in the state, enrolling 21 percent of the state's high school students, had free condom programs (Blake 2003). These numbers are small, but the announcement of a free condom program often stirs up a reaction among parents and other citizens in a community (see, for example, Ramos 1996).

Perhaps the most common objection to the practice of distributing condoms to students is that it violates religious beliefs of many citizens in the community. In March 2009, for example, Stonehill College in suburban Boston banned the distribution of condoms on campus. A spokesperson for the college said that the college's policy follows church teachings, and those teachings prohibit the use of contraceptive devices (Schworm 2009). Members of religious groups are also citizens of the community, and their beliefs and value systems should also be respected. Offering free condoms to teenagers is an affront to those beliefs and value systems and should not be permitted.

Opponents to this view point out that the United States is a nation where the interests of church and state are kept separate. It may be true that the distribution of condoms is offensive to some individuals, but if the practice contributes to good public health (by way of reduced rates of unwanted pregnancy and sexually transmitted infections), then it should be instituted for the general well-being of society.

Critics of free condom distribution also argue that a program of this kind only makes the problems it attempts to solve worse because it encourages adolescents to become more sexually active. If you teach a boy or girl how to use a condom, they say, that person will be more likely to become engaged in sexual activities, with a potential increase in the rate of sexually transmitted infections and unplanned pregnancies (Focus on the Family 2009a; also see Limbaugh 2007).

Proponents of condom distribution point out that numerous studies have now been conducted on the correlation (if any) between condom distribution and extent of sexual activity. In studies of such programs in two large cities—New York and Philadelphia—researchers found that students from schools with free condom-distribution programs were no more sexually active than students in comparable schools. In the New York case, the percentage of students who were sexually active in New York City, which has a distribution program, and Chicago, which does not, was essentially the same, about 60 percent. In Philadelphia, the rate of sexually active teenagers was slightly less in schools with distribution programs (56%) than in schools without such programs (Guttmacher et al. 1997; Furstenberg, Frank F., Jr., et al. 1997; also see Schuster et al. 1998; Zabin et al. 1986; Rabb 1998).

An additional argument against condom distribution programs has recently been developed by those opposed to such programs, namely that condoms are unreliable devices for protecting against unwanted pregnancies and sexually transmitted infections. Critics often quote failure rates of up to 20 percent or more, indicating that knowledge of how to use a condom does not in and of itself guarantee protection against sexually transmitted infections or unwanted pregnancies. A position paper on this topic from Focus on the Family, an evangelical Christian organization, claims that

> studies have found condom failure rates in protecting against pregnancies for teens to be as high as 22.5 percent. As for protecting against STDs, in 2001 several government health agencies together released a report on

condom effectiveness. The report found evidence that condoms are about 85 percent effective in preventing the spread of HIV/AIDS. (Is 85 percent good enough in protecting your child against a deadly and incurable virus?) The report also found condoms to be somewhat effective in protecting men (but not women) from gonorrhea. But the prominent scientists who prepared the report found no conclusive evidence that condoms protect against any other STD, including HPV, the primary cause of cervical cancer, which kills more women than AIDS does. (Focus on the Family 2009a; also see Limbaugh 2007; Christian Contraception 2009)

Proponents of condom distribution respond to this argument by explaining that condoms are safe anywhere from 85 to 99 percent of the time, depending on a number of factors, including the quality and age of the condom and the skill with which it is used. They base these arguments on information provided by the Centers for Disease Control and Prevention and the American College of Obstetrics and Gynecology (American College of Obstetrics and Gynecology 2009; Centers for Disease Control and Prevention 2009a). Clearly, each side of this argument has a legitimate position in that the effectiveness of condoms depends very much on a number of factors, such as quality of product and skill in use, and ultimately the decision to use one depends on the risk one is willing to take in avoiding infection and pregnancy given the stated rates of failure.

Homosexuality

Another topic that generally receives widespread support for inclusion in sex education programs, but among the lowest level of support of all topics, is homosexuality. In its 2004 survey of public attitudes about sex education, for example, the National Public Radio/Kaiser Family Foundation/John F. Kennedy School of Government Poll found that 73 percent of respondents found it appropriate for sex educators to talk about homosexuality and sexual orientation at either the junior high (80% approval) or senior high (73% approval) level, with 25 percent saying the topic was not appropriate for either age group (NPR/Kaiser/Kennedy School Poll 2004b, 13). While this level of support appears to be significant, the topic of homosexuality ranks 16th out of 18 topics in the NPR/KFF/JFK poll, followed only by oral sex (72% approval) and obtaining of contraceptives by girls without parental consent (71% approval) (NPR/Kaiser/Kennedy School Poll 2004a). These nationwide results have been confirmed in a number of local polls on the same topic, the appropriateness of various topics for sex education classes. In Alabama, for example, a state in which respondents might be expected to take a somewhat less supportive view of the subject, respondents to a recent poll expressed approval for the inclusion of homosexuality in sex education courses by almost the same margin as in the NPR/KFF/JFK poll. In the Alabama poll, 72 percent of respondents approved discussions of issues about homosexuality, provided they were presented in a neutral and unbiased manner (Center for Governmental Services at Auburn University 2005, 1). A similar study of a much smaller population produced very similar results. That study, conducted by the University of North Florida, asked respondents about topics they deemed appropriate for sex education classes in both middle and high schools. Researchers found that 75.8 percent of respondents thought the topic was suitable for middle school (8%), high school (23.5%), or both levels (44.3%), while 21.5 percent thought the subject was not appropriate for either level (Public Opinion Research Laboratory. University of North Florida 2006, 24).

In spite of the apparently widespread support for discussions of issues related to homosexuality in sex education courses, that topic has been the focus of a significant number of complaints in schools throughout the nation. One of the concerns of some individuals is that mention of same-sex relationships in a sex education class is, in fact, an excuse for promoting homosexuality and encouraging more students to become interested in and, perhaps, involved in homosexual relationships. Such programs are, these individuals say, a way of recruiting boys and girls to the homosexual movement. For example, Louis Sheldon, chairman of the Traditional Values Coalition, has written a special report on programs for the recruitment of children by public schools. In this report, Sheldon argues that "[Gay and lesbian] activists use issues of 'safety,' 'tolerance,' and 'homophobia' as tactics to promote homosexuality in our nation's schools." He goes on to say that these "militants" are "pushing for aggressive recruitment programs in public schools. If you want children, what better place to find them than in the public schools? After all, since homosexual couples can't reproduce, they will simply go after your children for seduction and conversion to homosexuality" (Sheldon [n.d.], 1). One of the most articulate spokespersons for this position has been Judith A. Reisman, president of the Institute for Media Education. In 2002, she wrote a long article describing, among other points, how she believes that gay and lesbian activists are using schools to promote homosexuality and to recruit boys and girls to becoming gay and lesbian. She concludes that "it has taken organizational commitment, planning, and effort to cultivate and initiate the current crop of bisexual and homosexual youth. However, on the other hand, homosexuality (bisexuality and transgendered sexuality) is the only extant sexuality cult receiving both tax dollars and direct access to school children, with laws protecting PROJECT 10 type teachers. The advisor, guide, teacher, or 'helping hand' aids recruitment and limits potential escapees during all stages of initiation of children into homosexuality" (Reisman 2002, 327; also see MissionAmerica.com 2007).

A second reason for concern about the inclusion of topics dealing with same-sex relationships in schools is similar to that for the topic of condoms, namely that many individuals have strong religious or personal objections to homosexual practices and do not believe that schools should present views in opposition to their beliefs. This kind of issue has traditionally been a difficult one for public schools. The American public undoubtedly has a wide range of views on almost any topic taught in public schools. Some people, for example, do not believe in the biological theory of evolution and, instead, accept the view of life on Earth offered under the rubric of "intelligent design." Such individuals object to having their children taught about evolution, unless alternative views (such as intelligent design) are taught concurrently. Other people may not believe that the Holocaust ever occurred or may not subscribe to explanations as to how the Civil War began or accept explanations of the fall of Communism presented in history textbooks. The objections that could be raised to a variety of school subjects because they offend the personal beliefs of one parent or one group of parents are almost endless. As judges in one of the cases involving the issue of homosexuality in sex education classes have written, "Public schools often walk a tightrope between the many competing constitutional demands made by parents, students, teachers, and the schools' other constituents," after which they enumerated some of those "competing demands" (United States Court of Appeals for the First Circuit 2007).

Perhaps the most common expression of parents' wishes to protect their children from unacceptable ideas has traditionally been efforts to have objectionable books removed from school libraries or the school curriculum. Among the books most commonly challenged over the past half century are works generally classified as classics, such as *The Great Gatsby, Catcher in the Rye, The Grapes of Wrath, To Kill a Mockingbird, 1984, Of Mice and Men, Brave New World, As I Lay Dying, A Farewell to Arms, Gone with the Wind, One Flew over the Cuckoo's Nest, All the King's Men*, and *Rabbit Run* (American Library Association 2009).

Schools are faced with the challenge of accommodating the wishes of individual parents or groups of parents, even though those individuals and groups represent only a small minority of residents of a district. One of the most common methods for handling this issue is by offering a so-called opt-out option to parents. This provision allows parents to choose to have students *not* attend certain classes, read certain books, or participate in certain school activities that they see as antithetical to their own views. Of course, opt-out provisions are generally not made available across the board in most systems because of the chaos they might produce if individual students were to decide which topics they were going to study in school and which they were going to ignore with an opt-out letter from their parents.

Because of the fundamentally controversial aspect of many topics in sex education, opt-out options are probably more common in this field than in any other part of the public school curriculum. The most recent survey of state policies on sex education, for example, found that 20 states and the District of Columbia require the teaching of sex education at some level of instruction. Most other states have no such requirement, but do have specific policies about the manner in which contraception and abstinence are taught. A much larger number of states—35 states and the District of Columbia—require that some form of education about HIV/AIDS be included in the curriculum. The issue of parental involvement in sex education is the subject of legislation in 38 states and the District of Columbia. In three of those states—Arizona, Nevada, and Utah—written consent from parents is required in order for students to attend a sex education class. In 36 states and the District of Columbia, students are allowed to opt out of sex education instruction by presenting a letter from parents (Arizona has both of these provisions) (Guttmacher Institute 2009).

The question of whether teachers may discuss issues related to homosexuality both in formal sex education classes and in any other kind of instructional setting has now been reviewed by U.S. courts at a number of levels and with regard to a variety of specific complaints. Although court decisions have varied, the general trend appears to be that exposure of students to topics dealing with homosexuality is not unconstitutional (Walsh 1996). As an example, the case of *Brown v. Hot, Sexy, and Safer Productions* (68 F.3D 525) in 1995 raised the question of whether an assembly dealing with HIV/AIDS, which included some graphic presentations, invaded the privacy rights of students and subjected them to sexual harassment because they were required to attend the assembly. The suit by students was dismissed by the district court on March 5, 1995, a decision that was upheld by the U.S. Court of Appeals for the First District on October 23, 1995. The appeals court concluded that

> the facts alleged here are insufficient to state a claim for sexual harassment under a hostile environment theory. The plaintiffs' allegations are weak on every one of the Harris factors, and when considered in sum, are clearly insufficient to establish the existence of an objectively hostile or abusive environment. (United States Court of Appeals for the First Circuit 1995)

Two other cases dealt with the more informal mention of homosexuality in schools. In *Godkin v. San Leandro School District*, parents complained that their constitutional rights had been violated because a teacher made pro-gay statements in a class. In *Berrill v. Houde*, parents argued that one of the complainant's children had been subjected to "gay recruiting" because the teacher had prohibited the use of derogatory language about gays and lesbians in her classroom. California district courts rejected both arguments (Stewart 2001, 242–43).

One of the most recent cases involving a discussion of homosexuality in schools is *Parker v. Hurley*, in which two sets of parents sued a number of employees of the Lexington (Massachusetts) school district (including superintendent William Hurley) for exposing their first- grade children to stories about same-sex relationships without having notified parents in advance of this activity. The parents argued that their religious tradition found that homosexual relationships were repugnant and immoral, and that the school's actions were, therefore, an affront to their religious beliefs. The parents' suit was dismissed by the district court and then again by the court of appeals. The latter court ruled that

> public schools are not obliged to shield individual students from ideas which potentially are religiously offensive, particularly when the school imposes no requirement that the student agree with or affirm those ideas, or even participate in discussions about them. . . . On the facts, there is no viable claim of "indoctrination" here. Without suggesting that such showings would suffice to establish a claim of indoctrination, we note the plaintiffs' children were not forced to read the books on pain of suspension. Nor were they subject to a constant stream of like materials. There is no allegation here of a formalized curriculum requiring students to read many books affirming gay marriage. . . . The reading by a teacher of one book, or even three, and even if to a young and impressionable child, does not constitute "indoctrination." (United States Court of Appeals for the First Circuit 2007)

The status of the discussion of homosexuality in sex education classes in public schools cannot be considered a matter of settled case law at this point. Still, for parents who object to having their children exposed to this topic, an opt-out option, in which they can have their children excused from such classes, generally appears to be the most prudent way of avoiding having to deal with this issue in the courts.

A topic increasingly mentioned in connection with same-sex relationships is the issue of gender identity. Over the past decade, gay, lesbian, and bisexual groups have more frequently been including transgendered individuals and issues in their work. Concurrent with that change has been the effort to include instruction about transgender issues in school sex education programs.

Thus far, relatively little progress has been made in this effort, at least partly because of the dominance of abstinence-only education in many of the nation's schools. In the NPR/KFF/JFK survey discussed above, no mention was made of transgender issues, so no information is available from that source about the occurrence of transgender issues in schools or how the general public feels about including this topic in sex education programs.

Some data are available from another source, however, the 2008 GENIUS Index (Gender Equality National Index for Universities and Schools), conducted by the Gender Public Advocacy Coalition (GenderPAC). According to that study, seven states have enacted policies to protect students from bullying and harassment on the basis of gender identity. Overall, the study found that more than 4,250,000 students in 1,115 high schools, 1,142 middle schools, 3,131 elementary schools, and 320 preschools are covered by antiharassment policies established by states or local school systems. Included among these policies are antiharassment protections adopted by 8 of the nation's 25 largest school systems: New York City Public Schools, Houston Independent School District, Hillsborough County School District, Philadelphia City Schools, Detroit City School District, Montgomery County Public Schools, Prince George's County Public Schools, and Memphis City School District (2008 GENIUS Index). This studies provides no information about the inclusion of gender identity in sex education courses, data which apparently does not currently exist.

Abortion

There is probably no issue related to human sexuality—and probably no issue in modern American society—more controversial than abortion. That topic deserves far more extensive and detailed attention than can be provided in this book (but see McBride 2007). The question can be asked, however, how the topic of abortion is integrated into programs of sex education and how parents, teachers, students, and the general community feel about this allotment of time and attention to such a controversial subject. Surprisingly, relatively little information is available on any of these questions, especially in view of the extensive research that has been done about other possible topics for sex education classes, such as sexually transmitted infections, contraception and pregnancy, and sexual orientation and gender identity. One study provides a hint as to the reason for this situation. In 2000, researchers at the Guttmacher Institute reported on changes that had taken place in sex education programs in the United States between 1988 and 1999. One of the trends they found was that some controversial issues in sexuality were receiving significantly less attention at the end of that period than at the beginning. Discussion of topics such as abortion, condom use, and sexual orientation had decreased by anywhere from 14 to 20 percent between 1988 and 1999. Even though significant majorities of sex education teachers thought these topics were important (89%, 81%, and 78%, respectively), they were less like to be included in sex education classes at the end of the study period than at the beginning. The actual percentage of classes in which each of the three topics was covered was 62 percent, 52 percent, and 50 percent, respectively, representing a difference of 27 percent, 29 percent, and 28 percent, respectively, in the attention teachers *thought* they should give a subject from the amount they *did* give to the subject (Dailard 2001). An important factor in this trend appears to be fears among teachers of community reaction against the inclusion of such topics in sex education courses. According to the Guttmacher study, more than a third of all teachers interviewed expressed such concerns (Dailard 2001). Interestingly enough, these fears may not reflect the interests and concerns of most community members, as expressed in studies such as the NPR/KFF/JFK survey discussed earlier. In the single question about abortion asked in that survey, 85 percent of respondents said that they thought that abortion topics are a legitimate subject for inclusion in sex education programs at either the middle school or high school level, or both. By contrast, 13 percent of respondents felt that abortion was not a suitable topic in sex education courses for students at either level (NPR/Kaiser/Kennedy School Poll 2004b, 12).

An even more powerful influence in the decreased attention paid to abortion and other controversial topics may have been the increasing emphasis on abstinence-only education that developed during the period covered by the Guttmacher study. That study found that the fraction of teachers who offered abstinence-only courses increased from 2 percent in 1988 to 23 percent in 1999 (Darroch, Landry, and Singh 2000, 204). Such courses may be less likely than comprehensive sex education programs to mention abortion.

Of even greater concern, perhaps, is the finding produced by one important study that abortion information that *is* provided by abstinence-only education programs may be biased or incorrect. In its 2004 study of 13 widely used abstinence-only education programs, for example, the Special Investigations Division (SID) of the House Committee on Government Reform noted that most abstinence-only programs are explicitly antiabortion and, perhaps for that reason, subject to providing erroneous information. The SID listed a number of statements and assertions provided in abstinence-only programs and pointed out how these statements and assertions differ from generally accepted scientific information (Special Investigations Division 2004, i, 13–14).

In any case, specialists in the field of sex education have given considerable thought to the presentation of abortion topics in school classes and have devised a number of suggestions for such curricula. One of the most detailed of these studies is one conducted by the Sexuality Information and Education Council of the United States (SIECUS). In its 2004 publication, *Guidelines for Comprehensive Sexuality Education*, SIECUS suggests two dozen concepts about abortion that can be presented at any one of four development levels: middle childhood (ages 5 through 8), preadolescence (ages 9 through 12), early adolescence (ages 12 through 15), and adolescence (ages 15 through 18). These concepts cover not only factual information about abortion, but also legal, ethical, social, and psychological issues related to the procedure (National Guidelines Task Force 2004, 61–62).

What Should Schools Teach about Sex?

The question of what schools should teach about human sexuality appears to be one that concerns citizens in almost every part of the United States. A recent survey of Web sites devoted to discussions about sex education curricula in public schools on Google found many descriptions of debates taking place on the content of programs in a variety of districts, including Winston-Salem/Forsyth County, North Carolina; Montgomery County, Maryland; Palm Beach County, Florida; Guilford County, North Carolina; Pittsburgh, Pennsylvania; Milwaukee, Wisconsin; El Paso, Texas; Sangamon County, Illinois; and St. Lucie County, Florida. In virtually all cases, parents and other interested stakeholders were arguing about the appropriate place of instruction on abortion, same-sex relationships, condom use, and other topics discussed earlier in this chapter.

Some national organizations have attempted to develop model curricula that can be adopted in whole or that can be adopted to fit local school situations. One of the best known of these recommendations can be found in *Guidelines for Comprehensive Sexuality Education*, a report published by the Sexuality Information and Education Council of the United States (SIECUS). This publication was developed by a panel of experts from a number of organizations with an interest in sex education, including the American Medical Association, March of Dimes Birth Defect Association, National Education Association, National School

Boards Association, Planned Parenthood, and SIECUS itself, along with representatives of secondary schools and colleges and universities. The third edition of the guidelines was issued in 2004.

The *Guidelines* publication itself focuses on general principles, rather than providing specific lesson plans for sex education classes. The publication begins with a discussion of certain desirable behaviors of a "sexually healthy adult," including items such as "appreciate one's own body," "avoid exploitative and manipulative relationships," "take responsibility for one's own behavior," and "develop critical-thinking skills." The publication then moves on to list six key concepts that should drive an effective curriculum in sex education: human development, relationships, personal skills, sexual behavior, sexual health, and society and culture. Each of these key concepts is, in turn, subdivided into smaller subconcepts, such as reproductive and sexual anatomy and physiology, puberty, sexual orientation, marriage and lifetime commitments, raising children, assertiveness, negotiation, masturbation, sexual abstinence, contraception, abortion, sexual abuse, sexual assault, gender roles, and sexuality and religion (National Guidelines Task Force 2004, 18).

Although the *Guidelines* publication does not itself include specific recommendations for curricula, SIECUS does provide access on its SexEdLibrary Web site to more than 100 lesson plans, some of which it has developed itself, and some of which have been adopted from other sources, suitable for instruction in the 39 topics listed in the *Guidelines* (SexEdLibrary.org 2009).

Issues That Transcend School Programs

A number of issues with which young men and women have to deal transcend the formal school experience, although they may appear at some point within formal school sex education programs also. Two examples of such issues have to do with access to contraceptive materials and devices by adolescent girls, and vaccination against the human papillomavirus (HPV) for prepubescent girls.

Access to Contraceptive Devices

A number of schools and school systems have considered whether they should provide contraceptives to all students who ask for them. This issue is an expanded version of the question considered earlier with regard to the dispensing of free condoms to male students who request them. The two issues are not identical, at least partly, apparently, because the general public may have somewhat differing views about sexually active males (who might request condoms) and sexually active females (who might request oral contraceptives or other birth control materials and devices). According to recent polls, most Americans seem to approve of schools' providing contraceptive devices to young women. In a 2007 poll conducted by Ipsos Public Affairs, about a third of all respondents approved providing birth control devices to all students who ask for them (30%), another third approved the practice only if students have parental approval (37%), and another third do not approve of having schools dispense contraceptives under any circumstances (PollingReport.com 2009). On the question of how the availability of contraceptives might affect the sexual activity of teenagers, respondents were evenly split. Forty-nine percent of respondents said they did not believe that the availability of contraceptives would encourage adolescents to be more sexually active, while 46 percent had the opposite view, believing that access to birth control would make adolescents more likely to be sexually active. Finally, a significant majority of respondents felt that the availability of contraceptives would contribute to a reduction in the number of teenage pregnancies (62%), while smaller numbers thought that it would have no effect (22%) or would actually result in an increase in the number of pregnancies (13%) (PollingReport.com 2009).

The question of whether schools should dispense birth control devices became national news in October 2007, when school officials at King Middle School in Portland, Maine, announced a new policy of providing contraceptives to children of high school age who were still enrolled in middle school. The decision was apparently one of very few instances in the United States in which contraceptive-dispensing programs were available at the middle school level. School officials pointed out that only 5 of the school's 510 pupils would qualify for the program because of its age restrictions. They said that one motivating factor in providing the program was that there had been seven pregnancies among middle school students in Portland's three middle schools in the preceding five years. On the basis of reports by many students that they were, indeed, sexually active, the school had been handing out free condoms since 2000, but they had not had, and had not requested, the authority to issue oral contraceptives also (CBS News 2007).

A number of parents approved of the school's decision. One mother and school board member said that "as a parent, I would hope that my child would come to me first. But if she doesn't feel comfortable, then I know that there's somebody there, and a support system in place for them to be able to talk to somebody." Another parent said that she was elated with the school's decision, and that critics of the new program should "just get over it." A number of parents and other interested observers had a somewhat different reaction. The nine people who spoke against the proposal at the school board meeting had two major concerns. First, they thought that making birth control devices available to students would encourage them to become more sexually active. Second, they were troubled that parents would not be notified if students requested contraceptive devices and/or if the school provided such devices (Bouchard 2007). In any case, the school refused to retract its decision to offer contraceptives to King students, and six months later, only one student had taken advantage of the new program (Sharp 2008).

The administration of contraceptive-dispensing programs is most commonly the responsibility of school-based health centers, in-school programs most commonly operated by hospitals, medical schools, local health departments, or community health centers. In 2009, there were about 1,700 of these centers, representing about 6 percent of all schools in the United States (National Assembly on School-Based Health Care 2009; National Center for Education Statistics 2009, table 5). Of this number, about a third offered birth control devices to students ("Others Not Likely to Follow School's Contraception Move" 2007). In this respect, then, the number of students in the United States who have access to birth control devices through schools is very small, roughly 2 percent of all students in the nation, almost all of them high school students.

The question of whether or not schools should be permitted (or required) to distribute contraceptive devices has become a common topic on the Internet. Dozens of blogs debate the pros and cons of the issue, generally with the same arguments being made for and against the practice. Among the 17 respondents writing in favor of school distribution programs on the Helium Web site, the most common position was that teenagers are going to be sexually active in any case, so helping them to protect against sexually transmitted infections and pregnancy is an important challenge for schools. One blogger expressed her view as follows:

> Birth control should be available in schools because young people are not going to stop experimenting. Along with the birth control, should be expert advice on how to use it, and what the consequences are if they don't. . . . The sex drive is high on the list of human needs. In the teens, boys particularly are keen to try it out and not every girl will be able to refuse. While generally girls are blamed for getting pregnant, she is usually unfortunate and has possibly been pressured into having sex by the powerful urges of her contemporary males. (Redfern 2009)

A number of bloggers also emphasized the use of contraceptives as a way that teenagers can protect themselves against disease and pregnancy, especially when they have not been properly educated about sexual topics in their own homes or at school. In the Helium poll, Kerah Pierce writes that

> I don't think it is encouraging teenagers to have sex but to learn more about it. If high schoolers know how to protect themselves instead of doing what they think is right they would be better off. Many teenagers that experiment do not know the risks or the proper way to protect themselves from disease or possible pregnancy. . . . Parents who are shy about the topic have kids that learn about it from school and friends. Normally when a teen learns about this subject from friends it is not accurate statements. Teens need to learn the importance of protection but to be abstinent also. It is better that a teen use protection rather than nothing at all. (Pierceall 2009)

A common argument against allowing schools to distribute contraceptives is that the practice will provide legitimacy for teenagers to be more sexually active. As one Helium blogger expressed the view:

> If you start doing that at your school, your [sic] sending the wrong message to kids that it is okay to be having sex. I mean after all, schools do have sex education courses for this type of thing. Do we not stress enough

about teenage girls becoming pregnant to begin with? . . .
If you start firing away with birth control, kids will just
think it's really cool to have sex whenever they want.

So if a young person wants to get birth control, then
they need to get their own, and experience life their own
way. If you give them the birth control, your [*sic*] giving
them a gun that will take their life away. (Burton 2009)

A number of bloggers in the Helium poll acknowledged concerns
about the transmission of sexual infections and the possibility of
unplanned pregnancies. They simply did not believe that solving these problems was the business of schools. As one blogger
writes:

It is my very deeply held conviction that public schools
should never dispense birth control materials to teenagers. Never.

It is not the school's business to invade the private
lives of its students. The responsibility of the school is to
teach, and nothing more. It is not the responsibility of the
school to act as a surrogate parent. . . .

The use of birth control is a personal, family matter,
and decisions concerning its use should be made only by
a family, not by outsiders. (Parsons 2009)

Among the more than 500 adults and teenagers who participated
in the Helium poll, the majority (56%) opposed the practice of
schools handing out contraceptives. The poll was not, of course,
conducted scientifically and represented the views of only those
individuals who chose to participate (Helium 2009).

Access to Contraceptives outside of Schools

The issue of access to contraceptive devices transcends debates
about the role of schools. Such devices are, of course, also available
at pharmacies, family planning centers, and other facilities that
have nothing to do with the educational establishment. Generally
speaking the opportunity for buying male contraceptive devices,
such as condoms and spermicides, is somewhat easier than it is
for buying female contraceptives since the former are generally
available to boys and men of any age without a prescription. Female contraceptive devices, however, are generally available only

by prescription. One question, then, is whether and under what circumstances a medical professional might be prompted to write a prescription for a contraceptive device for an underage girl. In fact, such instances are probably rare and occur in most cases not for the purpose of providing contraception but to deal with other reproductive problems, such as irregular or difficult menstrual periods (Van Hooffet al. 1998). It has also been reported that one can order female contraceptive devices through the Internet from sources outside the United States (see, for example, 111DrugStore. com 2009).

The Controversy over Plan B

One of the most contentious issues about contraceptives for women in the past decade has been with regard to the approval of a form of emergency contraception (EC) known as Plan B. Plan B consists of two pills, each containing 0.75 milligrams of the hormone levonorgestrel to be taken within 72 hours of sexual intercourse. The pills prevent the release of a fertilized egg from the ovaries, thus interrupting the earliest stages of pregnancy. Plan B was approved as a prescription drug by the U.S. Food and Drug Administration (FDA) in May 1999. In April 2003, the drug manufacturers submitted a petition to the FDA to have the drug's status changed from a prescription product to an over-the-counter (OTC) drug. Eight months later, an FDA advisory committee voted 23 to 4 to approve the petition, but the FDA itself declined to accept that recommendation and kept Plan B on its prescription-only list.

Over the next 32 months, the FDA declined to change its position on the availability of Plan B, a period of time characterized by intense political lobbying by both proponents and opponents of changing the drug's status to OTC from prescription only. Toward the end of this period, the controversy became further complicated as the U.S. Congress declined to move forward on the nomination of Andrew von Eschenbach as commissioner of the FDA until the agency agreed to change its position on Plan B. Finally, on August 24, 2006, the FDA did just that, approving the use of Plan B for purchase by women and their male partners over the age of 18 (The Emergency Contraception Website 2009).

The FDA's decision did not end the controversy over Plan B, however, as proponents of the drug insisted that it should be available without prescription for women 17 and older, not 18 and older. Opponents argued that 17 is simply too young for a girl to be able to purchase contraceptive devices without the advice and approval of a physician and/or her parents. They also cited the slippery-slope argument, that dropping the age from 18 to 17 made it easier to drop the age even further—or perhaps eliminate the age provision entirely—at some time in the future (Galanos 2009).

For another 30 months, the FDA declined to change its position on the 17-year-old versus 18-year-old controversy. Finally, in March 2009, Judge Edward R. Korman, of the U.S. District Court for the Eastern District of New York, ordered the FDA to adopt the younger age standard and allow 17-year-old women and their male partners over the age of 17 to purchase Plan B over the counter (United States District Court. Eastern District of New York 2009). A month later, the FDA acted on that order and made the contraceptive available to women 17 and older (U.S. Food and Drug Administration 2009).

Pharmacist Choice in Filling Contraceptive Prescriptions

Yet another issue involving the furnishing of contraceptives to women has arisen in the past decade. That issue concerns the right of pharmacists who disagree with the use of contraceptives to decline to fill legally written prescriptions for such pharmacists. As an example: In January 2005, a mother of six children visited a Walgreens pharmacy in Milwaukee, Wisconsin, to have a prescription filled for emergency contraception because her husband's condom failed during an act of intercourse. The Walgreen pharmacist refused to fill the prescription, telling the woman that "You're a murderer. I will not help you kill this baby. I will not have the blood on my hands" (Chandrasekhar 2006). The woman's response that she was requesting emergency contraception, which does not produce an abortion, was rejected by the pharmacist.

The "freedom of choice for pharmacists" movement is based on the belief that an individual pharmacist who objects to abortion or the use of contraceptives because of his or her religious, moral, or ethical beliefs is justified in refusing to fill a prescription for a contraceptive. The public record is now replete with many examples of cases of this kind in almost every state of the union, ranging from local family-owned pharmacies to giants like those operated in Target, Walgreens, Winn Dixie, and Wal-Mart stores (Coyne 2005; also see Planned Parenthood Affiliates of New Jersey

2009). A representative of the Christian Legal Society's Center for Law and Religious Freedom, which defends pharmacists who take this position, has said that "more and more pharmacists are becoming aware of their right to conscientiously refuse to pass objectionable medications across the counter. We are on the very front edge of a wave that's going to break not too far down the line" (News Journal 2005).

The American Pharmaceutical Association (APhA) has taken a stance in support of the right of pharmacists to refuse to fill prescriptions that violate their personal beliefs. The APhA's official position is that

> APhA recognizes the individual pharmacist's right to exercise conscientious refusal and supports the establishment of systems to ensure patient's access to legally prescribed therapy without compromising the pharmacist's right of conscientious refusal. When this policy is implemented correctly, and proactively, it is seamless to the patient, and the patient is not aware that the pharmacist is stepping away from the situation. In sum, APhA supports the ability of the pharmacist to step away, not in the way, and supports the establishment of an alternative system for delivery of patient care.
>
> APhA policy does not support lecturing a patient or taking any action to obstruct patient access to clinically appropriate, legally prescribed therapy. APhA policy does not interject the pharmacist between the patient and the physician. (American Pharmacists Association 2008)

Not all medical professionals agree with the APhA. The American Medical Association (AMA), for example, has taken the position that pharmacists should not come between patients and the medical advice provided by their physicians. The association expressed concern about the actions of pharmacists who object to filling a prescription and then refuse to return the prescription to a patient, increasing the difficulty in having the prescription filled. The AMA House of Delegates passed a resolution at its 2005 meeting supporting the action of states and the federal government to ensure that patients are able to have legally written prescriptions filled whether or not a specific pharmacist has individual objections to the material required by a prescription (Adams 2005).

Both the state and federal government have begun to take legal action on the question of whether pharmacists have the right to refuse to fill prescriptions that offend their personal religious, ethical, or moral beliefs. The first regulation of this kind was adopted in Illinois in April 2005, when Governor Rod Blagojevich issued an emergency rule stating that pharmacies in the state that sell contraceptives are not allowed to refuse to fill prescriptions because of personal beliefs about contraception and abortion (Illinois Government News Network 2005). Since that action, just under a hundred bills have been filed in state legislatures regarding the rights of a pharmacist to refuse to fill prescriptions for contraceptives. Those bills fall into two general categories, those allowing pharmacists to take such actions with fear of reprisals for their decisions, and those prohibiting pharmacists from refusing to fill such prescriptions. As of May 2009, 11 bills had been enacted in California, Colorado, Florida, Georgia, Illinois, Maine, Mississippi, South Dakota, Tennessee, and Washington State. Eight of those laws reaffirm the right of a pharmacist to fill a prescription with which he or she does not agree, for whatever reason. Only the California, Illinois, and Washington legislation has the opposite force, requiring a pharmacist to fill any legally written prescription for a contraceptive (National Conference of State Legislatures 2009).

In June 2007, U.S. Representative Carolyn B. Maloney (D-NY) and Senator Frank Lautenberg (D-NJ) introduced a bill, H.R. 2596/S. 1075, to establish federal policy on the filling of prescriptions for contraceptives by pharmacists. The bill, known as the Access to Birth Control Act, had two major provisions. First, a pharmacist was not permitted to refuse to fill a legally written prescription on the basis of his or her personal objections to the use of contraceptives. If the prescribed medication was not available, a pharmacist would be required to take one of a number of possible actions to see that the prescription would be properly filled. Second, a pharmacist would not be allowed to "intimidate, threaten, harass customers," "interfere or obstruct" with filling of a prescription, "intentionally misrepresent or deceive customers" about a prescription, "breach medical confidentiality" in filling a prescription," or "refuse to return" a valid prescription (U.S. House of Representatives 2007).

Opponents of birth control and contraceptives argued that the bill imposed on their own religious and ethical beliefs. For example, an article in a newsletter published by the Concerned Women for America of Kansas argued that

> historically, the right to refuse to do something that violates one's conscience has been honored by civilized society. Only in the realm of despots are people forced to do something that is inherently wrong for them, particularly when it involves taking a life. . . .
>
> The FDA has been known to make mistakes in approving drugs, and doctors have made mistakes in prescribing. Pharmacists provide a line of defense to ensure that patients' lives and health are protected and can make patients aware of ethical concerns. Yet this bill would punish pharmacists up to $500,000 for acting on their ethical duty. (Concerned Women for America of Kansas 2007)

In any case, the debate over the Access to Birth Control Act of 2007 has become moot since the bill was never considered by the House committee to which it was referred, and it died at the end of the 100th Congress. The issue of pharmacists' right to fill or not refill prescriptions, however, is almost certainly not dead, and it may well appear in some future congressional debate.

Human Papillomavirus (HPV)

The term *human papillomavirus* refers to a group of viruses that cause warts and certain types of cancer. Some HPV viruses cause no symptoms whatsoever, and an individual with these viruses is unaware that she or he has been infected. More than 130 varieties of the human papillomavirus have been identified, about 40 of which can be transmitted by intimate or sexual contact. Sexually transmitted HPV viruses are classified as low-risk or high-risk. Low-risk viruses are responsible for an infection known as genital warts, which are soft, moist, pinkish warts that appear on the vagina, cervix, penis, or anus. They are uncomfortable and sometimes painful, but they represent no serious long-term medical threat to an individual. They can be removed by a physician, although the virus remains in the body and the warts may return at a later date. High-risk viruses can lead to cancer of the vulva, vagina, and anus in women and cancer of the anus and penis in men.

·Genital HPV infections are currently the most common sexually transmitted infection in the United States. The Centers for Disease Control and Prevention (CDC) estimates that about 20 million Americans are currently infected with one strain or another of HPV, and 6.2 million new infections occur every year. The CDC estimates that about 1 percent of all sexually active Americans have genital warts at any one time (Centers for Disease Control and Prevention 2009b).

By far the most serious issue with regard to HPV infections is the risk of cancer that some strains of the virus pose. The American Cancer Society has estimated that there will be 11,270 new cases of cervical cancer diagnosed in the United States in 2009 and 4,070 deaths from the disease during the same period. Comparable figures for other forms of HPV-related cancers are 3,580 new cases of vulvar cancer and 900 deaths; 2,160 new cases of vaginal cancer and 770 deaths; 1,290 new cases of penile cancer and 300 deaths; 5,290 new cases of anal cancer and 710 deaths (American Cancer Society 2009).

The treatments for HPV-related cancer are similar to those for other types of cancer, primarily chemotherapy and radiation. As with most medical problems, the best approach is to adopt behaviors that reduce the risk of contracting cancer. In the case of HPV infections, the most effective method of prevention is abstinence and/or restricting one's sexual activity to well-established long-term relationships with a person whose sexual history is known. Condoms also provide some measure of protection against HPV infections, although that protection is limited because condoms do not necessarily cover all regions of the body through which infection may spread.

In June 2006, the FDA gave its approval for the marketing of a new vaccine against four strains of HPV: HPV 6, HPV 11, HPV 16, and HPV 18. The first two of these strains are responsible for about 90 percent of all cases of genital warts, while the latter two are responsible for about 70 percent of all cases of cervical cancer, as well as some cases of anal cancer. The vaccine, called Gardasil, made by Merck & Company, is administered in a series of three injections over a period of six months. It is recommended for girls between the ages of 11 and 12, although it can be given as early as age 9 (Centers for Disease Control and Prevention 2007).

One might expect the availability of a vaccine against four dangerous strains of HPV to be enthusiastically supported by anyone interest in sexual health. And, in fact, most such groups are pleased that this new option for sexual health care is available. However, controversy has developed over some possible applications of the new vaccine. For example, in July 2008, the U.S. Citizenship and Immigration Services announced that women between the ages of 11 and 26 applying to immigrate to the United States would henceforth be required to be vaccinated against HPV (U.S. Citizenship and Immigration Services 2008). The agency's decision was met with objections from a number of women's groups, who argued that required vaccinations infringe on a woman's right to make important decisions about her own reproductive health. For example, the National Organization for Women (NOW) issued a press release saying that

> the new requirement violates a woman's basic right to self-determination, creates additional barriers for immigrant families seeking adjustment of status, and unfairly forces immigrant women to subject their bodies to a new treatment with known side effects. . . .
>
> The HPV vaccination requirement is essentially a surcharge applied only to young immigrant women that will effectively block them from immigrating to the U.S. or becoming U.S. citizens. Gardasil is the most expensive vaccine on the market, costing a person nearly $500. . . . This is and can be a lot of money for women seeking adjustment of immigration status. (National Organization for Women 2008)

Another area in which debate has developed over the use of the new HPV vaccine is the public school system. Some advocates for the vaccine have argued that its use is really a public health issue, similar to the use of vaccination to prevent other kinds of infectious disease. They recommend that vaccination of young girls be required as a condition of school entry, as is the case with vaccinations for diphtheria, tetanus, pertussis, hepatitis A, hepatitis B, polio, varicella, measles, mumps, rubella, and some other contagious diseases (although requirements differ by state). If society is able to prevent cervical cancer, anal cancer, and other devastating diseases, should it not do so, they ask?

Perhaps the strongest representation of this position occurred in 2007, when Governor Rick Perry of Texas issued an executive order requiring all girls to be vaccinated for HPV as a condition for entry into sixth grade in the state's schools. In announcing his order, Perry said:

> Never before have we had an opportunity to prevent cancer with a simple vaccine. While I understand the concerns expressed by some, I stand firmly on the side of protecting life. The HPV vaccine does not promote sex, it protects women's health. In the past, young women who have abstained from sex until marriage have contracted HPV from their husbands and faced the difficult task of defeating cervical cancer. This vaccine prevents that from happening. (Office of the Governor Rick Perry 2007)

Perry's executive order angered almost every group in the state, from women's rights activists to right-to-life supporters to members of both parties in the state legislature. Perry's own lieutenant governor, for example, noted that "I think while the HPV vaccine can play a very important role in preventing cervical cancer, I don't think government should ever presume to know better than the parents" (MacLaggan 2007). Two months after Perry issued his executive order, the Texas legislature voted overwhelmingly to overturn that order. It passed a bill (135 to 2 in the house and 30 to 1 in the senate) delaying the implementation of an HPV vaccination plan until at least 2011 (Blumenthal 2007).

The Texas debate over HPV vaccinations raised some more general questions about efforts by the drug's manufacturer, Merck, in trying to convince state governments to make such vaccinations mandatory for school children. Questions were raised about Merck's own role in Perry's decision and about its involvement in other states' consideration about the inclusion of HPV vaccination in state immunization programs. The company finally decided to issue a public statement that it would no longer pursue its efforts to convince states of the value of requiring HPV vaccinations for elementary school girls (Childs 2007).

In Conclusion

In some ways, the American public appears to have reached consensus on some fundamental issues relating to sexual health. There appears, first of all, to be widespread support for the principle that adolescents should receive some type of education about human sexuality in public schools. Furthermore, there is a significant consensus on the topics that ought to be included in such sex education programs, with general approval for a number of topics, especially those related to sexually transmitted infections and pregnancy and contraception. Other topics about which there has traditionally been some disagreement, such as sexual orientation and certain types of sexual behaviors, receive less enthusiastic support, but are still approved by about three quarters of the general population.

Some issues related to sexual health are still very controversial, however, and attempts to include them in public school programs tend to create sometimes fiery debate. The distribution of condoms and other contraceptive devices and the discussion of same-sex relationships are just two such topics. History suggests that reasoned discussion among those on all sides of an issue may eventually result in curriculum decisions that will help students have access to important information that they can use in building their own philosophy of human sexuality.

References

Adams, Damon. 2005. "AMA to Protect Patient Access to Medications." *AMNews*, July 11. http://www.ama-assn.org/amednews/2005/07/11/prsd0711.htm. Accessed on June 15, 2009.

American Cancer Society. 2009. "What Are the Key Statistics about Anal Cancer/Penile Cancer/Vaginal Cancer/Vulvar Cancer?" http://www.cancer.org/docroot/CRI/content/CRI_2_4_1X_What_are_the_key_statistics_for_Anal_Cancer_47.asp; http://www.cancer.org/docroot/CRI/content/CRI_2_4_1X_What_are_the_key_statistics_for_Penile_Cancer_47.asp; http://www.cancer.org/docroot/CRI/content/CRI_2_4_1X_What_are_the_key_statistics_for_Vaginal_Cancer_47.asp; http://www.cancer.org/docroot/CRI/content/CRI_2_4_1X_What_are_the_key_statistics_for_Vulvar_Cancer_47.asp. Accessed on June 16, 2009.

American College of Obstetricians and Gynecologists. "Contraception." Online brochure. http://www.acog.org/publications/patient_education/bp022.cfm. Accessed on June 8, 2009.

American Library Association. 2009. "Banned and/or Challenged Books from the Radcliffe Publishing Course Top 100 Novels of the 20th Century." http://www.ala.org/ala/issuesadvocacy/banned/frequentlychallenged/challengedclassics/reasonsbanned.cfm. Accessed on June 14, 2009.

American Pharmacists Association. 2008. "Issue Brief: Pharmacist Conscience Clause." http://www.pharmacist.com/AM/Template. cfm?Section=Home2&TEMPLATE=/CM/ContentDisplay. cfm&CONTENTID=15688. Accessed on June 15, 2009.

Blake, Susan M. et al. 2003. "Condom Availability Programs in Massachusetts High Schools: Relationships With Condom Use and Sexual Behavior." *American Journal of Public Health* 93 (6): 955–61.

Bleakley, Amy, Michael Hennessy, and Martin Fishbein. 2006. "Public Opinion on Sex Education in U.S. Schools." *Archives of Pediatric and Adolescent Medicine* 160 (11; November): 1151–56.

Blumenthal, Ralph. 2007. "Texas Legislators Block Shots for Girls Against Cancer Virus." *New York Times*, April 26. http://www.nytimes. com/2007/04/26/us/26texas.html?_r=2&oref=slogin. Accessed on June 16, 2009.

Bouchard, Kelley. 2007. "Middle School Adds Birth Control Options." *Portland Press Herald/Maine Sunday Telegram*, October 18. http:// pressherald.mainetoday.com/story.php?id=141436&ac=PHnws. Accessed on June 15, 2009.

Burton, Ryan. 2009. "Should Schools Give Teens Birth Control?" http:// www.helium.com/debates/161091-should-schools-give-teens-birth- control/side_by_side?page=4. Accessed on June 15, 2009.

CBS News. 2007. "Birth Control for Maine Middleschoolers." http:// www.cbsnews.com/stories/2007/10/18/national/main3379737.shtml. Accessed on June 15, 2009

The Center for Governmental Services at Auburn University. 2005. "Sex Education in Public Schools: What Alabama Thinks." *Ask Alabama* 2 (9; June): 1–3.

Centers for Disease Control and Prevention. 2007. "HPV (Human Papillomavirus): What You Need to Know." http://www.cdc.gov/ vaccines/pubs/vis/downloads/vis-hpv.pdf. Accessed on June 16, 2009.

Centers for Disease Control and Prevention. 2009a. "Genital HPV Infection—CDC Fact Sheet." http://www.cdc.gov/STD/HPV/STDFact- HPV.htm#common. Accessed on June 16, 2009.

Centers for Disease Control and Prevention. 2009b. "Unintended Pregnancy Prevention: Contraception." http://www.cdc.gov/ ReproductiveHealth/UnintendedPregnancy/Contraception.htm. Accessed on June 8, 2009.

Chandrasekhar, Cahru A. 2006. "Rx for Drugstore Discrimination: Challenging Pharmacy Refusals to Dispense Prescription Contraceptives under State Public Accommodations Laws." *Albany Law Review* 70 (1; Winter): 55–115.

Childs, Dan. 2007. "Political Intrigue in Merck's HPV Vaccine Push." ABCNews Health. http://abcnews.go.com/Health/story?id=2890402 &page=1. Accessed on June 16, 2009.

Christian Contraception. 2009. "Male Condoms." http://www. christiancontraception.com/condoms.php. Accessed on June 13, 2009.

Concerned Women for America of Kansas. 2007. "Bridging the Gap." http://www.cwfa.org/images/content/fc2007-06-21.pdf. Accessed on June 15, 2009.

Coyne, Brenda. 2005. "More Pharmacists Refusing to Fill Emergency Contraception Orders." *New Standard*. http://newstandardnews.net/content/index.cfm/items/2522. Accessed on June 15, 2009.

Dailard, Cynthia. 2001. "Sex Education: Politicians, Parents, Teachers and Teens." http://www.guttmacher.org/pubs/tgr/04/1/gr040109. html. Accessed on June 14, 2009.

Darroch, Jacqueline E., David J. Landry, and Susheela Singh. 2000. "Changing Emphases in Sexuality Education in U.S. Public Secondary Schools, 1988–1999." *Family Planning Perspectives* 32 (5; September–October): 204–11, 265.

Dawson, Deborah Anne. 1986. "The Effects of Sex Education on Adolescent Behavior." *Family Planning Perspectives* 18 (5; September–October): 162–70.

The Emergency Contraception Website. 2009. "Plan B and the Bush Administration." http://ec.princeton.edu/pills/planbhistory.html. Accessed on June 15, 2009.

Fass, Paula S., ed. 2004. *Encyclopedia of Children and Childhood: In History and Society*. New York: Macmillan Reference. http://www.faqs.org/childhood/Re-So/Sex-Education.html. Accessed on June 11, 2009.

"Few Americans Favor Abstinence-only Sex Ed." 2006. http://www. msnbc.msn.com/id/15603764. Accessed on June 13, 2009.

Focus on the Family. 2009a. "Condoms and Abstinence: Separating Truth From Myth." http://www.citizenlink.org/FOSI/abstinence/A000002137.cfm. Accessed on June 13, 2009.

Focus on the Family. 2009b. "Is Sex Ever Really 'Safe'?" http://www. troubledwith.com/ParentingTeens/A000000529.cfm?topic=parenting%20 teens%3A%20sexual%20activity. Accessed on June 13, 2009.

Furstenberg, Frank F., Jr., et al. 1997. "Does Condom Availability Make a Difference? An Evaluation of Philadelphia's Health Resource Centers." *Family Planning Perspectives* 29 (3; May–June): 123–27.

Furstenberg Frank F., Kristin Moore, and James L. Peterson. 1986. "Sex Education and Sexual Experience among Adolescents." *American Journal of Public Health* 75 (11):1331–32.

Galanos, Mike. 2009. "Commentary: Plan B Risky for 17 Year-old Girls." CNNHealth.com. http://www.cnn.com/2009/HEALTH/04/30/ galanos.plan.b/index.html. Accessed on June 15, 2009.

Guttmacher, Sally et al. 1997. "Condom Availability in New York City Public High Schools: Relationships to Condom Use and Sexual Behavior," *American Journal of Public Health*. 87 (9; September): 1427–33.

Guttmacher Institute. 2009. "State Policies in Brief as of June 1, 2009: Sex and STI/HIV Education." http://www.guttmacher.org/statecenter/ spibs/spib_SE.pdf. Accessed on June 14, 2009.

Helium. 2009. "Should Schools Give Teens Birth Control?" http://www. helium.com/debates/161091-should-schools-give-teens-birth-control. Accessed on June 15, 2009.

Illinois Government News Network. 2005. "Gov. Blagojevich Takes Emergency Action to Protect Women's Access to Contraceptives." http://www.illinois.gov/PressReleases/ShowPressRelease. cfm?SubjectID=3&RecNum=3805. Accessed on June 15, 2009.

Jayson, Sharon. 2009. "Obama Budget Cuts Funds for Abstinence-only Sex Education." *USA Today.* http://www.usatoday.com/news/ health/2009-05-11-abstinence-only_N.htm. Accessed on June 13, 2009.

Jensen, Robin E. 2007. "Using Science to Argue for Sexual Education in U.S. Public Schools: Dr. Ella Flagg Young and the 1913 'Chicago Experiment.'" *Science Communication* 29 (2): 217–41.

Kirby, Douglas B., and Nancy L. Brown. 1996. "Condom Availability Programs in U.S. Schools." *Family Planning Perspectives* 28 (5; September–October): 196–202.

Limbaugh, Rush. 2007. "Condoms: The New Diploma." In *Current Issues and Enduring Questions: A Guide to Critical Thinking and Argument, with Readings,* ed. Sylvan Barnet and Hugo Bedau, 426–30. New York: Bedford/St. Martin's.

MacLaggan, Corrie. 2007. "Perry's HPV Vaccine Order Draws Backlash from GOP," February 6,. http://www.statesman.com/news/content/ region/legislature/stories/02/06/6hpv.html. Accessed on June 16, 2009.

Marsiglio William, and Frank L. Mott. 1986. "The Impact of Sex Education on Sexual Activity, Contraceptive Use and Premarital Pregnancy among American Teenagers." *Family Planning Perspectives* 18 (4): 151–61.

McBride, Dorothy E. 2007. *Abortion in the United States: A Reference Handbook.* Santa Barbara, CA: ABC-CLIO.

MissionAmerica.com. 2007. "The Dirty Dozen Checklist: Does Your School Promote Homosexuality?" http://www.missionamerica.com/ agenda.php?articlenum=67. Accessed on June 14, 2009.

Moran, J. P. 1996. "'Modernism Gone Mad': Sex Education Comes to Chicago, 1913." *Journal of American History* 83 (2): 481–513.

Mueller, Trisha E., Lorrie E. Gavin, and Aniket Kulkarni. 2008. "The Association between Sex Education and Youth's Engagement in Sexual Intercourse, Age at First Intercourse, and Birth Control Use at First Sex." *Journal of Adolescent Health* 42 (1; January): 89–96.

National Abstinence Education Association. 2008. http://www.abstinenceassociation.org/docs/action_alerts/2008_Letter_to_Harkin_Specter.pdf. Accessed on June 12, 2009.

National Abstinence Education Association. 2009. "President's Budget Eliminates Funding for Effective Abstinence Education Programs." http://www.abstinenceassociation.org/newsroom/pr_051109_presidents_budget_eliminates_funding.html. Accessed on June 13, 2009.

National Assembly on School-Based Health Care. 2009. http://www.nasbhc.org/site/c.jsJPKWPFJrH/b.2561543/k.C944/advocacy.htm. Accessed on June 14, 2009.

National Center for Education Statistics. 2009. "Digest of Education Statistics." Table 5. http://nces.ed.gov/programs/digest/d08/tables/dt08_005.asp. Accessed on June 14, 2009.

National Conference of State Legislatures. 2009. "Pharmacist Conscience Clauses: Laws and Legislation. Updated May 2009." http://www.ncsl.org/default.aspx?tabid=14380. Accessed on June 15, 2009.

National Guidelines Task Force. 2004. *Guidelines for Comprehensive Sexuality Education*, 3rd edition. New York: Sexuality Information and Education Council of the United States.

National Organization for Women. 2008. "National Coalition for Immigrant Women's Rights Statement: HPV Vaccination Requirement Discriminates Against Immigrant Women," September 29. http://www.now.org/issues/diverse/nciwr/100108immigrationhpv.html. Accessed on June 16, 2009.

News Journal. 2005. "Pharmacists War over Contraceptives." http://news.dcealumni.com/461/280305-pharmacists-war-over-contraceptives/. Accessed on June 15, 2009.

NPR. 2004. "Sex Education in America." http://www.npr.org/templates/story/story.php?storyId=1622610. Accessed on June 12, 2009.

NPR/Kaiser/Kennedy School Poll. 2004a. "Sex Education in America." http://www.kff.org/newsmedia/upload/Sex-Education-in-America-Summary.pdf. Accessed on June 12, 2009.

NPR/Kaiser/Kennedy School Poll. 2004b. "Sex Education in America: General Public/Parents Survey." http://www.kff.org/newsmedia/

upload/Sex-Education-in-America-General-Public-Parents-Survey-Toplines.pdf. Accessed on June 12, 2009.

Office of the Governor Rick Perry. 2007. "Statement of Gov. Rick Perry on HPV Vaccine Executive Order," February 5. http://governor.state.tx.us/news/press-release/2291/. Accessed on June 16, 2009.

111DrugStore.com. 2009. "Buy Female Hormones, Contraceptives Online Without Prescription." http://www.111drugstore.com/topselling.php?catnum=10. Accessed on June 15, 2009.

"Others Not Likely to Follow School's Contraception Move." 2007. *USA Today.* http://www.usatoday.com/news/health/2007-10-17-middle-school-birth-control_N.htm. Accessed on June 14, 2009.

Parsons, Tom. 2009. "Should Schools Give Teens Birth Control?" http://www.helium.com/debates/161091-should-schools-give-teens-birth-control/side_by_side?page=13. Accessed on June 15, 2009.

Pierceall, Kerah. 2009. "Should Schools Give Teens Birth Control?" http://www.helium.com/items/1021068-should-schools-give-teens-birth-control. Accessed on June 15, 2009.

Planned Parenthood Affiliates of New Jersey. 2009. "Refused at the Counter: Personal Stories." http://www.plannedparenthoodnj.org/library/topic/pharmacy_refusal/refused_at_the_counter. Accessed on June 15, 2009.

PollingReport.com. 2009. "Abortion and Birth Control." http://www.pollingreport.com/abortion.htm. Accessed on June 14, 2009.

Public Opinion Research Laboratory. University of North Florida. 2006. "Sex Education Survey. Kids Connected by Design. St. Lucie County, Florida." http://www.stluciecountyhealth.com/hiv_aids/sex_ed_report.pdf.

Rabb, Marian. 1998. "Condom Availability in High School Does Not Increase Teenage Sexual Activity but Does Increase Condom Use." *Family Planning Perspectives* 30 (1; January–February): 48–49.

Ramos, Pilar S. 1996. "The Condom Controversy in the Public Schools: Respecting a Minor's Right of Privacy." *University of Pennsylvania Law Review* 145 (1; November): 149–92.

Redfern, Rosemary. 2009. "Should Schools Give Teens Birth Control?" http://www.helium.com/debates/161091-should-schools-give-teens-birth-control/side_by_side?page=4. Accessed on June 15, 2009.

Reisman, Judith A. 2002. "Crafting Bi/homosexual Youth." *Regent University Law Review* 14 (2; Spring): 283–342.

Rosenbaum, Janet Elise. 2009. "Patient Teenagers? A Comparison of the Sexual Behavior of Virginity Pledgers and Matched Nonpledgers." *Pediatrics* 123 (1; January): e110–20.

Schuster Mark A. et al. 1998. "Impact of a High School Condom Availability Program on Sexual Activities and Behaviors." *Family Planning Perspectives* 30 (2; March–April): 67–72, 88.

Schworm, Peter. 2009. "Catholic College Bars Student's Free Condoms." *Boston Globe*, March 5. http://www.boston.com/news/local/ massachusetts/articles/2009/03/05/catholic_college_bars_students_ free_condoms/. Accessed on June 13, 2009.

Science Daily. 2007. "Sex Education Linked to Delayed Teen Intercourse, New Study Says." http://www.sciencedaily.com/ releases/2007/12/071220231428.htm. Accessed on June 11, 2009.

SexEdLibrary.org. 2009. "Over One Hundred Lesson Plans in One Place." http://www.sexedlibrary.org/. Accessed on June 16, 2009.

Sexuality Information and Education Council of the United States. 2008. "No More Money: Funding Chart." http://www.nomoremoney.org/ index.cfm?fuseaction=page.viewpage&pageid=1004. Accessed on June 12, 2009.

Sharp, David. 2008. "AP Exclusive: 6 Months Later, 1 Student Got Contraceptives," April 18. http://www.boston.com/news/local/ maine/articles/2008/04/18/ap_exclusive_6_months_later_1_student_ got_contraceptives/. Accessed on June 15, 2009.

Sheldon, Louis P. [n.d.] "Homosexuals Recruit Public School Children." *Traditional Values* 18 (11): 1–8.

Special Investigations Division. December 2004. Minority Staff of the Committee on Government Reform. *The Content of Federally Funded Abstinence-only Education Programs.* [n.p.].

Stewart, Chuck. 2001. *Homosexuality and the Law*. Santa Barbara, CA: ABC-CLIO.

Trenholm, Christopher et al. April 2007. *Impacts of Four Title V, Section 510 Abstinence Education Programs.* Princeton, NJ: Mathematic Policy Research.

2008 GENIUS Index. "Gender Equality National Index for Colleges and Schools." http://74.125.95.132/search?q=cache:lYDSnjkFTSEJ:www. gpac.org/genius/2008.pdf+2008+genius+index&cd=1&hl=en&ct=clnk &gl=us. Accessed on June 15, 2009.

Tyack, David, and Elisabeth Hansot. 1990. *Learning Together: A History of Coeducation in American Public Schools.* New Haven, CT: Yale University Press.

Underhill Kristen, Don Operario, and Paul Montgomery. 2007. "Abstinence-only Programs for HIV Infection Prevention in High-income Countries." *Cochrane Database of Systematic Reviews.* http:// www.google.com/search?hl=en&q=underhill+operario&aq=f&oq=& aqi=. Accessed on June 13, 2009.

United States Code. 2009. http://www.gpoaccess.gov/uscode/index.html. Accessed on June 12, 2009.

United States Court of Appeals for the First Circuit. 1995. *Ronald C. Brown, et al., Plaintiffs—Appellants, v. Hot, Sexy and Safer Productions, Inc., et al., Defendants—Appellees.* http://www.ca1.uscourts.gov/cgi-bin/getopn.pl?OPINION=95-1275.01A. Accessed on June 14, 2009.

United States Court of Appeals For The First Circuit. 2007. *Parker v. Hurley.* 474 F. Supp. 2d 261 (D. Mass 2007), 37–43. http://caselaw.lp.findlaw.com/cgi-bin/getcase.pl?court=1st&navby=docket&no=071528. Accessed on August 28, 2009.

United States District Court. Eastern District of New York. 2009. *Annie Tummino et Al.,—Against—Frank M. Torti.* http://www.nyed.uscourts.gov/pub/rulings/cv/2005/05cv366mofinal.pdf. Accessed on June 15, 2009.

U.S. Citizenship and Immigration Services. 2008. "USCIS Changes Vaccination Requirements to Adjust Status to Legal Permanent Resident." http://www.uscis.gov/portal/site/uscis/menuitem.5af9bb95919f35e66f614176543f6d1a/?vgnextoid=902252b10f45b110VgnVCM1000004718190aRCRD&vgnextchannel=1958b0aaa86fa010VgnVCM10000045f3d6a1RCRD. Accessed on June 16, 2009.

U.S. Department of Health and Human Services. Health Resources and Services Administration. 2000. "Maternal and Child Health Federal Set-Aside Program; Special Projects of Regional and National Significance; Community-Based Abstinence Education Project Grants." http://frwebgate.access.gpo.gov/cgi-bin/getdoc.cgi?dbname=2000_register&docid=00-29425-filed.pdf. Accessed on June 12, 2009.

U.S. Department of Health and Human Services. Office of Public Health and Science. Office of Population Affairs. 2009. "Adolescent Family Life." http://www.hhs.gov/opa/familylife/. Accessed on June 12, 2009.

U.S. Food and Drug Administration. 2009. "Updated FDA Action on Plan B (levonorgestrel) Tablets." http://www.fda.gov/NewsEvents/Newsroom/PressAnnouncements/ucm149568.htm. Accessed on June 15, 2009.

U.S. House of Representatives. 2007. "A Bill to Establish Certain Duties for Pharmacies to Ensure Provision of Food and Drug Administration-approved Contraception, and for Other Purposes." http://maloney.house.gov/documents/reproductivechoice/alpha/041707ABCbill.pdf. Accessed on June 15, 2009.

Van Hooff, Marcel H. A. et al. 1998. "The Use of Oral Contraception by Adolescents for Contraception, Menstrual Cycle Problems or Acne." *Acta Obstetricia et Gynecologica Scandinavica* 77 (9): 898–904.

Walsh, Mark. 1996. "Parent-Rights Cases Against Schools Fail to Make Inroads." *Education Week,* April 10. http://www. edweek.org/login.html?source=http://www.edweek.org/ew/ articles/1996/04/10/29rights.h15.html&destination=http://www. edweek.org/ew/articles/1996/04/10/29rights.h15.html&levelId=1000. Accessed on June 14, 2009.

Zabin, Laurie S. et al. 1986. "Evaluation of a Pregnancy Prevention Program for Urban Teenagers." *Family Planning Perspectives* 18 (3; May–June): 119–26.

Zelnick, M., and Y. J. Kim. 1982. "Sex Education and Its Association with Teenage Sexual Activity, Pregnancy and Contraceptive Use." *Family Planning Perspectives* 14 (3; May–June): 117–19, 123–26.

3

Worldwide Perspective

Generalizing about the status of the sexual health of adolescents in various countries around the world is a challenging task. Life in Great Britain is so different from life in Saudi Arabia, or Japan, or Honduras, or Fiji that it is difficult to describe the knowledge that young people have about issues in sexuality, the sexual issues they face in their everyday lives, the sources and kinds of information available to them about sexuality, and the ways and extent to which they are able to make use of such information. There is no doubt that pregnancy and contraception have always been and still are issues of extreme importance to most women—and, probably, many men—in nations around the world. In many countries, women still face the dilemma of how they will deal with the birth of a sixth, seventh, or eighth child, just as their ancestors have done for hundreds or thousands of years. Throughout most of time, they and their male partners have had to rely on folk remedies, such as the array of pessaries described in Chapter 1 of this book.

But new issues have begun to arise over the past century also. One factor in the changing face of human sexuality has been a demographic change. As more people move from rural to urban settings, they often lose contact with traditional sources of information about human biology, such as direct contact with farm animals and instruction by parents and other close relatives. Although the information gained from these traditional sources may not always be accurate or helpful, it may sometimes be better than no information at all. In addition, access to information from outside one's home neighborhood, state, or homeland through sources such as films, radio, television, and the Internet have exposed young people in almost every part of the world to ideas and images about which they would have known next to nothing in the past. Finally, the terrible pandemic of the HIV/AIDS crisis may have been the single most powerful force in driving nations to increase their attention to sex education than any single event in the past. The overall consequence of factors such as these is that countries in every part of the world have begun to think more seriously about the kind of instruction in human sexuality that young people need. The answer to that question differs, of course, depending on a host of factors, including dominant religious values, traditional ethical systems, community attitudes and beliefs, specific needs within a community or nation, and resource availability. This chapter reviews some of the issues with which individuals, families, neighborhoods, and nations are dealing in the area of human sexuality.

Sex Education

With almost 200 separate and distinct nations in the world, it is clearly impossible to make generalizations about any aspect of sex education. Arguably the single best source for information on this subject—and on almost any other topic in the area of human sexuality—is a publication, *The Continuum Complete International Encyclopedia of Sexuality*, which has detailed descriptions of the status of many sexuality-related topics in 62 countries of the world (Francoeur and Noonan 2004). Readers are referred to this invaluable source for far more detailed information than can be provided here.

Europe

The term *sex education* can refer to any number of situations, ranging from personal "birds and bees" talks between parents and children to formal classes in schools devoted solely to this topic. Every conceivable variation on these methods can be found somewhere in the world. Probably the most formal approaches to sex education are to be found in the most developed nations of the world: Europe, the United States, Australia, and New Zealand. In these nations, educators and sexologists have been thinking for almost a century about formal methods by which students can be taught about essential topics in the area of human sexuality.

Today, in most of those nations, sex education is either required as part of the standard school curriculum, or sex education courses are a normal part of that curriculum. Some examples of this situation are as follows.

Denmark: Sex education has been part of Danish schools since the early 1900s, but it became a required subject in 1970. Rather than existing as a separate course, the subject is typically integrated into other subjects, so that students can raise a question about sexuality in any class at any time. While this arrangement may have some advantages, it has also proved to be one of the weak spots in instruction about human sexuality. The major problem is that many teachers do not feel competent to deal with questions about human sexuality, so they avoid discussing them in their classes. In a survey conducted in 2005, the Danish Family Planning Association (Dansk familieplanlægning forening) found that instruction in sexuality was "simply too uneven and random as regards hours spent on the subject and teachers' knowledge" (Sex and Samfund 2009). In an effort to deal with that issue, the association has been attempting to increase the amount of attention paid to sex education for future teachers during their college training. As a result of these efforts, the Danish government made it mandatory as of January 2007 for all teachers colleges to offer a course in sex education, although students are not required to attend those courses (Wellings and Parker 2006, 38). The deficiencies in the Danish model appear to be apparent when students are asked about their experiences in schools. Fewer than half thought that their instruction in sexual issues was both "relevant and sufficient" (Francoeur and Noonan 2004, Denmark).

Netherlands: The approach to sex education in the Netherlands has been called a model for the rest of the world. That praise comes at least in part because the Dutch have the lowest pregnancy rate among teenagers of any developed country in the world (Valk 2000). Although sex education is not required by the national government, it is offered in almost every school in the country, usually as a part of a biology class. Given the nation's long tradition of local autonomy in education, it is not surprising that instruction in sexuality varies significantly from school to school and from teacher to teacher. As might be expected, topics that are taught and the approaches used in teaching them tend to reflect a particular teacher's own expertise and biases. The topics most commonly included in the Dutch curriculum include physical and emotional development; human reproduction;

relationships; sexual behavior; masturbation; sexual problems; safer sex, and sex, culture, and religion (Wellings and Parker 2006, 67). Overall, almost no data exist describing the status of sex education programs in the country (Francoeur and Noonan 2004, Netherlands).

Poland: The situation in Poland is significantly different from that in Denmark and the Netherlands. Under Communist rule in the 1970s, the Polish government introduced an approach to sex education called Preparation for the Life in the Socialist Family, which included some mention of topics traditionally covered in sex education courses. With the fall of Communism, the Roman Catholic Church reasserted its authority in a number of fields, including education, and all types of sex education were banished from schools. Sex education is now an independent part of the curriculum in Poland under the rubric of Education for Family Life (EFL), which represents exclusively the Roman Catholic view of human sexuality. All schools are required to offer Education for Family Life programs, but students are not required to attend such classes. In fact, parents must sign a letter of agreement authorizing a child to attend an EFL class, an agreement that he or she may abrogate at any time in the future for any specific lesson (Wellings and Parker, 71–72).

Spain: The character of sex education in Spain is strongly influenced by the nature of the national government, which shares power with 17 autonomous communities and 2 autonomous cities. The country's approach to sex education is made somewhat more confusing by the fact that, although Spain is traditionally a strongly Roman Catholic nation, it has recently adopted a number of liberal social policies with regard to human sexuality, including a recognition of same-sex marriage and the loosening of regulations on abortion. The national government has no formal policy or regulation on sex education, and instructional policies developed by local communities range from across the board instruction in schools to stand-alone lessons outside the formal school setting run by independent agencies and organizations. Overall, one report has concluded that

> sexuality education in Spain is said to be inadequate and almost non-existent, particularly in rural areas, and its provision needs to be better evaluated. Attitudes of young people are conditioned by stereotypes, myths and erroneous beliefs about sexuality, although

recently some observers have noted an increase in the official commitment to sexuality education. (Wellings and Parker 2006, 78)

United Kingdom

As is the case in most countries around the world, the status of sex education in the United Kingdom has undergone a significant evolution over the past few decades. The guiding principle today is provided under a rubric known as Personal, Social, Health, and Economic Education (PSHE), which originated in the 1990 National Curriculum statement as Personal Social Education (PSE). The fundamental components of PSE, as outlined in the 1990 document, were economic and industrial understanding, career education and guidance, health education, education for citizenship, and environmental education (Macdonald 2009, 10). In 2000, the government adopted a modified form of PSE in a new national framework described as "Preparing Young People for Adult Life: Personal, Social and Health Education (PSHE)." The framework was a recommendation to local school districts, but was not made a statutory requirement.

In September 2008, PSHE was again modified, this time with the addition of two additional topics, personal well-being, and economic well-being and financial capability. The new guidelines kept their former acronym of PSHE, which now stood for Personal, Social, Health, and Economic Education. A month later, the government announced plans to make PSHE compulsory in all public schools in the country, and asked Alasdair Macdonald, headmaster of the Morpeth school in East London, to conduct a review of these plans. Macdonald announced the results of his review in April 2009, which included 20 recommendations for the implementation of the government's new policy. The first recommendation was that the government should, indeed, proceed with its plans to make PSHE mandatory in all primary and secondary schools, for students age 5 through 16. Macdonald also recommended that individual schools be permitted to determine how best to implement the government's general guidelines in their own specific situations. In what was to become the most controversial of the recommendations, Macdonald also suggested that religious schools be allowed to include topics in addition to those in the national curriculum, such as the evils of same-sex behavior and the importance of abstinence as the sole acceptable method of contraception (Macdonald 2009, 7–9; Curtis 2009). As had previously been the case, parents were also to be given the right to have their children opt out of any sex education classes with which they disagreed.

Although received favorably by many parts of British society, a number of questions were raised about the government's new approach to sex education. Christian groups in particular were especially disturbed about requirements that schools teach subjects of which they disapproved, such as contraception and same-sex relationships. For example, Norman Wells of the Family Education Trust said that "Making PSHE a statutory part of the national curriculum could be used as a vehicle to promote positive images of homosexual relationships. It is difficult to see how teaching children as young as 11 about same-sex relationships and civil partnerships fits in with a study of personal wellbeing, and many parents will be very concerned about the prospect of such lessons being imposed over their heads." A similar view was expressed by Simon Calvert, of the Christian Institute, who said that "pressing the virtues of homosexuality" could lead to more experimentation, which could be "harmful" to children. "What we don't want to see," he continued, "is vulnerable young people being exploited by outside groups which want to normalise homosexuality" (The Christian Institute 2009).

By contrast, other observers found other problems with the Macdonald report. A number of gay and lesbian organizations, for example, objected to the fact that the report apparently legitimized the stigmatization of young gay men and lesbians by religious schools. George Broadhead of the Pink Triangle Trust, for example, wrote to the schools secretary Ed Balls that "it is surely unacceptable that a large proportion of our schools should be allowed to tell pupils (in line with the teaching in their holy books) that homosexual relationships are morally wrong, with the inevitable consequence that anti-gay bullying will increase." That theme was echoed by David Christmas, secretary of the Gay and Lesbian Humanist Association. "If the government wants a generation of young gay people to grow up who feel isolated, embittered, and alienated from the rest of society," he said, "then they are going the right way about it. Ideally, state funding of religious schools should be phased out. Failing this, the least that we as taxpayers should expect is that schools be required to offer relevant education and support to all of their pupils, including those who are, or may be, gay and lesbian" (Geen 2009).

Asia and Australasia

Sex education policies and practices in other countries around the world mirror the diversity seen in European nations. Some examples from Asia and Australasia include the following:

Japan: Japan is a very centralized nation, with many national policies and practices set, sometimes in great detail, by the national government. In education, those policies and practices are set out in the *Course of Study*, which is revised about once every 10 years. The *Course of Study* does not provide for any specific course in sex education, but, instead, indicates that topics in human sexuality are to be covered in relevant courses, such as biology, health, domestic science, and sociology. Recommendations for ways of achieving this goal are provided in a publication, *Sex Education Guidelines*, developed by the Japanese Association for Sex Education. In recent years, a number of factors have led to reconsideration of the approach to sex education in Japan. Among these factors are the spread of HIV/AIDS around the world and in Japan, a continued increase in the rates of sexually transmitted infections and unplanned pregnancies, a greater demand for abortions among unmarried young women, and a significant decrease in the age of first menses (by about two years) among Japanese girls (The Body 2004).

China: Traditionally, human sexuality has been a taboo subject in China. As recently as 2002, for example, a survey of 1,500 families in Beijing found that 74 percent of all parents provided no sex education at all to their children, two-thirds of whom said they were simply too embarrassed to raise the subject. Only 3 percent of respondents said that they provided complete and detailed information about sexuality to their children (Francoeur and Noonan 2004, China). Yet, for some time, Chinese educators have experienced significant pressure to offer some kind of instruction about sexuality. A number of factors have been responsible for this change, including the growing Chinese population, demanding better information about contraception; increases in the rate of unplanned teenage pregnancy and sexually transmitted infections; an increase in problems of sexual dysfunction among adults; and demands for greater sexual freedom as a result of exposure to Western ideas and practices with regard to sexuality. As a result of these pressures, a number of school districts in China have begun to develop new educational textbooks and other materials on human sexuality for use within and outside of schools. A lead organization in the new approach to sex education is the China Family Planning Association, which is developing sex education curricula that focus on "sex in the context of personal relationships" (China Development Brief 2005).

India: Plans to expand formal sex education programs in India's school have recently experienced a reversal in fortunes. Although the country has traditionally had little or no instruction about human sexuality in schools, that situation appeared to be about to change in 2004 when a group of governmental agencies jointly developed a new program called the Adolescence Education Program (AEP), with the objective of teaching Indian children fundamental facts about sexually transmitted infections, pregnancy and contraception, and related topics. At least one factor in the decision to establish the program was the fact that India currently has the largest number of HIV/AIDS cases of any Asian nation.

Plans to implement the AEP program ran into a roadblock, however, in May 2007, when a petition was filed with the Indian parliament's Committee on Petitions, requesting a review of the AEP program. Petitioners claimed that the proposed program would "corrupt Indian youth and lead to a collapse of the education system, transform student-teacher relations into that of a man and woman, lead to the creation of immoral society and growth in single-parent families." It would, they continued, "promote promiscuity of the worst kind" (Rajalakshmi 2009; also see Vishnoi and Thacker 2009).

After an extended review of the petition, the Committee on Petitions announced its decision in April 2009. It agreed with petitioners that there was no place in Indian schools for a discussion of human sexuality. The only place topics of this nature might be mentioned, the committee said, was in biology classes for students who are not going to continue their education after high school graduation. Committee members made their case strongly. They said that:

> a message should be given to schoolchildren that there should be no sex before marriage, which is immoral, unethical and unhealthy

> the new curriculum should include appropriate material on the lives and teachings of our great saints, spiritual leaders, freedom fighters and national heroes so as to inculcate in children our national ideals and values, which would

neutralise the impact of cultural invasion from various sources

school syllabi should cater to the needs and requirement of our society and culture

our country's social and culture ethos are such that sex education has absolutely no place in it.

The committee concluded that the AEP was "a cleverly used euphemism whose real objective was to impart sex education to schoolchildren and promote promiscuity" (Rajalakshmi 2009). Finally, the committee scolded the governmental agencies that had developed the curriculum in the first place, saying that it was shocking to note how so many agencies of the government could come

together, conceptualise a syllabus, provide all kinds of justification to it, spend substantial amount [sic] of money in the printing of the material and then circulate it throughout the country with the avowed aim of providing scientific information and knowledge to the adolescents whereas the reality was that the AEP volumes were highly objectionable and bound to be rejected lock, stock and barrel. (Rajalakshmi 2009)

The Committee on Petitions' decision is only a recommendation to government agencies, but as an expression of parliamentary attitudes, it may well have significant influence on the direction of sex education (if it is to exist at all) in India over the near future.

Australia: The Australian government has traditionally taken a laissez-faire attitude toward sex education. There are essentially no national guidelines or requirements, and individual schools decide whether or not to teach about human sexuality and, if so, what topics to include in courses. Currently, most teenagers get information about sexual topics from friends, on the Internet, through the media, from pornographic materials or Web sites, or from special groups organized to provide accurate information on the subject (Milburne 2009). That situation may be changing. One force for greater emphasis on sexuality education in the schools is a growing body of research providing a clearer understanding of the status of adolescent sexuality in Australia. One of the most recent studies found that about a third of Australian teenagers had become sexually active at the age of 14 or younger, but less than half felt that they could talk about sexual issues with their parents. More than 90 percent of teenagers reported having had some form of sex education in schools, but more than two-thirds (69%) of those respondents thought that that experience had been only average or below average in quality. More than half (56%) of parents interviewed expressed a similar view. In addition, teens generally reported not having instruction in a number of topics that sex educators regard as essential elements in any good sex education program, such as sexual decision-making and dealing with non-consensual sex. Overall, 66 percent of teenagers and 75 percent of adults expressed a desire for mandatory sex education classes in their schools (Quantum Market Research and Marie Stopes International 2008, 3). Although some discussion in the Australian parliament has occurred about developing some form of mandatory sex education program for the country, no action has as yet been taken.

The Muslim World

This section will be short. Sex education outside the home is not permitted by the Islamic tradition. No evidence exists that sex education in schools is available anywhere in the Muslim world. In fact, leaders of the faith speak clearly about the necessity of keeping instruction about sexual issues strictly within the home environment. In his book, *Sex Education: An Islamic Perspective*, Shahid Athar, Clinical Associate Professor of Internal Medicine and Endocrinology at the Indiana University School of Medicine in Indianapolis, writes that

> Islamic sex ed should be taught at home starting at an early age. Before giving education about anatomy and physiology, the belief in the Creator should be well established. As Dostoevsky put it, "Without God, everything is possible," meaning that the lack of belief or awareness of God gives an OK for wrongdoing.
>
> A father should teach his son and a mother should teach her daughter. In the absence of a willing parent, the next best choice should be a Muslim male teacher (preferably a physician) for boys and a Muslim female teacher (preferably a physician) for a girl at the Islamic Sunday school.

The curriculum should be tailored according to age of the child and classes be held separately. Only pertinent answers to a question should be given. By this I mean that if a five year old asks how he or she got into mommie's stomach, there is no need to describe the whole act of intercourse. Similarly it is not necessary to tell a fourteen year old how to put on condoms. This might be taught in premarital class just before his or her marriage. (Athar 2009)

Surveys of sex education programs around the world tend to confirm this view. Entries for Islamic countries reviewed in the *Continuum Complete International Encyclopedia of Sexuality,* for example, report that any sex education that takes place occurs exclusively within the home or under the instruction of a religious leader (Francoeur and Noonan 2004; see Bahrain, Egypt, Indonesia, Iran, and Morocco, as examples). Deviations from this theme are rare and apparently of minimal impact. For example, Turkey now has a long history as a secularized Islamic nation, which is more amenable to Western-style sex education programs (Francoeur and Noonan 2004, Turkey). But even here, formal sex education programs appear to be rare, especially in less urban regions where religious influences are still strong ("Degree Project Studies Sex Education in Iranian and Turkish Schools" 2006). Nigeria has the potential to be another exception. The pressures of population growth and a skyrocketing rate of sexually transmitted infections and deaths from abortions have prompted the nation to consider making sex education more generally available through formal means, such as primary and secondary schools. Even here, however, the problem is made more difficult for religious reasons because, as one writer has noted, "Both Christianity and Islam do not see the need for sexuality education in Nigeria" (Adepoju 2005, 11).

Latin America

The situation for sex education in Latin America and the Caribbean is similar to, but a mirror image of, sex education in Muslim nations. In this case, it is the Roman Catholic Church that provides the greatest force preventing schools from teaching about human sexuality. In its reviews of the status of sex education in Argentina, Brazil, Colombia, Costa Rica, and Mexico, the *Continuum Complete International Encyclopedia of Sexuality* consistently reflects the view that national governments may develop broad guidelines for instruction in human sexuality, but those guidelines are almost never expressed in actual programs in primary and secondary schools (Francoeur and Noonan 2004). In 2003, the United Nations Population Fund conducted a study of the status of sex education programs in Latin America and the Caribbean, and found that viable programs existed in only four countries: Brazil, Colombia, Cuba, and Mexico (although research by this author does not confirm these results as of 2009; Cevallos 2006). An indication of the opposition of the Catholic Church to sex education in schools was expressed in 2006 by José Guadalupe Martín, president of the Mexican bishops' conference, in response to an effort by the Mexican senate to expand sex education programs in the nation. "It is a misguided concept," Bishop Martín said, "that the state can decide what should or should not be done in the field of sex education, as if the state had begot those children" (Cevallos 2006).

Cuba: The one country that stands out in Latin America and the Caribbean with regard to sex education is Cuba, probably because it is the most free of Roman Catholic influences traditional in the rest of the region. Since 1959, the nation has emphasized sex education programs on both a formal and informal level for all children and adults. Some elements of Cuba's sex education program in recent years include

> 48 television programs on various aspects of human sexuality developed by the National Center of Sexual Education (CENESEX), the Young Communist Union (UJC), and the Cuban Radio and Television Institute

> more than 30 community intervention programs on human sexuality topics for people of all ages, such as "The Family, a Place for Human Development," "Growing During Adolescence," "Discovering Roads," "Values and Sexuality," "Comprehensive Adolescent Care," and "Responsible Motherhood and Fatherhood"

> a Program for a Responsible Sexual Behavior, developed by the Ministry of Education, in collaboration with CENESEX and the United Nations Population Fund, used by an estimated 12,000 educational institutions and over 2 million people, including children, adolescents, mothers, fathers, and teachers (Francoeur and Noonan 2004, Cuba; also see Olson and Dickey 2002; Feinberg 2007)

Africa

The available evidence suggests that sex education is essentially absent from formal education programs in most of Africa. Religious proscriptions, by both Islamic and Christian faiths, appear to be a strong factor banning the mention of topics related to human sexuality in schools across the continent. One observer has described the situation in Ghana, which may well represent the overall status of sex education throughout Africa:

> Theoretically, sex education should be covered, but in practice few schools have a comprehensive program on family life education. Policymakers, perhaps for the fear of arousing religious opposition, are ambivalent on issues concerning sex education. On the one hand, sex education is part of the school curricula in order to acknowledge official interest, yet on the other hand, most officials feel unconcerned that it is not effectively taught, thus pacifying the moral and religious critics. (Francoeur and Noonan 2004, Ghana)

(A 2003 update on this article suggests that, despite efforts by health and sex educators from Ghana and the United Nations, this situation has changed very little, if at all.)

Sex education in most parts of Africa appears to be largely the same as it has been for centuries, with whatever instruction that is available coming from parents, other adults, or nonscientific procedures. In Tanzania, for example, the primary means by which boys gain knowledge about their sexuality is probably the initiation rites through which many (although not all) boys must pass as they become men (Francoeur and Noonan 2004, Tanzania).

The situation for Africa has, it must be said, undergone a fairly significant change over the past two decades, primarily because of the spread of the HIV/AIDS epidemic, a point that will be discussed later in this chapter.

New Issues of Concern in Human Sexuality

Education about human sexuality has undergone some significant changes in the past two decades for three major reasons.

First, the HIV/AIDS pandemic has made it essential for governments in some nations to develop some form of education about sexually transmitted diseases in order to deal with the appalling rates of the disease in their countries. Second, the availability of new contraceptive devices has made it possible, for the first time in history, for women to have access to safe, reliable methods of contraception. Third, the increased visibility of alternative sexual lifestyles has forced societies to at least consider how they will deal with such lifestyles and what message they will send young people. The rest of this chapter will explore the ways in which nations around the world are dealing with these new challenges.

The HIV/AIDS Pandemic

The HIV/AIDS pandemic has become one of the great health issues in the history of the world. Not all nations have been equally affected by the disease, but few countries have been spared the scourge. Today, the region most seriously affected by the disease is Africa, especially sub-Saharan Africa. According to the best estimates available, 22 million people were living with HIV/AIDS in sub-Saharan Africa at the end of 2007, the last year for which data are available. An additional 1.9 million people were diagnosed with the disease during that year. An estimated 1.5 million people had already died of the disease, leaving behind more than 11 million orphans (Avert 2009a). Even in sub-Saharan Africa, some nations apparently have been largely spared by the disease. Infection rates are less than 1 percent in Senegal and Somalia, but greater than 20 percent in other nations, such as Botswana (23.9%), Lesotho (23.2%) and Swaziland (26.1%).

Dismissal and Denial

Some nations have chosen to ignore the threat posed by HIV/AIDS to their people. The South African government has famously declined to accept current medical explanations for the disease and refused to adopt modern technology for dealing with it. For many years, then-president Thabo Mbeki consistently refused to admit that HIV/AIDS is caused by a virus. In an interview with the South African edition of *Time* magazine in 2000, for example, he said that

> a whole variety of things can cause the immune system
> to collapse. Now it is perfectly possible that among those

New Issues of Concern in Human Sexuality **89**

things is a particular virus. But the notion that immune deficiency is only acquired from a single virus cannot be substained [sic]. Once you say immune deficiency is acquired from that virus your response will be antiretroviral drugs. But if you accept that there can be a variety of reasons, including poverty and the many diseases that afflict Africans, then you can have a more comprehensive treatment response. (Transaction Campaign News, September 8, 2000)

Mbeki was supported in his view of HIV/AIDS by his minister of health, Dr. Manto Tshabalala-Msimang, whose recommended treatment for the disease was a mixture of garlic, lemon, and beetroot (Blandy 2006).

As a result of Mbeki's policies, very few people with HIV/AIDS received the retroviral drugs that could have helped them. According to one estimate, only 4 percent of those individuals with HIV/AIDS received retrovirals in 2004, with that rate increasing slowly to 15 percent in 2005, 21 percent in 2006, and 28 percent in 2007 (UNAIDS 2008, 271). In retrospect, the failure of the South African government to use modern drugs for the treatment of HIV/AIDS, may have been responsible for as many as 300,000 deaths in the country (Boseley 2008).

South Africa is by no means the only nation to have hesitated in developing programs to deal with the HIV/AIDS pandemic. A similar situation obtains in Swaziland, the nation with the largest percentage of infected adults in the world. According to a counselor quoted in one report on the status of AIDS education in the country, "Sex education for young people in Swaziland is very shallow. Young people have never been exposed to sex education resulting in young people having problems when they have to take decisions pertaining to sex." Another observer was quoted as saying that "AIDS education clubs in most schools in the community have died a natural death, even though they used to exist in the past. Teachers do not seem to be motivated to assist pupils to form and sustain these activities" (United Nations Population Fund 2009b, Swaziland). According to another report, the government has spent about a quarter of 1 percent of its annual budget on HIV/AIDS prevention programs and has admitted a "lack of seriousness" in dealing with the crisis (Avert 2009b).

An even more extreme reaction to the HIV/AIDS crisis than that found in South Africa and Swaziland, where at least the pandemic is acknowledged, can be found in some countries that deny the disease even exists in their nation. For many years, China was the classic example of this situation. Until the early 2000s, the Chinese government denied that HIV/AIDS was present in the country and that stories to the contrary were a fabrication of Western media. Officials claimed that the disease was caused by "capitalist decadence," so that citizens of their own Communist country were safe from the disease. Only in the first years of the 21st century did the Chinese government begin to acknowledge that the disease was, in fact, present in the country and to ask the U.S. Centers for Disease Control and Prevention for assistance in dealing with the problem ("Continuing Denial Helps AIDS Spread" 2001; also see Rosenthal 2000). As of the end of 2007, officials estimate that there are 700,000 people living with AIDS in China, of whom 39,000 died in that year (Avert 2009c).

China's next-door neighbor, Myanmar, has long taken a similar stance. In 2001, health minister Major General Ket Sein told a meeting of the World Health Organization that his nation had no cases of HIV/AIDS because the people in Myanmar do not misbehave sexually, so there is no way for the disease to spread. Prevention programs in any case would have limited value since the sale and distribution of condoms is illegal in the country ("Continuing Denial Helps AIDS Spread" 2001).

Programs of Prevention and Treatment

Far more common throughout the world than nations that deny the existence of the HIV/AIDS pandemic or that dismiss its importance as a public health issue are countries that have proactively and aggressively developed programs for educating children, adolescents, and adults about the diseases and about methods by which it can be prevented. In many cases, these programs have been incorporated into existing sex education classes in public and, sometimes, private, schools. In the United States, for example, teaching about HIV/AIDS ranks very high among priorities of parents and other adults for inclusion in sex education classes. The 2004 NPR/Kaiser Family Foundation/JFK School of Government poll found that 98 percent of all respondents felt that the topic was an essential part of sex education classes, with 78 percent saying it should be taught at both the high school and middle school levels (NPR/Kaiser/Kennedy School Poll 2004). In countries where sex education classes do not exist or are not common, governments, international agencies, nongovernmental organizations, and other groups have developed programs that can be incorporated on a stand-alone basis in schools, as part of the school curriculum, or in settings outside formal educational institutions. Some examples of these programs are as follows:

Tanzania: The African Medical and Research Foundation (AMREF) has developed a program called MEMA Kwa Vijana, which means "good things for young people" in the native language of Kiswahili. The program is aimed at increasing the understanding among young people between the ages of 12 and 19 of sexually transmitted infections, contraception, and related issues. In the period between January 2004 and December 2007, the program trained 630 teachers in the fundamentals of sexual health, trained 227 health care workers in methods for providing assistance to young people in the fields of sexually transmitted infections and contraception, and worked to raise awareness of local government officials about issues related to adolescent sexual health (AMREF 2009).

Dominican Republic: Education about human sexuality in public schools has largely been absent in rural areas of the Dominican Republic because parents have traditionally believed that such topics should be taught in the home. The problem is that few parents have the knowledge or skills to teach very much beyond the basic fundamentals of human biology (if that), and they are almost certainly unqualified to teach about HIV/AIDS and its prevention. In 1998, Mujeres en Desarrollo Domiciano (MUDE), an organization concerned with women's health and development, initiated a program in which they sought the active participation of parents and teachers in the development of materials for making available information about HIV/AIDS to high school students in rural areas. By enrolling adults during the earliest stages of the project, it eventually received the "enthusiastic support" of adults who conceived the effort as their own as much as that of MUDE (Alvarez 1998).

Cambodia: Cambodia has had a very successful sex education program that emphasizes HIV/AIDS prevention at the secondary level for many years. In May 2009, the government announced that it would be extending that program to the primary level. It pointed out that many Cambodian children leave school after primary school, so do not have access to instruction offered at the secondary level. The primary program will mirror that of the secondary program and include the same topics as those taught at the higher level, including "knowledge about HIV/AIDS and life skills, such as negotiation skills, how to say 'no,' goal setting, and how to provide care and support to people living with HIV/AIDS" (Kunthear 2009).

India: In a nation where the government has essentially refused to deal with the HIV/AIDS pandemic, the only source of information about the disease can be nongovernmental groups of one kind or another. In 2001, the Church of North India, a collaboration of six Protestant and Anglican denominations, announced that it was expanding a trial program of HIV/AIDS education for adolescents in all 26 of its dioceses, which cover two-thirds of the nation. Surveys had shown that up to 60 percent of women interviewed in the nation were unfamiliar with the disease, suggesting that some form of instruction of young people had become urgent. Administrators of the program pointed out that they were being approached not only by churches within the denomination, but also by public school educators whose students had no other access to information about the diseases (Akkara 2001).

Argentina: Argentina is typical of some Latin American countries in that sexuality is a prominent feature of the media and many public events, but sex education in schools and other formal settings is strongly discouraged. The government has no policy or program for sex education in the schools. Recognizing the deficiency of information for teenagers about many sexual issues, a number of nongovernmental organizations have been working for well over a decade to find other ways of providing crucial information about human sexuality to Argentina's adolescents. One approach has been to develop programs of peer education, in which teenagers are trained to teach each other about human sexuality, including issues such as HIV/AIDS prevention. In 1999, these efforts led to the formation of Nacional de Adolescentes en Salud Sexual y Reproductiva (National Network of Adolescents for Sexual and Reproductive Health) by the most dedicated adolescent participants in earlier programs. The Network has since provided a mechanism by which concerned teenagers can interact and exchange ideas and techniques for teaching about human sexuality. One of the network's first projects was a daylong event held at Parque Avellaneda, in Buenos Aires, a popular hangout for local adolescents. The theme for the event was HIV/AIDS prevention and included information about condom use and other topics related to sexuality, HIV/AIDS, and reproduction (Correra 2000).

Evaluation

These examples illustrate the vast array of approaches the nations and nongovernmental groups are taking to HIV/AIDS education. One question that has been of interest to researchers is how effective such programs are and which programs and which elements are more effective than others. A considerable amount of research has been devoted to answering this question. One of the most exhaustive of these studies was conducted by the UNAIDS Interagency Task Team on Young People in 2006. Researchers carefully examined all published reports on the effectiveness of HIV/AIDS education program and selected 22 that met a number of criteria for accuracy, reliability, validity, and other criteria. They then measured the effectiveness of these 22 studies on their effectiveness in measuring 55 sexual behaviors.

The review found that, overall, the 22 programs significantly improved a total of 21 of the 55 sexual behaviors measured. Of these programs, 16 significantly improved 5 of the behaviors most essential to HIV/AIDS prevention: a delay in the age of first sexual intercourse, reduction in the frequency of sexual activity, decrease in the number of sexual partners, increase in the use of condoms or contraceptives, and reduction in the incidence of unprotected sex. Of all programs studied, only one (a peer-run program) resulted in an increase in sexual behavior, frequency of sexual activity. On the basis of this study, researchers developed a system for recommending or not recommending certain types of programs for HIV/AIDS that they classified as "Steady, Ready, Go," ranging from programs that did not meet criteria for success ("Steady"), to those that met some criteria, but not others ("Ready"), to those that met all criteria ("Go"). Of the top four programs that met researchers' "Go" criteria, one was a school-based program, one a health-agency-based program, and two were media programs (Ross, Dick, and Ferguson 2006, 103–50).

A similar study on the effectiveness of HIV/AIDS education programs was conducted in 2008 by ETR Associates for the Interagency Youth Working Group of Family Health International. This study was somewhat broader than the 2006 WHO study in that it considered 83 programs, of which only 18 were from developing nations. The study found that, in the majority of cases, educational programs had no measurable effect on any of the 10 behaviors measured. Those measures included delay of initiation of sex, reduced frequency of sex, reduced number of partners, increased condom use, increased use of other contraceptives, reduced sexual risk-taking, reduced pregnancy (self-report and laboratory tests), and reduced rate of sexually transmitted infections (self-report and laboratory tests). The areas in which programs were most effective were reduced risk-taking (14 positive [i.e., successful] programs; 14 not significant; 0 negative [increase in negative behavior]); increased condom use (26 positive; 28 not significant; 0 negative); and increased use of other contraceptives (6 positive; 8 not significant; 1 negative) (Kirby, Laris, and Rolleri 2005, 17).

Perhaps the most useful part of this study was the identification of 17 characteristics that seemed to make for an effective curriculum in HIV/AIDS education. Among those characteristics were the involvement of individuals with a wide range of backgrounds in the development of the curriculum; the provision of a safe environment in which young people could participate in the program; a focus on clear and specific goals related to sexually transmitted infections and HIV/AIDS; the use of methods and messages that are appropriate to a participant's cultural background, sexual maturity, and developmental age; and the obtaining of at least minimal support from relevant educational and other agencies (Kirby, Laris, and Rolleri 2005, 27).

Other Sexually Transmitted Infections

Although it is undoubtedly the most serious of all sexually transmitted infections, HIV/AIDS is certainly not the only such disease with which world health agencies are concerned. Of those diseases, chlamydia is the most common treatable bacterial infection, affecting about 92 million people worldwide in 1999. (World statistics on sexually transmitted infections are currently being updated, but 1999 is presently the latest year for which comprehensive data are available.) The rate of infection varies widely around the world with one of the highest rates occurring in Cape Verde, where 13 percent of all pregnant women are infected with chlamydia. The highest infection rate regionally is in sub-Saharan Africa, where the rate is about 119 per 1,000 adults. The lowest rate is in East Asia and the Pacific, with a rate of about 7 adults per 1,000 (Avert 2009d).

Gonorrhea and syphilis are two other STIs for which worldwide data are available. There were an estimated 62.35 million cases of gonorrhea worldwide in 1999, and an estimated 12.22 million cases of syphilis. Studies for individual countries have found the rate of gonorrheal infection ranging from a low of 0.02 percent among pregnant women in Gabon to a high of 7.8 percent in South Africa. For syphilis, the highest rate of infection among pregnant women has been found in Cameroon (17.4%) and South Africa (8.4%), with much lower rates in Morocco (3%) and Sudan (2.4%). Although the infection rates among adults for both gonorrhea and syphilis have been declining significantly in most developed nations, the one exception has been in the newly independent states of the former Soviet Union, where infection rates for syphilis have increased from about 5 to 15 cases per 100,000 in 1990 to 120 to 170 cases per 100,000 in 1996 (Avert 2009d).

Sexually transmitted infections worldwide are a matter of increasing concern to international health agencies. In 2000, the World Health Assembly asked the director general of the World Health Organization (WHO) to develop a worldwide strategy for dealing with the spread of HIV/AIDS and other sexually transmitted infections. As a result of that directive, WHO's Department of Reproductive Health and Research (RHR) spent a number of years developing such a strategy, which was released in late 2006. That document, *Global Strategy for the Prevention and Control of Sexually Transmitted Infections: 2006–2015*, outlined an overall philosophy for the prevention and treatment of STIs, along with a number of specific actions that WHO/RHR hoped to initiate in an effort to combat the spread of STIs. Among those actions were the following:

promotion of safer sexual behaviors

inclusion of STI diagnosis and treatment in all basic health services

development of special services for high-risk populations, such as long-distance truck drivers, military personnel, adolescents, and military personnel

improved access to quality condoms at affordable prices

promotion of early recourse to health services for people with STIs and their partners

screening of asymptomatic patients

involvement of all relevant stakeholders in the development and execution of programs for the prevention and treatment of STIs (World Health Organization 2006, chapter 3)

Contraception and Family Planning

One of the most troublesome pieces of data about the world situation in the 21st century is its continued increase in population. As recently as 1960, the world population was only just over three billion people. It took 14 years for the world to add another billion people, 11 years to add the next billion, and 12 years to add one more billion. Experts predict that world population will reach seven billion in 2012, eight billion in 2025, and nine billion in 2040. Although the rate of population growth has now been decreasing every year since 1970, it is still close to 1 percent annually, guaranteeing a growth in population for the foreseeable future (U.S. Census Bureau 2009).

National and international governmental and nongovernmental agencies have been concerned about the world's burgeoning population for at least three decades. A number of regional and international conferences have been held to assess population trends and to consider national and international policies to deal with apparently endless growth. One of the earliest of these conferences, the World Population Conference, was held in Bucharest, Romania, in 1974. Representatives to that conference produced a document, the World Population Plan of Action (WWPA), that stressed the importance of development, rather than family planning, as a way for countries to deal with their growing populations. Partly in respect of the many newly independent nations in Africa, the document also acknowledged that population control was essentially a national concern about which outside forces should not be concerned (Department of Economic and Social Affairs. Population Division 2002, 128).

The Bucharest conference was followed by two more major conferences on world population at 10-year intervals, one in Mexico City in 1984 and one in Cairo in 1994. At each of these worldwide conferences and at a number of regional conferences, a major shift of emphasis in population control began to appear, with greater emphasis on the need for family planning as a way of bringing population growth under control. The final Programme of Action approved by attendees at the Cairo conference not only made a stronger statement for the use of contraceptive technology in reducing births, but also took a much broader view of this topic, introducing a discussion of sex and sexuality (words that were not mentioned in the Bucharest or Mexico City documents); women's rights; gender-based disparities of income and social status; rape; pornography; and female genital mutilation (Department of Economic and Social Affairs. Population Division 2002, 129). In the decade following adoption of the Programme of Action, many nations had begun to take a more aggressive, contraception-focused approach to their population problems. For example, Gabon, Nigeria, South Africa, and Tanzania had all developed educational campaigns to inform the public of the threat posed by overpopulation. Côte d'Ivoire and Lesotho had established counseling services for women most at risk for unwanted pregnancies. And Mali had introduced a new program promoting the status of women (Department of Economic and Social Affairs. Population Division 2002, 129; the original document from which this information comes is available at http://www. uneca.org/search.htm: United Nations Economic Commission for Africa. *Report of the Fourth Meeting of the Follow-up Committee on the Implementation of the Dakar/Ngor Declaration (DND) and the Programme of Action of the International Conference on Population and Development (ICPD-PA), Yaounde, Cameroon, January 18–31*).

Research suggests that many nations are making progress in the development of family planning programs as a way of dealing with growing population issues (J. Ross 2002). However, a great deal more needs to be done. In 2009, the United Nations Population Fund estimated that there were at least 200 million women worldwide who wanted to use safe and effective contraceptives in order to manage their pregnancies, but were unable to do so because of lack of access either to the necessary information or to contraceptives themselves. The UNFPA predicted that this "unmet need" would grow by at least 40 percent over the next 15 years (United Nations Population Fund 2009a).

The question of how nations around the world will deal with their own population problems has been an important political issue in the United States for over 20 years. At the Mexico City conference in 1984, the United States delegation announced that the administration of President Ronald Reagan had adopted a new policy, one that would no longer permit the funding of nongovernmental family planning programs "which perform or actively promote abortion as a method of family planning" (Policy Statement of the United States of America at the United Nations International Conference on Population (Second Session) Mexico, D.F. August 16–13, 1984, [5]). Family planning organizations both within the United States and around the world were outraged at this decision, arguing that it dramatically inhibited the access of women around the world—especially in developing nations—to the contraceptive information and devices they so badly needed to control their own fertility. The policy remained in effect, however, until January 22, 1993, when newly elected President Bill Clinton rescinded the policy (White House. Office of the Press Secretary 1993). The election of George W. Bush as President in 2000 restored the Reagan philosophy on family planning to the White House, and on his first day in office, Bush restored the Mexico City policy (USAID 2001). Finally, with the election of Barack Obama as the nation's 44th President, the nation's policy on the funding of family planning programs in other nations reversed course yet again when Obama signed yet another memorandum to USAID, instructing them to "immediately waive such conditions" as were contained in the 1984 and 2001 policy statements (White House 2009). A last-ditch effort by the Republican party to restore the Mexico City policy came five days after President Obama's memorandum when Senator Mel Martinez (R-FL) introduced an amendment to an unrelated children's health insurance bill requiring reinstatement of the policy. The amendment failed by a vote of 37 to 60, apparently resolving the issue for at least as long as the Democratic party maintains its majority in both houses of Congress. (The debate over the Martinez amendment can be found in the *Congressional Record* for January 28, 2009, pages S955–60.)

Sexual Orientation and Gender Identity

As discussed in Chapter 2, teenagers in the United States who know that they are gay, lesbian, or bisexual or who question their sexual orientation or gender identity often face difficult challenges in coming to terms with that realization and working out their relationships with parents, other adults, and peers. Those problems tend to be, however, somewhat less serious than those faced by teenagers in many other parts of the world where same-sex relationships are regarded much more negatively than they are in the United States. In many countries, those teenagers face physical or emotional abuse, or even death, usually as a result of state-sponsored and legal prohibitions or because of religious or cultural beliefs and traditions. As of 2009, homosexual acts at any age are illegal in 80 nations (and legal in 115 countries), and are punishable by death in five Muslim countries: Iran, Mauritania, Saudi Arabia, Sudan, Yemen, and in Muslim regions of Nigeria and Somalia. Four countries—Belize, Lesotho, Swaziland, and Trinidad and Tobago—ban the entry of gay, lesbian, and bisexual individuals into their nations. In almost all nations of the world, discrimination in employment, housing, and other areas of life on the basis of sexual orientation are legal, with only 10 nations in the world having specific prohibitions against such forms of discrimination (Ottosson 2009, 48–54; see also Sanders 2005).

The risks faced by young GLBTQ men and women is anything but theoretical. In February 2006, for example, a 19-year-old South African lesbian, Zoliswa Nkonyana, was reportedly beaten with golf clubs and stoned to death by a group of teenagers because of her sexual orientation (Davis 2006). In addition to assaults and murders by individual criminals, state-sponsored executions of gay men and lesbians because of their sexual orientation have also been reported recently in a number of countries, such as Iraq, Nigeria, and Saudi Arabia (Gay Nigerian Sentenced to Death by Stoning 2001; Grew 2008; "Member of Iraqi Gay Group Pleads for Help 'Before It's Too Late' " 2009; "Saudi Arabia: Young Man Sentenced to Death for Being Gay" 2009).

In many countries with a less negative view about same-sex relationships, school authorities, public health officials, and others often struggle with the question of whether they should provide information for young women and men about such relationships. The debates over this issue often follow the same pattern as those that have occurred in the United States (see Chapter 2), with opponents arguing that the mention of same-sex relationships in classrooms ipso facto will increase students' interest in and participation in such activities. Proponents of the inclusion of discussions about same-sex relationships respond that simply talking about the subject will not make young people more likely to become gays or lesbians, and that information about all kinds of sexual topics is important in today's world.

Specific information about the inclusion of sexual orientation and gender identity in school and out-of-school programs in most nations of the world is very thin. One useful source of this information is a series of papers collected in preparation for a conference on Youth Sex Education in a Multicultural Europe held in Cologne, Germany, in November 2006. Sixteen nations prepared overview reports describing their efforts to provide teenagers with information about various aspects human sexuality. As expected, the treatment of instruction about sexual orientation and gender identity varied significantly from nation to nation. Table 3.1

TABLE 3.1
Youth Education on Sexual Orientation in 16 European Countries

Country	Schools	Health Services	General Counseling	HIV/AIDS Counseling	Other
Austria	Y	Y	Y	Y	—
Belgium	Y	Y	N	N	Y[1]
France	Y	N	Y	N	Y[2]
Germany	Y	—	—	Y	Y[3]
Hungary	N	N	N	N	N
Kyrgyz Republic	N	Y	—	Y	Y[4]
Latvia	Y	N	N	N	Y[5]
Netherlands	Y	Y	N	N	N
Portugal	N	N	N	N	Y[6]
Russia	N	Y	N	N	Y[7]
Sweden	Y	Y	—	Y	Y[8]
Switzerland	Y*	Y	Y	Y	Y[9]
Turkey	N	N	Y	Y	Y[10]
Ukraine	Y	Y	N	Y	N
United Kingdom	N	N	—	Y	Y[11]
Uzbekistan	Y	Y	N	N	Y[12]

Source: Country Papers, *Youth Sex Education in a Multicultural Europe*, 2006, http://english.forschung. sexualaufklaerung.de/3051.0.html#. Accessed on June 21, 2009.
— = No response for this category.
[1] Youth advice and family planning centers
[2] Youth and family planning services
[3] Pregnancy and family counseling
[4] Social services; religious organizations
[5] Universities and vocational training institutions
[6] Web sites and help line
[7] Social counseling centers
[8] RFSL (Swedish Association for Lesbian, Gay, Bisexual and Transgender Rights) centers
[9] Sex education services
[10] Universities; community and informal services
[11] Youth services; social services; community services
[12] Social services

summarizes the services available in each of these 16 countries on sexual orientation from a variety of possible sources.

Some of the specific comments made about educational efforts in various countries is instructive. The report from the Kyrgyz Republic, for example, says that no mention of sexual orientation is made in formal school settings "because homosexuality is not widely accepted considering national and cultural traditions in the Kyrgyz Republic." Instead, some instruction is provided through other resources, such as health clinics, HIV/AIDS counseling services, and religious organizations. The Kyrgyz report concludes that "[t]here is a great need to develop public programmes in this area" (Country Papers. Kyrgyz Republic 2006). Other nations, however, have developed a variety of ways of bringing to teenagers information about sexual orientation, using either formal or informal means. For example, sexual orientation is not specifically mentioned under national curriculum guidelines in France, but a number of nongovernmental organizations, most of them gay and lesbian organizations, have developed programs for helping teachers deal with the subject in their own classrooms (Country Papers. France 2006). Similar approaches are used in Germany, where assistance is provided by Lambda, a network of gay and lesbian organizations and in Sweden, where the group primarily involved is the Swedish Association for Lesbian, Gay, Bisexual and Transgender Rights (RFSL). In Belgium, sexual orientation is actually part of the national curriculum for sex education in schools, published under the rubric of "Good Lovers" (Country Papers. Germany 2006; Country Papers. Sweden 2006; Country Papers. Belgium 2006).

Although progress in the treatment of sexual orientation and gender identity in some developed nations of the world has obviously taken place, most teenagers around the world in Africa, Asia, the Middle East, and Latin America still have little or no access to information about these topics.

References

Adepoju, Adunola. 2005. "Sexuality Education in Nigeria: Evolution, Challenges and Prospects." Lagos, Nigeria: Understanding Human Sexuality Seminar Series 3, March. http://www.arsrc.org/downloads/uhsss/adepoju_sexed.pdf. Accessed on June 17, 2009.

Akkara, Anto. 2001. "Indian Church Steps Up Education Programs to Deal with Threat of AIDS." *Christianity Today*, August 1. http://www.christianitytoday.com/ct/2001/augustweb-only/8-13-54.0.html. Accessed on June 19, 2009.

Alvarez, R. R. 1998. "Introducing Participatory AIDS and Sexuality Education into a Reproductive Rural Health Project for Adolescents and Youths." http://gateway.nlm.nih.gov/MeetingAbstracts/ma?f=102227945.html. Accessed on June 19, 2009.

AMREF. 2009. "MEMA Kwa Vijana ("Good Things for Young People"), Mwanza, Tanzania." http://uk.amref.org/what-we-do/mema-kwa-vijana-good-things-for-young-people-mwanza-tanzania/. Accessed on June 19, 2009.

Athar, Shahid. 2009. "Sex Education: An Islamic Perspective." *Islam for Today.* http://www.islamfortoday.com/athar19.htm. Accessed on June 17, 2009.

Avert. 2009a. "HIV and AIDS in Africa." http://www.avert.org/aafrica. htm. Accessed on June 17, 2009.

Avert. 2009b. "HIV and AIDS in Swaziland." http://www.avert.org/ aids-swaziland.htm. Accessed on June 19, 2009.

Avert. 2009c. "South East Asian HIV & AIDS Statistics." http://www. avert.org/aidssoutheastasia.htm. Accessed on June 19, 2009.

Avert. 2009d. "STD Statistics Worldwide." http://www.avert.org/ stdstatisticsworldwide.htm. Accessed on June 21, 2009.

Blandy, Fran. 2006. " 'Dr Beetroot' Hits Back at Media over AIDS Exhibition." *Mail & Guardian Online,* August 16. http://www.mg.co.za/ article/2006-08-16-dr-beetroot-hits-back-at-media-over-aids-exhibition. Accessed on June 17, 2009.

The Body. 2004. "Japan: A New Spin on Sex Education for a Sexier New Generation." http://www.thebody.com/content/world/art26583.html. Accessed on June 16, 2009.

Boseley, Sarah. 2008. "Mbeki AIDS Denial 'Caused 300,000 Deaths.' " *Guardian.* http://www.guardian.co.uk/world/2008/nov/26/aids- south-africa. Accessed on June 17, 2009.

Cevallos, Diego. 2006. "Education-Latin America: Let's (Not) Talk About Sex." Inter Press Service, April 18. http://ipsnews.net/news. asp?idnews=32929. Accessed on June 17, 2009.

China Development Brief. 2005. "Sex Education Begins to Break Taboos." http://www.chinadevelopmentbrief.com/node/57. Accessed on June 16, 2009.

The Christian Institute. 2009. "Gay Lessons Obligatory for England's Schools." http://www.christian.org.uk/news/20090429/gay-lessons- obligatory-for-englands-schools/. Accessed on June 17, 2009.

"Continuing Denial Helps AIDS Spread." 2001. *Bangkok Post.* http:// www.aegis.com/news/bp/2001/BP010807.html. Accessed on June 19, 2009.

Correra, Ceclia. 2000. "Argentina's National Network of Adolescents Towards Free and Formed Sexual and Reproductive Lives." http:// www.accessmylibrary.com/coms2/summary_0286-28774107_ITM. Accessed on June 19, 2009.

Country Papers. Belgium. 2006. "Youth Sex Education in a Multicultural Europe." http://english.forschung.sexualaufklaerung.de/fileadmin/ fileadmin-forschung/pdf/country_papers_belgium.pdf. Accessed on June 21, 2009.

Country Papers. France. 2006. "Youth Sex Education in a Multicultural Europe." http://english.forschung.sexualaufklaerung.de/fileadmin/file admin-forschung/pdf/country_papers_france.pdf. Accessed on June 21, 2009.

Country Papers. Germany. Republic. 2006. "Youth Sex Education in a Multicultural Europe." http://english.forschung.sexualaufklaerung. de/fileadmin/fileadmin-forschung/pdf/country_papers_germany.pdf. Accessed on June 21, 2009.

Country Papers. Kyrgyz Republic. 2006. "Youth Sex Education in a Multicultural Europe." http://english.forschung.sexualaufklaerung.de/ fileadmin/fileadmin-forschung/pdf/country_papers_kyrgyz_republic. pdf. Accessed on June 21, 2009.

Country Papers. Sweden. 2006. "Youth Sex Education in a Multicultural Europe." http://english.forschung.sexualaufklaerung.de/fileadmin/ fileadmin-forschung/pdf/country_papers_sweden.pdf. Accessed on June 21, 2009.

Curtis, Polly. 2009. "Sex Education for Five-year-olds to Be Made Compulsory in Schools." *Guardian*. April 27. http://www.guardian. co.uk/education/2009/apr/27/sex-education-contraception-schools. Accessed on June 17, 2009.

Davis, Andrew. 2006. "South African Lesbian Murdered." *Windy City Times,* April 1. http://www.windycitymediagroup.com/gay/lesbian/ news/ARTICLE.php?AID=11154. Accessed on June 21, 2009.

"Degree Project Studies Sex Education in Iranian and Turkish Schools." 2006. http://www.mah.se/templates/ExternalNews____35690.aspx. Accessed on June 17, 2009.

Department of Economic and Social Affairs. Population Division. 2002. *Levels and Trends of Contraceptive Use as Assessed in 2002.* New York: United Nations.

Feinberg, Leslie. 2007. "Sex Education Campaign Battled Old Prejudices." *Workers World,* May 11. http://www.workers.org/2007/ world/lavender-red-97/. Accessed on June 17, 2009.

Francoeur, Robert T., and Raymond J. Noonan, eds. 2004. *The Continuum Complete International Encyclopedia of Sexuality.* New York and London: The Continuum International Publishing Group.

"Gay Nigerian Sentenced to Death by Stoning." 2001. Sodomy Laws. http://www.glapn.org/sodomylaws/world/nigeria/ninews003.htm. Accessed on June 21, 2009.

Geen, Jessica. 2009. "Gay Charities Express Concern over Faith School Sex Education Proposals." *Pinknews.* http://www.pinknews.co.uk/ news/articles/2005-12243.html. Accessed on June 17, 2009.

Grew, Tony. 2008. "55 Arrested During Raid on 'Gay Party' in Saudi Arabia." *Pinknews.* http://www.pinknews.co.uk/news/articles/2005-8544.html. Accessed on June 21, 2009.

Kirby, Douglas, B. A. Laris, and Lori Rolleri. 2005. *Impact of Sex and HIV Education Programs on Sexual Behaviors of Youth in Developing and Developed Countries.* Youth Research Working Paper No. 2. Research Triangle Park, NC: Family Health International.

Kunthear, Mom. 2009. "Govt Begins HIV Training for Teachers." *Phnom Penh Post,* May 19. http://www.phnompenhpost.com/index. php/2009051925925/National-news/Govt-begins-HIV-training-for-teachers.html. Accessed on June 19, 2009.

Macdonald, Alasdair. 2009. "Independent Review of the Proposal to Make Personal, Social, Health and Economic (PSHE) Education Statutory." [n.p] [April 24].

"Member of Iraqi Gay Group Pleads for Help 'Before It's Too Late.' " 2009. *UK Gay News.* http://www.ukgaynews.org.uk/Archive/09/ Apr/0601.htm. Accessed on June 21, 2009.

Milburne, Caroline. 2009. "Think Sex." *The Age.* http://www.theage. com.au/news/education-news/think-sex/2006/05/28/1148754861223. html. Accessed on June 17, 2009.

NPR/Kaiser/Kennedy School Poll. 2004. "Sex Education in America." http://www.kff.org/newsmedia/upload/Sex-Education-in-America-Summary.pdf. Accessed on June 12, 2009.

Olson, Beatriz R., and Richard A. Dickey. 2002. "Mass Health Education on Sex and Sexuality and Its Impact on Cuba: An Interview-Based Medical Report on the Development, Evolution, and Current Status of This Educational Program in Cuba, with Emphasis on Women's Health." *Journal of Women's Health* 11 (9; November): 767–71.

Ottosson, Daniel. 2009. *State-sponsored Homophobia: A World Survey of Laws Prohibiting Same Sex Activity Between Consenting Adults.* [Brussels]: International Lesbian, Gay, Bisexual, Trans, and Intersex Association.

"Policy Statement of the United States of America at the United Nations International Conference on Population (Second Session) Mexico, D.F. August 16–13 [*sic*], 1984. http://www.populationaction. org/Publications/Reports/Global_Gag_Rule_Restrictions/ MexicoCityPolicy1984.pdf. Accessed on June 19, 2009.

Quantum Market Research and Marie Stopes International. 2008. *Sex—Telling It Like It Is.* Melbourne: Marie Stopes International.

Rajalakshmi, T. K. 2009. "Rajya Sabha Committee sees 'Indian Culture' Threatened by Sex Education." Communalism Watch. http:// communalism.blogspot.com/2009/05/rajya-sabha-committee-sees-indian.html. Accessed on June 17, 2009.

Rosenthal, Elisabeth. 2000. "In Rural China, a Steep Price of Poverty: Dying of AIDS." *New York Times,* October 28. http://www.nytimes. com/2000/10/28/world/in-rural-china-a-steep-price-of-poverty-dying-of-aids.html?pagewanted=all. Accessed on June 19, 2009.

Ross, David A., Bruce Dick, and Jane Ferguson. 2006. *Preventing HIV/ AIDS in Young People: A Systematic Review of the Evidence from Developing Countries.* UNAIDS Inter-agency Task Team on Young People. Geneva, Switzerland: World Health Organization. WHO Technical Report Series No. 938.

Ross, John A. 2002. "Effort Measures for Family Planning Action Programs: Past Trends and Future Prospects." http://www.un.org/esa/population/publications/completingfertility/RevisedRosspaper.PDF. Accessed on June 19, 2009.

Sanders, Douglas. 2005. "Human Rights and Sexual Orientation in International Law." http://www.ilga.org/news_results.asp?LanguageI D=1&FileCategory=44&FileID=577. Accessed on June 21, 2009.

"Saudi Arabia: Young Man Sentenced to Death for Being Gay." 2009. *Hudson New York* (with link to original story in Arabic). http://www.hudsonny.org/2009/04/saudia-arabia-young-man-sentenced-to-death-for-being-gay.php. Accessed on June 21, 2009.

Sex and Samfund. 2009. "Sex Education." http://www.sexogsamfund. dk/Default.aspx?ID = 1605. Accessed on June 16, 2009.

Smith, Anthony et al. 2007. "Sex in Australia: A Guide for Readers." *Australian and New Zealand Journal of Public Health* 27 (2; September): 103–5.

Transaction Campaign News, September 8, 2000. http://www.tac.org. za/newsletter/2000/ns000908.txt. Accessed on June 17, 2009.

UNAIDS. 2008. "Country Progress Indicators." *2008 Report on the Global AIDS Epidemic.* http://data.unaids.org/pub/GlobalReport/2008/ jc1510_2008_global_report_pp235_324_en.pdf. Accessed on June 17, 2009.

United Nations Population Fund. 2009a. "Ensuring That Every Pregnancy Is Wanted." http://www.unfpa.org/rh/planning.htm. Accessed on June 19, 2009.

United Nations Population Fund. 2009b. "Report Card: HIV Prevention for Girls and Young Women. Swaziland." http://www.unfpa.org/hiv/docs/report-cards/swaziland.pdf. Accessed on June 19, 2009.

USAID. 2001. "Memorandum for the Administrator of the United States Agency for International Development." http://www.usaid.gov/whmemo.html. Accessed on June 19, 2009.

U.S. Census Bureau. 2009. "International Data Base." http://www.census.gov/ipc/www/idb/worldpop.html. Accessed on June 19, 2009.

Valk, Guss. 2000. "The Dutch Model." http://www.unesco.org/courier/2000_07/uk/apprend2.htm. Accessed on June 16, 2009.

Vishnoi, Anubhuti, and Teena Thacker. 2009. "No Sex Education in Schools, Leads to Promiscuity: House Panel." *Express India,* April 18. http://www.expressindia.com/latest-news/No-sex-education-in-schools-leads-to-promiscuity-House-panel/448353/. Accessed on June 17, 2009.

Wellings, Kay, and Rachel Parker. 2006. *Sexuality Education in Europe: A Reference Guide to Policies and Practices.* Brussels: IPPF European Network.

White House. 2009. "Memorandum for the Secretary of State; the Administrator of the United States Agency for International Development." http://www.whitehouse.gov/the_press_office/MexicoCityPolicy-VoluntaryPopulationPlanning/. Accessed on June 19, 2009.

White House. Office of the Press Secretary. 1993. "Memorandum for the Acting Administrator of the Agency for International Development." http://clinton6.nara.gov/1993/01/1993-01-22-aid-family-planning-grants-mexico-city-policy.html. Accessed on June 19, 2009.

World Health Organization. 2006. *Global Strategy for the Prevention and Control of Sexually Transmitted Infections: 2006–2015: Breaking the Chain of Transmission.* Geneva: World Health Organization. Also available online at http://www.who.int/reproductivehealth/publications/rtis/9789241563475/en/index.html.

"Youth and HIV/AIDS: Can We Avoid Catastrophe?" 2001. *Population Reports* 29 (3; Fall; Series L, No. 12): 1–39.

4

Chronology

Humans have struggled with issues related to sexual health for centuries at least, and probably as long as the race has existed. This chapter summarizes some of the important events in the history of sexually transmitted infections, contraception and family planning, the development of sexual orientation, and sexual identity.

ca. 3000 BCE	Egyptian temple drawings from this period suggest the availability of condoms, although the use to which they were put (ceremonial, to protect from sexually transmitted diseases, or as a contraceptive) or the materials of which they were made are unclear.
ca. 1850 BCE	Evidence suggests that women begin to use the pessary, a contraceptive device inserted into the vagina, to prevent pregnancy. A wide variety of materials were apparently used for the purpose, including honey, hot oil, wine, sodium carbonate, and even crocodile dung.
Seventh Century BCE	Explorers discover the first oral contraceptive, a plant known as silphion, near the city of Celene in North Africa, in the region that is now Libya. Once its contraceptive properties are recognized, the plant is in great demand among Greek women, such that it was harvested to extinction by about 100 CE.

Sixth Century BCE
Chinese women are said to use mercury as an abortifacient.

Fourth Century BCE
The Greek natural philosopher Aristotle (384–322) is credited with being the first person to recommend a variety of substances for use as a spermicide. He suggests that women spread oil of cedar, frankincense, olive oil, or other substances on their vaginas in order to avoid pregnancy.

Second Century CE
The Greek physician Soranus (98–138) writes a work that is regarded as the first medical text on birth control in the ancient world, a book entitled *Gynaecology.* He recommends a number of ways of preventing sperm from entering the womb, such as sneezing, standing up, or jumping backward seven times, or the use of a pessary by the woman.

ca. 1640
A collection of condoms made from the intestines of animals are discarded near an outhouse associated with Dudley Castle in England. Prior to that time, condoms had been made out of a wide array of materials, including linen fabric soaked in saline solution, silk paper, leather, and even tortoise shell (!).

ca. 1750
The Venetian adventurer and author, Giacomo Casanova, describes contraceptive methods he used in his numerous seductions of women, including condoms made of lamb intestine or linen for himself and a half lemon rind as a primitive cervical cap. Casanova and other men and women of the time were probably at least as concerned about the prevention of sexually transmitted infections as they were of preventing pregnancy with such devices.

ca. 1850
Massachusetts physician Charles Knowlton becomes the first person in the United States to be sentenced to prison for providing information about and advocating birth control. In 1832 he published a pamphlet of contraceptive advice entitled *Fruits of Philosophy.* He also recommended douching with a solution of salt, vinegar,

and zinc sulfite or aluminum potassium sulfite after sexual intercourse as the most effective means of birth control, a contraceptive technique that became widely popular for almost half a century.

1495   The first well-documented outbreak of syphilis occurs during the Italian War of 1494–1498. By the end of the war, the disease had become pandemic throughout Europe and begun to spread to India and China.

1610   The Virginia colony passes the first antisodomy law in the United States, requiring the death penalty for anyone convicted under the laws. Women are not included in the law's provisions.

1641   The Massachusetts Bay Colony enacts a new penal code that includes sodomy as a capital crime. The definition of sodomy is taken directly from Leviticus 20:13. By the end of the century, nearly all colonies had adopted similar laws against sodomy, requiring the death penalty for those convicted of the crime.

1786   Pennsylvania adopts a number of fundamental legal reforms, removing the death penalty for crimes such as burglary, robbery, sodomy, and buggery (sexual intercourse with animals). By the end of the century, a number of other states had followed suit and reduced the penalty for sodomy to loss of property, assignment to servitude, or some other punishment.

1838   A German gynecologist, Friedrich Wilde, invents the cervical cap, which he offers to his patients as a means of birth control. He first takes a wax impression of a woman's cervix, and then fashions a cup-shaped cap of uncured rubber. The cap becomes very popular in Europe, but not in the United States.

1844   American inventor Charles Goodyear patents a process for vulcanizing rubber, providing an ideal material from which to make condoms and giving them their perhaps most common slang name of "rubbers."

1870s	The Voluntary Motherhood movement emphasizes the naturalness and beauty of women's sexuality and rejects the use of contraceptives as unnatural and demeaning to women. The movement stresses instead the use of periodic or permanent abstinence as the primary means of birth control.
1873	The U.S. Congress passes the Comstock Act, a law prohibiting the transmission of "obscene, lewd, and/or lascivious" materials through the U.S. mails. The legislation included any and all contraceptive devices or information. Twenty-four states eventually passed similar legislation restricting the distribution of such materials and information within the states. These laws are collectively known as the Comstock laws.
1879	German physician Albert Ludwig Neisser discovers the bacterium that causes gonorrhea, a bacterium named in his honor as *Neisseria gonorrhoeae*.
Late 1870s	A German gynecologist by the name of Wilhelm Peter Johann Mensinga, writing under the pseudonym of Karl Hasse, describes the first "diaphragm pessary," a hollow hemispherical device made out of rubber that fits into the vagina. The device soon becomes very popular under the name of the Mensinga diaphragm or, more simply, the diaphragm.
1884– 1924	The simian immunodeficiency virus (SIV) found in monkeys is thought to have transmuted to a form transmissible to humans that eventually evolves to become human immunodeficiency virus (HIV), which causes acquired immunodeficiency syndrome (AIDS).
1889	Cecil Reddie, headmaster at the Abbotsholme School in England, is said to be the first person to offer a sex education course in a school setting. Reddie is quoted as saying that he hoped to "prevent mental illusions due to false ideas from within" and to "prevent false teaching from other fellows."
1898	At its first national convention, a year after being formed, the National Congress of Parent and Teachers

Association (PTA) includes a session on sex education in which the importance of training in the subject prior to puberty is emphasized.

1905   The German microbiologist Fritz Schaudinn (1871–1906) and the German dermatologist Erich Hoffmann (1868–1959) first describe the bacterium, *Treponema pallidum*, that causes syphilis.

1906   German bacteriologist August von Wassermann (1866–1925) develops a test for the diagnosis of syphilis, making it possible not only for early treatment of the disease, but also for prevention of its spread.

1909   German bacteriologist Paul Ehrlich (1854–1919) and his student, Sahachiro Hata (1873–1938), discover a cure for syphilis, the chemical compound arsphenamine, later marketed as Salvarsan and 606 (because it was compound number 606 in a long series of compounds being tested in their laboratory).

German gynecologist Richard Richter invents what is probably the world's first intrauterine device.

1912   The National Education Association (NEA) recommends that public school teachers be trained in the teaching of sex education topics.

A Special Committee on the Matter and Methods of Sex Education of the American Federation for Sex Hygiene presents a report before the 15th International Congress on Hygiene and Demography on the content and methodology of sex education classes for high school and college students.

1913   Japanese bacteriologist Hideyo Noguchi (1876–1928) demonstrates that syphilis is caused by the spirochete *Treponema pallidum*.

Superintendent of Chicago schools Ella Flagg Young institutes the first sex education program in the United States by requiring high school students to attend a series of lectures on sexual hygiene. The so-called

1913
(*cont.*)
Chicago Experiment lasts only a year when members of the board of education decide the subject is too controversial to continue.

1915
A group of women in New York City found the National Birth Control League, later to become the International Planned Parenthood Federation.

1916
Margaret Sanger establishes the first birth control clinic in the United States, in the Brownsville section of Brooklyn, New York. Nine days later, New York police officers close down the clinic. Sanger and her colleagues are arrested and found guilty of "maintaining a public nuisance," and Sanger is sentenced to 30 days in prison.

1918
The U.S. Public Health Service launches a national sex education campaign to educate all Americans about the risks of venereal diseases (sexually transmitted infections).

1921
Sanger founds the American Birth Control League, later to become the Planned Parenthood Federation of America.

1922
The U.S. Public Health Service publishes a book, *High Schools and Sex Education*, with suggestions for helping students develop "the proper information and attitudes about the place of sex in the life of a normal adult" through the usual courses offered in high school, such as biology, general science, home economics, social studies, and English.

1924;
1927
Japanese gynecologist Kyusaku Ogino (1882–1975) and Austrian gynecologist Hermann Knaus (1892–1970) independently devise the rhythm method of birth control, in which women refrain from intercourse during the fertile phase of their menstrual cycles.

1924
Bavarian immigrant Henry Gerber and a group of friends found the Society for Human Rights, the first gay rights group in the United States. The society survives only a brief time and is disbanded when the wife of one of its

directors reports the group's existence to the police. The organization publishes the first magazine for gay men in the United States, *Friendship and Freedom.*

1928   German gynecologist Ernst Gräfenberg introduces one of the world's first commercially available intrauterine devices, a flexible ring made of silk that, in a later formulation, was wrapped in silver wire. The device was popular in Germany for about a decade before being replaced by other contraceptive devices.

1929   The German Reichstag (parliament) removes Paragraph 175, the section criminalizing same-sex sexual acts, from the German Constitution. The law had first been adopted in 1871, and its repeal never took effect because of the rise of the Nazi party in Germany in the early 1930s. Instead, the Nazi-controlled parliament actually extended the provisions of Paragraph 175 in 1934 to include as criminal acts "a kiss, an embrace, even homosexual fantasies."

In his encyclical *Divini Illius Magistri*, issued on December 31, 1929, Pope Pius XI declares that sex education outside the home or the church is false and cannot be countenanced by practicing Roman Catholics. On March 21, 1931, the Holy See issued a decree (Educ. 306) clarifying the responsibility of Catholics to abide by the Pope's ruling on sex education, which remains in effect today.

1930   In an encyclical titled *Casti Canubi* (Of Chaste Marriage), Pope Pius XI declares that all artificial forms of contraception are a sin in the eyes of the Roman Catholic Church.

1933   Swedish sex educator and journalist Elise Ottesen-Jensen forms what was probably the world's first association to promote sex education in schools, the National League for Sex Education.

1936   In the case *United States v. One Package of Japanese Pessaries*, the U.S. Court of Appeals for the Second Circuit overturns the federal Comstock Act (see 1873).

1940   The U.S. Public Health Service once again argues for increased attention to sex education in schools, claiming that such instruction is an "urgent need."

1948   Alfred Kinsey, researcher at Indiana University, publishes *Sexual Behavior in the Human Male*, still considered by many authorities the best available data on sexual attitudes, feelings, and behaviors in American men.

The United Nations establishes the World Health Organization (WHO), an agency that has since been the primary organization responsible for public health issues such as sexually transmitted infections, pregnancy, and contraception worldwide.

1951   Three gay men, Henry Hay, Bob Hull, and Chuck Rowland, found the Mattachine Society in Los Angeles. The society is created to provide aid and comfort to gay men and lesbians and to educate the general public on gay issues.

1952   With the financial support and encouragement of John D. Rockefeller III, a group of scientists found the Population Council to assist countries around the world in attacking their own unique population problems in whatever manner they agree is best for them.

1953   The German government begins the rearrest of gay concentration camp survivors as "repeat offenders" when they refuse to renounce their intention of continuing to take part in homosexual acts.

Alfred Kinsey publishes *Sexual Behavior in the Human Female*, a companion volume to his 1948 book dealing with male sexuality.

The American School Health Association develops a national program of family life education for the nation's public schools, which includes a discussion of sex education topics.

1955   A joint committee of the American Medical Association and the National Education Association publishes five pamphlets on sex education for use in the nation's schools. The topics of the pamphlets are *Parents' Privilege* and *A Story about You* for upper elementary students, *Finding Yourself* for middle school students, *Learning about Love* for high schoolers, and *Facts Aren't Enough* for adults.

1959   The American Law Institute proposes a model penal code for state laws dealing with abortion. The code would legalize abortion for reasons of physical or mental health of the mother, pregnancy due to rape and incest, and fetal deformity.

The Cuban government decides that courses in human sexuality are to be a part of the nation's formal educational program. That decision has remained in effect ever since, with the government providing sex education both in primary and secondary schools, but also in a number of other settings, including health clinics and the media.

1960   The U.S. Food and Drug Administration approves the use of Enovid as the first oral contraceptive.

1961   Illinois becomes the first state to decriminalize homosexual acts between consenting adults in private.

1964   Mary Calderone and colleagues found the Sexuality Information and Education Council of the United States (SIECUS) to serve as an advocate for sex education, sexual health issues, and sexual rights in the United States.

1965   In *Griswold v. Connecticut*, the U.S. Supreme Court strikes down the state of Connecticut Comstock Act prohibiting the use of contraceptives as a violation of the petitioners' constitutional right to privacy. The court's decision applies only to married couples (also see 1972).

1969   The Canadian parliament decriminalizes homosexual acts between consenting adults in private.

The Stonewall riots of June 27 and 28 in New York City mark the symbolic beginning of the gay rights movement in the United States. Triggered by a police raid on the Stonewall, a popular gay bar in Greenwich

1969
(*cont.*) Village, the riots begin in and around the bar and soon spread throughout lower Manhattan.

A group of individuals working for the repeal of state abortion laws and legitimizing a woman's right to choose with regard to pregnancy forms the National Association for the Repeal of Abortion Laws (NARAL), now known as NARAL: Pro-Choice America.

1971 In its decision in the case of *United States v. Vuitch*, the U.S. Supreme Court upholds a District of Columbia law that permits abortions only for the purpose of saving a woman's life or health, which the court acknowledges as referring to both her physical and mental health. The decision is taken by some to mean that the court regards abortion as permissible for virtually any reason.

1972 In *Eisenstadt v. Baird*, the U.S. Supreme Court extends its *Griswold v. Connecticut* decision (1965) to void the ban on the use of contraceptive materials among unmarried couples.

Outraged by seeing her son being beaten at a gay pride parade in New York City, Jeanne Manford organizes Parents and Friends of Lesbians and Gays, the first group to provide support for parents and to advocate for gay and lesbian civil rights.

1973 In the case of *Roe v. Wade*, the U.S. Supreme Court announces a decision that has been the law of the land ever since, essentially banning any prohibition on abortion during the first trimester of pregnancy, but allowing states to impose restrictions on abortions in the second and third trimesters.

Largely in response to the Supreme Court's decision in *Roe v. Wade*, a number of pro-life groups meet in Detroit to establish the National Right to Life Committee.

1974 The United Nations sponsors the first international conference on world population issues, held in Bucharest, Romania. The conference issues the World Population Plan of Action, which emphasizes development as the primary solution to population problems faced by (primarily) developing nations.

1976   The FDA approves the first intrauterine device for sale in the United States. The device is a T-shaped object that must be inserted by a doctor and that can be left in place for up to 10 years.

1978   California's Proposition 6 (the "Briggs Initiative") provides for the firing of all gay and lesbian teachers and all teachers who allude to homosexual behavior positively in the classroom. The initiative is eventually defeated, to some extent because of the strong objections from Governor Ronald Reagan.

1980   In Providence, Rhode Island, gay teenager Aaron Fricke sues his high school to allow him to bring a male date to the senior prom. He wins his suit and is accompanied by Paul Guilbert to the school dance. Fricke later writes of these events in a popular book, *Reflections of a Rock Lobster.*

        Georgetown University, run by Jesuits of the Roman Catholic Church, expels its gay student group from campus, forbidding it to use any university facilities. The student group takes the university to court and wins its case eight years later.

        New Jersey becomes the first state to mandate sex education in all public schools at all grade levels.

1981   The Council of Europe adopts a resolution supporting gay rights legislation in member nations. Three years later, the European Parliament adopts a similar resolution, 114 to 45.

        Wisconsin becomes the first state to pass a law prohibiting discrimination against gay men and lesbians in employment, housing, and public accommodations.

        The U.S. Congress passes the Adolescent Family Life Act, Title XX of the Public Health Service Act. The act is designed to encourage adolescents to postpone sexual

1981   activity until marriage and to emphasize chastity and
(*cont.*)   self-discipline in their sexual lives. The act also pro-
        vides support for pregnant or parenting teens and their
        families.

        The first cases of HIV infection and AIDS are reported
        among gay men and, later, intravenous drug users in
        California and New York.

1982   HIV and AIDS cases are first reported among Haitians
        and hemophiliacs.

1983   Linda Conway, a West Virginia kindergarten teacher,
        is fired from her job because her superiors think she
        looks like a lesbian, in spite of Conway's insistence that
        she is not a lesbian. Three years later, the state supreme
        court confirms the school board's right to dismiss Con-
        way because of her appearance.

        HIV and AIDS cases are first reported among women,
        children, and heterosexuals.

        German virologist Harald zur Hausen (1936–) dis-
        covers a link between the human papillomavirus and
        cervical cancer, an accomplishment for which he was
        awarded a share of the 2008 Nobel Prize in Physiology
        of Medicine.

1984   French virologist Luc Antoine Montagnier (1932–)
        and American virologist Robert Gallo (1937–) inde-
        pendently discovery that HIV infection is caused by
        the human immunodeficiency virus, which gives the
        disease its name. Priority for the discovery becomes a
        matter of contention over the next decade, with many
        authorities now giving Montagnier credit for discov-
        ery of the virus and Gallo for demonstrating its being
        the causative agent in the disease.

        President Ronald Reagan announces that it shall be
        the policy of the United States not to provide funding
        for any nongovernmental organization that performs
        or promotes abortion as a part of its family planning

program. The policy becomes known as the Mexico City Policy because it was announced at the 1984 United Nations International Conference on Population held in that city.

1986   Pope John Paul II issues a papal letter declaring that homosexuality is "intrinsically disordered" and calling for all Catholics to oppose civil rights legislation for lesbians and gay men.

1987   Researchers at the Burroughs Wellcome company and the U.S. National Cancer Institute discover that the drug zidovudine, also known as azidothymidine (AZT) or Retrovir, is effective in the treatment of HIV infections.

1989   In the case of *Webster v. Reproductive Health Services*, the U.S. Supreme Court rules that governmental agencies are not required to allow the use of public facilities to provide abortion services. Some observers see the ruling as the court's first step back from its more expansive view of abortion as expressed in *Roe v. Wade*.

1990   Seventy gay and lesbian educators found the Gay and Lesbian Independent School Teachers Network (GLSTN), later to be renamed the Gay, Lesbian, and Straight Education Network (GLSEN).

Experts estimate that about eight million people worldwide are living with AIDS.

1991   A superior court judge in Los Angeles rules that the Boy Scouts of America may legally prohibit an Eagle Scout from becoming a scoutmaster because of his sexual orientation.

1992   In *Planned Parenthood of Southeastern Pennsylvania v. Casey*, the U.S. Supreme Court issues a complex and very divided opinion on abortion rights, essentially affirming its 1973 ruling in *Roe v. Wade*, but modifying some fundamental aspects of that ruling.

1993   The FDA approves the injectable drug Depo Provera as an extended contraceptive for use over three month periods.

President Bill Clinton rescinds the Mexico City Policy on family planning originally announced in 1984 by President Ronald Reagan.

Twenty-one-year-old Brandon Teena is raped and murdered in Lincoln, Nebraska, by two friends who have learned that she/he is a transgendered person. The case becomes the subject of an Academy Award winning film, *Boys Don't Cry*.

1994   The United Nations sponsors the third international conference on worldwide population issues, held in Cairo, Egypt. The Programme of Action adopted by the conference emphasizes for the first time the importance of contraceptive technology in dealing with problems of overpopulation throughout the world, but especially in developing nations.

1995   Penny Culliton, a teacher in New Ipswich, New Hampshire, is fired for listing as voluntary reading two gay-themed books, *Maurice*, by E. M. Forster, and *The Education of Harriet Hatfield*, by May Sarton.

The United Nations establishes the Joint United Nations Programme on AIDS (UNAIDS) as the lead UN agency for dealing with the HIV epidemic around the world.

1996   South Africa becomes the first nation in the world to prohibit discrimination on the basis of sexual orientation as part of its national constitution.

In the case of *Nabozny v. Podlesny* heard before the Seventh Circuit Court of Appeals, a jury awards Jamie Nabozny $962,000 because administrators at his Wisconsin high school failed to protect him from antigay harassment. The case is important because of the precedence it establishes in similar cases of antigay harassment in schools throughout the nation.

The U.S. Congress passes the Welfare Reform Act, Title V of the Welfare Reform Act of 1996, which provides funding for abstinence-only sex education programs that meet certain specific criteria (eventually known as the A–H criteria).

Medical researchers begin to make use of a combination antiretroviral treatment, consisting of three different drugs, for the treatment of HIV infections.

1998   In one of the most famous hate crimes of modern times, college student Matthew Shepard is murdered near Laramie, Wyoming.

The FDA approves the first emergency contraceptive product, PREVEN Emergency Contraceptive Kit, made by the Gynétics corporation in Belle Mead, New Jersey.

1999   The Queer Youth Alliance (now the Queer Youth Network) is founded in Great Britain as the world's first gay-rights organization for gay and lesbian youth.

The state of California passes three gay-rights bills, one providing for a domestic partnership registry, one outlawing harassment of gay youth in schools, and one banning discrimination in housing, employment, and public accommodation.

The FDA approves production and sale of the first single-hormone emergency contraceptive product, Plan B, made by the Women's Capital Corporation of Bellevue, Washington.

2000   The FDA approves two new contraceptive devices. The first is a monthly injectable contraceptive, Lunelle, which contains a combination of estrogen- and progestin-related hormonal products. In October 2004, Pharmacia Corporation announced a recall of the product citing questions as to its efficacy in preventing pregnancies. The drug is currently not available in the United States. The second approved product is Mirena, a T-shaped intrauterine device effective for up to five years.

2000
(*cont.*)
In amending Title XI of the Social Security Act, the U.S. Congress establishes a competitive grant program for abstinence-only sex education programs, the Special Projects of Regional and National Significance–Community-Based Abstinence Education (SPRANS–CBAE), which expands upon similar legislation adopted in 1981 and 1996.

2001
The FDA approves applications for two new contraceptive technologies. The first is the birth control patch Ortho Evra, a product that delivers two hormones, estrogen and progestin, transdermally during three of each four-week cycle of use. The second device is called NuvaRing, a vaginal contraceptive ring that also delivers two forms of estrogen and progestin on a monthly basis.

President George W. Bush reinstates the Mexico City Policy on family planning originally announced by President Ronald Reagan in 1984 and rescinded by President Bill Clinton in 1993.

Myanmar health minister Ket Sein tells a meeting of the World Health Organization that his nation has no cases of HIV/AIDS because the people in Myanmar do not misbehave sexually, so there is no way for the disease to spread.

Attahiru Umar, a gay Nigerian man, is sentenced to death by stoning by a Nigerian court because of his sexuality (gay).

2002
On January 1, Saudi Arabia beheads three men found guilty of "engaging in the extreme obscenity and ugly acts of homosexuality."

2003
The FDA approves Seasonale, a birth control pill that alters a woman's menstrual cycle so that she has only four periods per year, but still provides the same pregnancy protection as a conventional oral contraceptive pill.

2004
A study conducted by the Special Investigations Division of the Minority Staff of the Committee on Government Reform of abstinence-only sex edu-

cation programs finds that four in five national abstinence-only programs contain "false, misleading, or distorted information about reproductive health."

2005   New Zealand becomes the first country in the world to outlaw hate crime and discrimination on the basis of gender identity.

Illinois governor Rod Blagojevich issues an order prohibiting pharmacies in the state from refusing to fill prescriptions for contraceptives because of a pharmacist's personal ethical or religious beliefs.

2006   The FDA approves Gardasil, a prophylactic vaccine against the human papillomavirus. The vaccine appears to be effective against types 16 and 18 of the virus, which together account for about 70 percent of all cases of cervical cancer, and against types 6 and 11, which cause 90 percent of all cases of genital warts. The U.S. Centers for Disease Control and Prevention recommends that all females between the ages of 11 and 26 be vaccinated with the product.

Nineteen-year-old Zoliswa Nkonyana is beaten with golf clubs and stoned to death by a group of teenagers because of her sexual orientation (as a lesbian). The act is only one of a number of violent attacks on lesbians and gay men in South Africa during the first decade of the 21st century.

2007   Experts estimate that about 33 million people worldwide are living with AIDS.

Senator Frank Lautenberg (D-NJ) introduces the Responsible Education about Life Act, outlining a comprehensive approach to sex education in U.S. schools that departs significantly from the abstinence-only philosophy of sex education supported by the federal government over the preceding decade. The act did not pass.

Governor Rick Perry (R-Texas) issues an executive order requiring all girls to be vaccinated for the HPV virus

2007
(*cont.*)

for admission to the sixth grade. Two months later, the state legislature overturns the executive order.

Representative Carolyn B. Maloney (D-NY) introduces legislation to make it illegal for pharmacists to fill prescriptions with which they disagree. The legislation is necessitated by the decisions of some pharmacists not to fill prescriptions for emergency contraceptives for women and minor girls. Maloney's bill is never considered by committee and dies at the end of the 110th session of the Congress.

The Portland (Maine) public school system makes national news when it announces that free contraceptives will be provided to students at the King Middle School who are legally old enough to engage in sexual intercourse.

2008

The U.S. Citizenship and Immigration Services issues a new directive requiring that all women between the ages of 11 and 26 entering the United States be vaccinated against the human papillomavirus. Some women's groups object to the new ruling claiming that it takes essential decisions about a woman's reproductive health out of the hands of individuals.

2009

President Barack Obama rescinds the Mexico City Policy on family planning introduced by President Ronald Reagan in 1984, rescinded by President Bill Clinton in 1993, and reinstated by President George W. Bush in 2001.

President Obama announces a drastic cutback in funding of abstinence-only education programs in his 2010 federal budget. He says that funds previously used for abstinence education would be going instead to teen pregnancy prevention programs.

Representative Barbara Lee (D-CA) reintroduces the Responsible Education about Life Act (see 2007).

Judge Edward R. Korman orders the U.S. Food and Drug Administration (FDA) to reconsider its rule limiting Plan B emergency contraception to men and women 18 and older. He orders that the agency reduce the age limitation to 17 and older. The FDA complies with the ruling.

The English government announces plans to make sex education mandatory in all public and private schools at both primary and secondary level. Religious schools are to be allowed to add topics that reflect their own theological biases about sexual issues in addition to those included in the national curriculum.

The Committee on Petitions of the Indian parliament releases a report saying that instruction in human sexuality has no place in Indian schools. The only exception is for discussions of the topic in biology classes designed for students who do not continue with their education beyond secondary level.

Swaziland member of parliament Timothy Myeni suggests compulsory HIV testing for every person in the country, to be followed by tattooing everyone who tests positive on his or her buttocks.

Reports say that more than 200 men in Iran are sentenced to death for a variety of reasons, one of them being their sexuality (gay).

5

Biographical Sketches

O ver the centuries, many women and men have contributed to the development of modern methods of contraception and family planning, to the conquest of sexually transmitted infections, and to the education of adults and young people about issues surrounding sexual orientation and gender identity. These individuals represent a wide range of professions, from the sciences to politics to advocacy in one's daily life. The sketches in this chapter provide a review of the lives and contributions of only some of these individuals.

Mary Steichen Calderone (1904–1998)

Calderone was an outspoken advocate for the teaching of sexuality in schools. She served for many years as medical director of the Planned Parenthood Federation and founded and served as president and executive director of the Sex Information and Education Council of the United States.

Mary Calderone was born as Mary Steichen on July 1, 1904, in New York City to Edward Steichen, a photographer and painter, and Clara (Smith) Steichen. The Steichen family spent many years in France, returning to the United States just after the onset of World War I. Mary graduated from the Brearley School in New York City in 1921 and then enrolled in a premedical curriculum at Vassar College. She soon became disillusioned with this field, however, and changed her concentration to theater arts, music, and English. Her bachelor's degree, awarded in 1925, was, however, in chemistry. Still, after leaving Vassar, she decided to give the theater a try, and spent three years in New York City working to gain roles on the stage. At the end of that time, she abandoned her plans and settle in with her marriage to actor Lon Martin. Calderone reached the nadir of her life in 1933 when her husband and eldest daughter died. After a period of counseling and testing, she decided to return to school to work for her M.D. She entered the Rochester University School of Medicine in 1934, at the age of 30, and received her M.D. five years later. After completing her internship at Bellevue Hospital in New York, Calderone enrolled at the Columbia University School of Public Health, where she earned her master's degree in public health in 1942. At Columbia, she met and married her second husband, Frank Calderone, with whom she was to have two children. During the early years of her marriage, she worked part-time as a family physician in Great Neck, New York.

In 1953, Calderone was offered a position as medical director at the Planned Parenthood Federation of America (PPFA). During her 11-year tenure with PPFA, Calderone revolutionized the organization's approach to contraception and family planning education, expanding its mission to include a broad range of issues related to human sexuality. In 1964, Calderone left PPFA to found the Sex (later, Sexuality) Information and Education Council of the United States (SIECUS) because she had become convinced that "handing out condoms was not enough." She served as executive director of SIECUS from 1964 to 1975 and as president from 1975 to 1982. During this period, she arguably had more influence on the character and direction of sex education in the United States than any person in the field. She made SIECUS into an umbrella organization that included sex educators, school administrators, physicians, social activists, and parents interested in developing programs of sex education in which human sexuality was presented as a positive force in one's life.

In 1982, Calderone retired from SIECUS and took a position as adjunct professor of human sexuality at New York University, a post she held until 1988. Faced with the onset of Alzheimer's disease, she then retired to a Quaker community in Kennett Square, Pennsylvania, where she died on October 24, 1998. Calderone was a prolific writer, whose best known works included *Abortion in the United States, Release from Sexual Tensions, Manual of Family Planning and Contraceptive Practices, Sexual Health and Family Planning, Sexuality and Human Values, Questions and Answers about Love and Sex, The Family Book about Sexuality* (with Eric Johnson), and *Talking with Your Child about Sex.* She received many awards and honors, including honorary doctorates from Woman's Medical College of Pennsylvania, Newark State College, Adelphi University, Kenyon College, Worcester Foundation for Experimental Biology, Brandeis University, Harvard University, Hofstra University, and Dickinson College.

Min-Chueh Chang (1908–1991)

Chang was part of a research team, that included John Rock and Gregory Pincus, responsible for the development of the first oral contraceptive, a product sometimes known simply as The Pill. He was also a prolific and highly respected researcher in the field of reproductive biology with 347 scholarly papers to his credit, 112 of which he authored by himself, and 38 more of which he was the senior author.

Min-Chueh Chang (sometimes known as M. C. Chang) was born in the village of Dunhòu, Shanxi province, China, on October 10, 1908. He attended Tsing Hua University in Peking, from which he received his bachelor's degree in animal psychology in 1933. He then stayed on at Tsing Hua as a teacher of psychology until 1938, when he entered a national competition for a few high-prestige foreign scholarships. He was successful in that competition and chose to continue his studies in agricultural science at the University of Edinburgh, in Scotland. By this time, Chang's scholarly interests had begun to evolve, and he had become more interested in the subject of animal reproductive biology than animal psychology. At the conclusion of his year at Edinburgh, he accepted an offer to continue his studies at Cambridge University, where he earned a Ph.D. in animal breeding in 1941.

At the conclusion of World War II, Chang was faced with the decision of where he would continue his research: in Great Britain, back at home, or in some other location. He eventually decided to accept an offer to spend a year with Gregory Pincus at the newly established Worcester Foundation for Experimental Biology. He had not been there long when he realized that he and Pincus were kindred spirits with a passion for hard work and a common interest in learning more about the reproductive biology of animals, with the rabbit as their organism of choice for study. When Margaret Sanger and Katherine McCormick approached Pincus in 1953 with a proposal for the development of an oral contraceptive pill, Chang was an obvious choice to join the research team since his specialty at the time was the study of the effect of various orally administered hormones on reproductive patterns in the rabbit. Along with Pincus and John Rock, Chang is given credit for having developed what may well have been the most significant medical breakthrough in the control of reproduction in women in history.

Chang remained at Worcester for the rest of his academic career. After development of the pill, he turned his attention to in vitro fertilization and accomplished the first artificial reproduction of a rabbit by this means in 1959 and of a rodent five years later. Chang died of heart failure in Worcester on June 5, 1991. Among his many honors and awards were the Albert Lasker Award, Ortho Medal and Award of the American Fertility Society, Hartman Award by the Society for the Study of Fertility, Frances Amory Prize by the American Academy of Arts and Sciences, and Wippman Scientific Research Award by the Planned Parenthood Federation of America. In 1990, he was elected to membership in the National Academy of Sciences.

Anthony Comstock (1844–1915)

Comstock was a strong opponent of all forms of behavior that he regarded as immoral. As secretary of the New York Society for the Suppression of Vice, he worked for the passage of federal and state laws prohibiting the distribution of obscene materials which at the time were given a very broad interpretation. These laws eventually became known as Comstock laws and have been enforced throughout most of the 20th century and, in some cases, into the 21st century.

Anthony Comstock was born in New Canaan, Connecticut, on March 7, 1844, to Polly and Thomas Anthony Comstock, a well-to-do family who had 10 children, 7 of whom survived childhood. Young Anthony enlisted in the army and served in the American Civil War from 1863 to 1865. After the war he opened a dry goods store in New York City, but soon became more interested in issues of morality. He was strongly opposed to the distribution of lewd, obscene, immoral, and indecent material which, at the time, might describe a very wide array of artistic, live, and written productions. In 1873, Comstock founded the New York Society for the Suppression of Vice (NYSSV) and convinced the Young

Men's Christian Association (YMCA), where he was employed, to finance the new organization. As secretary of the NYSSV, Comstock began to lobby the U.S. Congress to pass new legislation strengthening an earlier antiobscenity act passed in 1864. When the new law was passed in 1873, Comstock was appointed Special Agent of the Post Office with the authority to carry out the act's provisions. He has been said to have confiscated "194,000 obscene pictures and photographs, 134,000 pounds of books, 14,200 stereopticon plates, 60,300 rubber articles, 5,500 sets of playing cards, and 31,500 boxes of aphrodisiacs" during the first six months in his new office and to have boasted later in life that "he had been responsible for the criminal conviction of enough people to fill a 61-coach passenger train—over 3,600 people" and to have been responsible for "at least 15 suicides" (A. Bates 1995, 159). A vast amount of the material seized by Comstock as obscene included contraceptive and family planning information which today is regularly available to the general public through any number and variety of outlets.

Comstock remained active in the campaign against obscenity for the rest of his life. He died on September 21, 1915 in New York City.

Paul Ehrlich (1854–1915)

Ehrlich was a German bacteriologist who was awarded a share of the 1908 Nobel Prize in Physiology or Medicine for his research on autoimmunity, the process by which a body develops immune responses against its own tissues, cells, or other components. In the area of sexual health, he is best known for his discovery of the first safe and effective treatment for syphilis, one of the most terrible diseases in human history.

Paul Ehrlich was born in Strehlen, Silesia, then a part of Prussia, a city now known as Strzelin, in modern Poland. He completed his secondary education at the Breslau Gymnasium (high school), and then studied medicine at the universities of Breslau, Strasbourg, Freiburg, and Leipzig, from which he received his medical degree in 1877. His doctoral dissertation dealt with the staining of cells, a topic that was to remain a centerpiece of his research for the rest of his life. In 1878, Ehrlich accepted an appointment as a researcher at the Berlin Medical Clinic, where he later had an opportunity to work with the famous Robert Koch on the tubercle bacillus responsible for tuberculosis. During this research, Ehrlich caught a mild case of the disease and traveled to Egypt for two years in order to live and work in a more amenable climate. Some biographers have surmised that this experience was a seminal factor in the development of Ehrlich's overall view to the search for methods of treating disease. He envisioned finding a magic bullet, some compound that would attack disease-causing microorganisms only, without affecting beneficial organisms or an animal's body. His work on staining suggested that some compounds must exist, compounds that recognize and attach themselves only to specific microorganisms. His goal was to find compounds that were effective in bonding to bacteria and other disease-causing microorganisms and then attach to the stain a poison that would kill the organism.

Over the years, Ehrlich methodically worked his way though hundreds of potential stains that might be used as a magic bullet. In 1909, one of his assistants, Sachahiro Hata, returned to a compound that had already been tested and rejected, called compound 606 because it was the 606th compound to have been tested. (At this point, Ehrlich was already working on compounds 900+.) Hata found that the compound was very effective in killing the spirochete that causes syphilis, *Treponema pallidum*. In 1910 the compound was made generally available to physicians under the name of salvarsan. It, along with a related drug called neosalvarsan, were the only safe and effective drugs for the treatment of syphilis until penicillin became generally available for this purpose in the 1940s.

Kevin Jennings (Dates unavailable)

In May 2009, Jennings was appointed Assistant Deputy Secretary in the Office of Safe and Drug Free Schools in the U.S. Department of Education. He is a founder of the Gay, Lesbian, and Straight Education Network (GLSEN) and has worked for many years to make schools safe environments for gay, lesbian, bisexual, transgender, and questioning (GLBTQ) youth.

Kevin Jennings was born in Winston-Salem, North Carolina, and graduated from Harvard College in 1985, where he gave the Harvard Oration at his graduation ceremonies. His first teaching position was in the history department at the Moses Brown School in Providence, Rhode Island, after which he took a job as teacher and chair of the history department at the Concord Academy in Concord, Massachusetts. In 1988, he became faculty adviser to the school's first Gay-Straight Alliance. Two years later, he was a founding member of GLSEN, a volunteer group of parents, teachers, and other adults concerned with issues faced by GLBTQ youth in the Boston area. The organization has since grown to a staff of 40 members who support the efforts of more than 10,000 students engaged in more than 4,300 gay-straight alliance groups around the nation.

In 1992, Jennings was appointed co-chair of the Education Committee of the Governor's Commission on Gay & Lesbian Youth by Massachusetts Governor William Weld. He was principal author of the commission's final report, "Making Schools Safe for Gay & Lesbian Youth." In 1993, he left the Boston area to become Joseph Kingenstein Fellow at Columbia University, from which he received his master's degree in 1994. He then became executive director of GLSEN, a post he held until October 2008. In 1999, he also earned his M.B.A. from the New York University Stern School of Business. Jennings is the author of six books, including *Telling Tales Out of School* and *Mama's Boy, Preacher's Son*.

Alfred Kinsey (1894–1956)

Kinsey was perhaps the most influential sex researcher in the world during his lifetime. He published two classic research studies on the nature of human sexuality, *Sexual Behavior in the Human Male* and *Sexual Behavior in the Human Female*, and also founded the Institute for Research in Sex, Gender, and Reproduction (now the Kinsey Institute for Research in Sex, Gender, and Reproduction) at Indiana University.

Alfred Charles Kinsey was born in Hoboken, New Jersey, on June 23, 1894, to Alfred Seguine Kinsey, a professor of engineering at Stevens Institute of Technology, and Sarah Ann (Charles) Kinsey. After graduating from Columbia High School in Hoboken, Kinsey enrolled at Stevens to study engineering, primarily because of his father's insistence. At the end of two years, he realized that engineering was not a field for which he was suited, and, with his father's acquiescence, he transferred to Bowdoin College, in Brunswick, Maine, where he majored in biology. After earning his B.S. in biology and psychology in 1916, Kinsey enrolled in a doctoral program in zoology at Harvard University. He received his Sc.D. from Harvard in 1919, and then took a position in the department of zoology at Indiana University, where he remained for the rest of his life.

By the mid-1930s, Kinsey had already achieved a reputation in his specialized field of entomology, the study of gall wasps, a subject about which he was regarded as the leading authority in the world. At the same time, he was increasingly interested in a topic that had concerned him for many years, education in sexuality. An opportunity to act on this interest occurred in 1938 when the Indiana student newspaper, *Daily Student*, published an editorial demanding that the university provide better information about and testing for venereal diseases, a health problem then sweeping the nation. Kinsey took this call as an opportunity to request permission to teach a noncredit course on marriage, in which a number of issues related to sexuality would be presented. The course was well received the first year it was offered, with 98 students enrolling, even though the university administration had stipulated that the course could not be announced or advertised publicly.

Before long, Kinsey had largely abandoned his research on gall wasps and focused his attention on human sexuality. In 1942, he received funding from the Rockefeller Foundation and the National Research Council for the creation of the Institute for Research in Sex, Gender, and Reproduction at Indiana. It was through the institute that Kinsey conducted the interviews (5,300 white males and 5,940 white women and girls) on which he based his classic books. The book on male sexuality was published in 1948 and eventually sold more than a half million copies, while the female version was released five years later with significantly smaller sales numbers (because the text was then available from a number of other sources).

Kinsey's work essentially came to an end after the publication of *Sexual Behavior in the Human Female*. His work had outraged large segments of the American population and efforts were made at all levels to ensure that he would write no more about the topic. Under pressure from the U.S. Congress, Dean Rusk, then president of the Rockefeller Foundation, ended the fund's support of the institute. Kinsey was unable to find funding from other sources, and he gradually withdrew from active participation in sexuality research. The institute eventually survived and continues to thrive as an independent organization within the purview of Indiana University. Kinsey died on August 25, 1956, as the result of an embolism caused by bruising his leg in a fall a few days earlier.

Charles Knowlton (1800–1850)

Knowlton is perhaps best known for being the first person in the history of the birth control movement in the United States to be imprisoned for his efforts on behalf of contraception. He was sentenced to three months of hard labor in Cambridge in 1833 because of a book he had written called *The Fruits of Philosophy, or the Private Companion of Young Married People by a Physician.*

Charles Knowlton was born on May 10, 1800, in Templeton, Massachusetts, to Stephen and Comfort (White) Knowlton. He attended local schools in Worcester County and the New Salem Academy, about 40 miles west of the city of Worcester. Knowlton's biographers note that, as a young man, Knowlton was somewhat mystified by and very concerned about the "wet dreams" that are a normal part of male adolescence. He apparently worried enough that his health was affected, and he even went to the extreme of submitting to electric shocks as a cure for his disorder. When he fell in love with and married the daughter of the man who administered the shocks, he was (not surprisingly today) completed cured of his malady.

Perhaps because of this early problem, Knowlton became interested in medical matters as a young man and enrolled for a series of lectures at Dartmouth Medical College, from which he received his M.D. in 1824. He then opened a medical practice in Hawley, Massachusetts, where he decided to supplement his medical knowledge by digging up recently buried corpses for dissection and study. When he was discovered pursuing these studies, he was arrested and sentenced to two months in jail. While serving his time in the Worcester County jail, Knowlton developed his general philosophy of life, a materialistic and atheistic view of the world, which he outlined in a book called *Modern Materialism*. Although he believed that the book would sell widely and bring him fame, he sold almost no copies. He eventually gave up on the book and returned to medical practice in Ashfield, Massachusetts.

At about this time, Knowlton had also become increasingly interested in issues of family planning. He had become convinced that the pattern of uncontrolled pregnancies among young women common at the time was both economically and medically harmful to families, especially to women. He began providing contraceptive advice to his patients, eventually setting down this advice in his book, *The Fruits of Philosophy, or the Private Companion of Young Married People by a Physician*. When word got out about the book, he was fined in 1832 and imprisoned for three months in 1833. The government's attempt to silence Knowlton actually had the reverse effect, arousing instead in the public an interest in the book and its subject. It eventually sold more than 10,000 copies and became widely popular throughout the United States, where the last edition was published in 1877.

Knowlton remained active as a traveling physician covering about 30 towns in western Massachusetts until his death on February 20, 1850, in Winchendon, Massachusetts.

Beverly LaHaye (1929–)

LaHaye founded Concerned Women of America in 1979 to promote Christian values in development of national policy in six major areas: sanctity of life, definition of the family, the fight against pornography, education, religious liberty, and national sovereignty.

Beverly LaHaye was born Beverly Jean Ratcliffe on April 30, 1929. She attended Bob Jones University, where she met her future husband, Tim LaHaye, later to become a well-known and influential evangelical minister and author of the *Left Behind* series of apocalyptic fiction novels. When the couple was married in 1947, Beverly left Bob Jones to become a full-time housewife and mother. The couple eventually had four children. LaHaye dates her interest in political issues to the day in 1979 when she saw Barbara Walters interviewing feminist Betty Friedan. LaHaye realized, she later said, that the ideas Friedan was expressing did not represent her or any of the women she knew (S. Bates 1993, 102). As a result, she decided to form a new organization, Concerned Women of America (CWA), that *did* more closely reflect her own views on a number of important social issues. LaHaye has remained as chairman of the CWA ever since.

LaHaye is a popular guest on a number of radio and television programs, including *CBS Evening News*, *NBC Nightly News*, *ABC's World News Tonight*, and *Nightline*. In 1990 she started her own radio program, *Beverly LaHaye Live*, which was later renamed *Concerned Women Today*. The program ceased production in 2004.

LaHaye is perhaps best known for the 16 books she has authored and coauthored, including *The New Spirit Controlled Woman*, *The Act of Marriage*, *Spiritual Power for the Family*, *and A Woman's Path to True Significance* (with Janice Crouse). LaHaye has received a number of awards and honors for her work, including the Christian Woman of the Year award (1984), given by the association of the same name; Religious Freedom Award (1991) of the Southern Baptist Convention, Thomas Jefferson Award (2001) of the Council for National Policy; American Association of Christian Counselors' Caregiver Award (2003), and Extraordinary Woman of the Year Award (2006) from the Extraordinary Women ministry. In 1992, she was awarded an honorary doctorate of humanities by Liberty University.

Hideyo Noguchi (1876–1928)

In 1911, Noguchi discovered the agent that causes syphilis, the spirochete bacterium called *Treponema pallidum*.

Noguchi was born Seisaku Noguchi on November 24, 1876, in Inawashiro, Fukushima prefecture, Japan. At the age of one and a half years, he fell into a fireplace, badly burning his left hand. The injury was to have significance on a number of occasions later in life. For example, when the damage to his burned fingers was finally repaired, he was so deeply impressed that he decided to become a physician himself. He apprenticed himself to the doctor who had repaired his hand and eventually passed the medical examination which earned him his M.D. in 1897. A year later, he changed his name from Seisaku to Hideyo because of a novel he had read about a physician with less than desirable qualities who had the same name as his own birth name.

In 1900, Noguchi took a research position at the University of Pennsylvania, reportedly because prospective employers in Japan were concerned about patient reactions to a doctor with such a badly damaged hand. Noguchi found research a very satisfying career, and later moved from Pennsylvania to a similar position at the Rockefeller Institute in New York City. It was at Rockefeller that Noguchi found the *T. pallidum* bacterium in the brain of a patient with late-term syphilis, providing the evidence that the bacterium was responsible for the disease. For his work in this area, Noguchi was nominated for a Nobel prize on nine occasions, although he was never given the award.

Beginning in 1918, Noguchi developed a growing interest in yellow fever, and he traveled extensively in South and Central America to test his hypothesis that the disease is caused by a spirochaete bacteria like *T. pallidum* rather than by a virus, as most researchers thought (Noguchi was wrong in this hypothesis). While working in Accra, Gold Coast, (now Ghana) in 1928, he fell ill with the disease he was studying, and died there on May 21, 1928. He received a number of honors during his lifetime, including the Order of Dannebrog (Denmark), Order of Isabella the Catholic (Spain), Order of the Polar Star (Sweden), and Order of the Rising Sun, 4th class (Japan); as well as honorary doctorates from the University of Quito, University of Guayaquil, and Yale University. In July 2006, the Japanese government established the Hideyo Noguchi Africa Prize for outstanding research on infectious diseases in Africa.

Elise Ottesen-Jensen (1886–1973)

Ottesen-Jensen was a politically active journalist and sex educator who was one of the founding members of the Riksförbundet för Sexuell Upplysning (RFSU; Swedish Association for Sexuality Education), one of the first organization's of its kind in the world. She was also an outspoken advocate for the rights of women and an active member of Sveriges Arbetares Centralorganisation (Central Organization of the Workers of Sweden), a far left political group.

Ottesen-Jensen was born Elise Ottesen in Høyland (now part of Sandnes) in Rogaland county, Norway, on January 2, 1886. She was the 17th of 18 children. Her life was strongly influenced when she learned at an early age that her younger sister had been sent to Denmark to bear a child so that she would be forced to give up the child for adoption. Ottesen adopted her hyphenated last name when she married a political organizer, Albert Jensen, although she was almost universally known by her nickname of Ottar. She had planned to become a dentist, but lost two fingers to an accident in her high school chemistry class, making that career impossible. Instead, she chose to become a journalist and political organizer. One of the first things she learned when she started to organize women was that they seemed to have more questions about sexuality than they did about politics. After she and her husband left Norway for Sweden (because of his political activities), she was introduced to the diaphragm by a doctor friend, and was soon traveling across the country teaching women about its use. She also agitated for more and better education about sexual health, advocated for abortion rights for women, and worked for civil rights for gay men and lesbians. In 1953, Ottesen-Jensen was one of the founders of the International Planned Parenthood Foundation. In her honor, the RFSU has named its newsletter *Ottar*. She died in Stockholm on September 4, 1973.

Robert Parlin (1963–)

Parlin was cofounder of the Gay, Lesbian and Straight Education Network (GLSEN) and established the first public school Gay/ Straight Alliance at Newton South High School, in Newton, Massachusetts, in 1989. He continues to be adviser to that group.

Robert Parlin was born in Grafton, Massachusetts, on August 1, 1963. He attended Harvard College, from which he received his B.A. in history and literature in 1985. He then continued his studies at the Harvard Graduate School of Education (HGSE), from which he received his M.Ed. in 1987. After graduating from HGSE, he accepted a job teaching history at Newton South, where he has remained ever since. In 1989, he was cofounder of the Gay and Lesbian School Teacher Network (GLSTN), which was later renamed the Gay, Lesbian, and Straight Education Network (GLSEN). In addition to his regular teaching assignments at Newton South, Parlin helped write the ninth grade sexuality and health curriculum for the Newton school system. He has also been a trainer on lesbian, gay, bisexual, and transgender (LGBT) issues in the New England region and has worked for the Massachusetts Department of Education's Safe Schools Program for Gay and Lesbian Students.

Parlin was elected to the HGSE Alumni Council in 2004 and was appointed to the Cambridge (Massachusetts) GLBT Commission in 2005. In 2007, Parlin created and taught a course on the history of gay/straight alliances at Wheelock College in Boston through the Stonewall Center for Lifelong Learning. In 1998, Parlin and his partner, Bren Bataclan, had the first gay commitment ceremony ever held at Harvard University's historic Memorial Church. In 2004, they were legally married in Cambridge.

Paul VI (1897–1978)

As the person acknowledged to be the representative of God on Earth, the head of the Roman Catholic Church espouses views on all matters of morality that members of the church are expected to understand and follow. Pope Paul VI clarified the church's position on a number of sexual issues, including birth control, in various of his writings, one of the most important of which was the encyclical *Humanae vitae* (Of human life), issued on July 25, 1968. In that encyclical, the pope confirmed a long-held position that all forms of artificial birth control are to be "absolutely excluded."

Paul VI was born Giovanni Battista Enrico Antonio Maria Montini on September 26, 1897, in the village of Concesio, in Lombardy, Italy. His mother was Giudetta (Alghisi) Montini, and his father, Giorgio Montini, was a nonpracticing lawyer, journalist, and member of the Italian parliament. He attended a Jesuit-run elementary school, Cesare Arici, and a state-operated secondary school, Arnaldo da Brescia, from which he received his diploma in 1916. He then entered the seminary to study to become a Roman Catholic priest, and was ordained in that office on May 29, 1920. After his ordination, Montini was sent to Rome to study at the Gregorian University, the University of Rome, and the Accademia dei Nobili Ecclesiastici. He was then assigned as attaché to the papal nunciate in Warsaw for one year. After returning to Rome in 1924, he held a number of posts in the Vatican hierarchy, including chaplain to the Federation of Italian Catholic University Students and substitute for ordinary affairs under Cardinals Pacelli and Maglione, secretaries of state, and, eventually, directly under the pope himself. In this office, Montini was responsible for organizing relief work and care of political refugees during World War II.

In 1954, Montini was named archbishop of Milan, the most senior post outside the Vatican. His work in revitalizing the diocese brought him worldwide attention and he was widely recognized as "the archbishop of the workers." Upon the death of Pope John XXIII on June 21, 1963, Montini was elected to become the new leader of the church, whereupon he took the name of Paul VI. Early in his papacy, Paul decided to issue encyclicals on two controversial topics, celibacy in the priesthood (*Sacerdotalis caelibatus*; June 24, 1967) and birth control (*Humanae vitae*; July 25, 1968). These encyclicals evoked widespread controversy from individuals both within and outside of the church. That controversy eventually overshadowed many aspects of the rest of Paul's work in the church, but never deterred Paul from his beliefs. Ten years after issuing *Humanae vitae*, he again reiterated his strong stand against the use of birth control devices by the faithful, a position that remains official doctrine today for Catholics. He died on August 6, 1978, at Castel Gandolfo, in Rome.

Gregory Goodwin Pincus (1903–1967)

Pincus is one of the three individuals responsible for the development of the first oral contraceptive to be approved for use in the United States, often referred to simply as The Pill. Late in his life, he also worked on the production of a morning-after pill that could be taken some hours or days after sexual intercourse.

Gregory Goodwin Pincus was born on April 9, 1903, in Woodbine, New Jersey, to Joseph and Elizabeth (Lipman) Pincus. Later in life, he credited his father and uncle, both agricultural scientists, with his own early interest in scientific research. Pincus attended Cornell University, from which he received his B.S. in agriculture in 1924. He then remained at Cornell to complete his master's and doctoral degrees in zoology in 1927. He did his postdoctoral studies in reproductive biology at Cambridge from 1927 to 1930 before accepting a post as instructor in biology at Harvard University, where he remained until 1937. At Harvard, Pincus's research dealt with hormonal systems in animals, especially the rabbit. He achieved a remarkable breakthrough in 1934 when he was able to achieve reproduction in a rabbit using in vitro fertilization. Although that accomplishment was scientifically significant, it came at a time when the general public was becoming increasingly concerned about scientific efforts to create life artificially, and Pincus was labeled as a "Frankenstein" by some members of the general public. Instead of confirming his scientific status, his rabbit experiment is said to have prevented his receiving tenure at Harvard.

In 1937, Pincus returned once more to Cambridge for a year before accepting an offer to become professor of experimental zoology at Clark University, in Worcester, Massachusetts. Although prominent in some fields, Clark was not then widely recognized as a scientific research institution of the first rank. Pincus struggled there to continue his research on animal hormones on a very limited budget. Over time, Pincus built up the research program at Clark and, in 1944, was able to establish the Worcester Foundation for Experimental Biology, for many years a center of research on animal (including human) endocrinology.

In 1953, Margaret Sanger and Katharine McCormick approached Pincus with a proposal that he begin research on the development of an oral contraceptive pill for women. Working with a colleague, Min-Chueh Chang, Pincus began to explore the use of progesterone to prevent ovulation. Pincus and Chang later found that a combination of progesterone and estrogen was even more effective than progesterone alone in preventing ovulation with the least risk to users. In 1956, joined by Harvard researcher John Rock, Pincus and Chang began testing their oral contraceptive in Puerto Rico. Based on the results of those tests, the U.S. Food and Drug Administration approved the new drug's use for certain menstrual disorders and miscarriages and in 1960 as an oral contraceptive.

After The Pill had been approved, Pincus and Chang turned their attention to research on a so-called morning after pill that could be taken as a contraceptive a few days after sexual intercourse. This research was interrupted, however, when Pincus died on August 22, 1967, in Boston, of bone cancer. The disease is thought to have been caused by Pincus's long-term exposure to carcinogenic substances during his work in the laboratory. Among the awards Pincus received are the Albert D. Lasker Award in Planned Parenthood, the Modern Medicine Award for Distinguished Achievement, and the American Medical Association Scientific Achievement Award.

John Rock (1890–1984)

Rock, along with colleague Gregory Pincus, developed the technology used in the first contraceptive pill approved for use by the U.S. Food and Drug Administration in 1960.

John Rock was born in Marlborough, Massachusetts, on March 24, 1890. He attended the High School of Commerce in Boston, from which he graduated in 1909, with the goal of having a career in business. His first job was as an accountant on a banana plantation in Guatemala, after which he took a similar position with an engineering firm in Woonsocket, Rhode Island. These experiences made him realize that he was not really suited to a career in business, and he applied for admission to Harvard College, from which he received his bachelor's degree in 1915. He then continued his studies at the Harvard Medical School,

earning his M.D. in 1918. He was originally interested in special-
izing in diseases of the nervous system, but eventually changed
his mind and decided to concentrate on gynecology and obstetrics. He completed his internship at the Massachusetts General
Hospital in 1919 and his residency at the Boston Lying-In Hospital
a year later. He then began a private practice, but abandoned that
occupation a year later to accept an appointment as assistant in
obstetrics at the Harvard Medical School.

Although himself a devout Roman Catholic, Rock was also
a fervent advocate for greater availability of contraceptive devices and methods for married women. He included a discussion of birth control in the classes he taught at Harvard (virtually
unheard of in medical schools at the time) and, in 1931, joined a
campaign (the only Catholic to do so) for the overturn of the Massachusetts law banning the sale of contraceptives. In 1939, when
the Vatican approved the use of the so-called rhythm method of
birth control, Rock opened the first clinic in the United States to
teach the method to women.

In 1952, Rock was asked by a colleague, Gregory Pincus, to
work with him on the development of an oral hormonal-based
contraceptive pill. Both men had been working on ovulation and
conception for many years, Pincus in rabbits and Rock in humans,
and the collaboration appeared to be a natural one, especially
since Pincus was not licensed as a physician and could not, therefore, conduct human trials with the new product. After almost a
decade of development and testing, the new product, to become
widely known as simply The Pill, was approved for use in the
United States by the Food and Drug Administration in 1960. After
this momentous step, Rock spent many years trying to convince
the Vatican that The Pill represented a form of natural birth control and that the pope should approve its use as a contraceptive
tool for women. In that effort, of course, he ultimately failed.

In 1969, Rock retired from active work and moved to a farm
in Templeton, New Hampshire. He died in nearby Peterborough
on December 4, 1984.

John D. Rockefeller III (1906–1978)

One of the wealthiest men in the world, Rockefeller became
very interested in issues of population during the 1950s, when
population growth appeared to be perhaps the single most

important issue facing nations around the world. In 1952, he provided $100,000 for the founding of the Population Council for the purpose of conducting research on population issues and developing programs for bringing a halt to the seemingly out-of-control population growth then under way.

John D. Rockefeller III was born in New York City on April 21, 1906, the grandson of oil magnate John D. Rockefeller and the son of John D. Rockefeller, Jr. He was educated at the Loomis Institute, in Windsor, Connecticut, and at Princeton University, from which he received his B.S. in industrial relations in 1929. As an heir to one of the world's great fortunes, Rockefeller spent his life in a variety of philanthropic activities, serving as a trustee of the Rockefeller Foundation from 1931 to 1970.

As is the case with many young men and women born to wealth, Rockefeller was exposed at an early age to a number of organizations and individuals with a variety of social and political special interests. In 1928, for example, he was appointed to the board of directors of the Bureau of Social Hygiene, a research institute created by the Rockefeller Foundation in 1911 for the study of the causes and control of crime. Four years later, he was appointed chairman of the Delinquency Committee of the Boys Bureau of New York City. In posts such as these, he began to develop an intimate knowledge of the difficult problems of everyday life faced by ordinary citizens with whom he might not otherwise have ever had contact.

By the early 1950s, Rockefeller had become especially interested in issues of population control. Evidence was beginning to accumulate that run-away population growth, especially in Asia, was likely to result in economic, social, and political problems of unprecedented significance. Rockefeller attempted to interest his fellows trustees in making population issues an important focus of the Rockefeller Institute's work, but failed. Instead, he made a grant from his own sources to make possible the founding of the Population Council as an instrument for research on the world's population problems, as well as those of the United States. (The council continues to exist today with an interest in a variety of population-related issues.) The council rapidly became an important force in the study of population issues worldwide and in the development of programs to bring population growth under control. In 1954, it helped to fund the United Nation's first World Population Conference in Rome. During the early 1960s, the council also supported research on an implantable intrauterine device that could be distributed to and easily used by women around the world as a primary means of family planning and birth control.

In 1970, Rockefeller was appointed chairman of the Commission on Population Growth and the American Future by President Richard M. Nixon. In its report, that commission recommended universal access to reproductive information and universal coverage for all patient costs related to maternity, abortion, and voluntary sterilization. Rockefeller was killed in an automobile accident in Mt. Pleasant, New York, on July 10, 1978.

Margaret Sanger (1879–1966)

Sanger was a nurse and birth control activist who worked relentlessly for the right of women to have control over their own sexuality. She founded the American Birth Control League, which later became the Planned Parenthood Federation of America, along with a number of other birth control and family planning organizations. She also wrote a number of books, pamphlets, brochures, and other materials with information about contraception and other aspects of women's sexual lives.

Sanger was born Margaret Higgins in Corning, New York, on September 14, 1879. Her mother was a devout Roman Catholic who experienced 18 pregnancies and 11 live births, of which Margaret was the sixth. Her father was a stonemason and an advocate for equal rights for women and socialistic principles. Margaret attended Claverack College and the Hudson River Institute, but left after two years to care for her ailing mother, who died in 1899. She was then able to resume her schooling, enrolling in a nursing program at the White Plains Hospital. Toward the end of that program, she spent some time interning at the Manhattan Eye and Ear Clinic in 1902, during which she met her husband-to-be William Sanger. They were married on August 18, 1902, after having known each other for six months.

When Margaret developed tuberculosis, the Sangers moved to Saranac, New York, where they lived until 1912. When they returned to New York City, she began working with poor women on the Lower East Side who commonly experienced multiple pregnancies and who, to avoid that fate, often attempted to abort themselves when they found that they were pregnant once again. Sanger was very troubled by what she saw and determined to do whatever she could to relieve the condition in which these women found themselves. In 1914, for example, she began to produce a monthly newsletter providing information about contraception and encouraging women to take responsibility for their own sexual health. The publication prompted the U.S. Postal Service to put out a warrant for Sanger's arrest on the grounds that she had violated the Comstock law against the distribution of obscene literature (the birth control information). Sanger fled the United States to avoid prosecution, but returned in 1915 emboldened to continue her efforts in aiding women, assisted by a vast amount of new information about contraception garnered during her stay in Europe.

On October 16, 1916, Sanger opened a family planning clinic at 46 Amboy Street in Brooklyn, the first facility of its kind in the United States. Nine days later, New York City police officers raided the clinic; Sanger was tried for operating a "public nuisance," and she was sentenced to 30 days in prison. Her experience did not deter her from her goal of educating women about contraception, and she spent the rest of her life in that task. In 1921, for example, she cofounded the American Birth Control League, not only to continue educating women and the general public about family planning, but also to conduct research and to be an advocate for legislation that would allow women greater reproductive freedom. In 1923, she opened the Clinical Research Bureau which, despite its name, was primarily the first legal birth control clinic in the United States. In the same year, she also founded the National Committee on Federal Legislation for Birth Control. She continued as an active advocate for birth control and family planning for the remaining 40 years of her life, organizing committees, chairing organizations, speaking at meetings, writing pamphlets, and attending national and international conferences. She was the author of a number of important books and pamphlets, including *Family Limitations, The Case for Birth Control: A Supplementary Brief and Statement of Facts, Woman and the New Race, What Every Girl Should Know, What Every Mother Should Know, The Pivot of Civilization,* "The Case for Birth Control," and *My Fight for Birth Control.* Sanger died in Tucson, Arizona, on September 6, 1966.

Matthew Shepard (1976–1998)

Shepard was a 21-year-old gay man who died of severe head injuries on October 12, 1998, after being attacked and assaulted a few nights earlier by two young men near Laramie, Wyoming. He has become an icon for individuals and organizations working to extend hate crime legislation in the United States to gay men, lesbians, bisexuals, and transgendered individuals.

Matthew Shepard was born in Casper, Wyoming, on December 1, 1976, the son of Judy and Dennis Shepard. He attended Crest Hill Elementary School, Dean Morgan Junior High School, and Natrona County High School for his freshman and sophomore years. He completed his secondary education at the American School in Switzerland, from which he graduated in 1995. He then returned to the United States where he briefly attended Catawba College, in North Carolina, and Casper College, in Wyoming, before moving to Laramie and enrolling at the University of Wyoming as a political science major.

On the evening of October 7, 1998, Shepard was offered a ride home from a Laramie bar by 21-year-old Russell Arthur Henderson and 22-year-old Aaron James McKinney. Instead of taking Shepard home, the two men drove him to a deserted field, tied him to a fence, pistol-whipped him, and left him for dead. Shepard was found alive, but in a coma, 18 hours later. He lived five more days before dying of his injuries. Henderson and McKinney offered a number of defenses during their trial, claiming at first a "gay panic" response to their contact with Shepard, during which they were temporarily insane, and later, that they had only intended to rob him, and not to do him serious physcial harm. They were eventually found guilty of felony murder and kidnapping charges, and both are currently serving two consecutive life sentences. Shepard's death has inspired a variety of responses, ranging from the writing and production of a play about the murder, *The Laramie Project*, which is often the source of controversy in communities where it is performed, to at least four films about Shepard's life and death, to any number of poems and songs about the episode. The latest effort to include gay men, lesbians, bisexuals, and transgendered individuals in the federal hate crimes law, which has yet to pass the U.S. Congress, is commonly known as the Matthew Shepard Act. (Wyoming also has no hate crimes legislation.) In December 1998, Judy and Dennis Shepard founded the Matthew Shepard Foundation to commemorate Matthew's life and to support diversity in education and to work to pass hate crimes legislation that includes lesbians, gay men, bisexuals, and transgendered people.

Marie Stopes (1880–1958)

Stopes was trained as a paleobotanist, but spent much of her life working for women's causes and for the promotion of family planning. She opened the first birth control clinic in Great Britain in 1921.

Marie Stopes was born in Edinburgh, Scotland, on October 15, 1880, the daughter of Charlotte Stopes, an active participant in the suffragette and women's rights movements, and Henry Stopes, a brewer with an amateur interest in archaeology. Although women had not yet been given the right to attend university classes, Charlotte Stopes had been awarded a certificate (essentially equivalent to a degree) by passing her final examinations at university level. Although she had no formal education herself until the age of 12, Marie Stopes proved to be an apt student and earned a scholarship to University College, London, at the age of 19. There she majored in botany and geology and earned her bachelor of science degree with first class honors in 1902. She then traveled to the University of Munich for further study, earning her Ph.D. in paleobotany in 1904. She then returned to University College and earned her D.Sc., making her the youngest person in history to have done so. After completing her studies, she spent a year doing research in Japan, was fellow and lecturer at University College, and lectured in paleobotany at the University of Manchester, where she was the first woman on the faculty.

After a series of unhappy relationships, Stopes married a fellow scientist, Reginald Ruggles Gates, in 1911. The couple had sexual problems from the outset (which turned out to be the result of Gate's impotence), and three years later they were divorced. During the marriage, Stopes spent many hours at the British Library, attempting to pinpoint the reason for the couple's sexual problems. After the divorce, she wrote a book summarizing her research, *Married Love: A New Contribution to the Solution of the Sex Difficulties*, a work for which she was to become famous. The theme of her book was that it was possible to combine a happy marriage with a fulfilling sexual life, while avoiding pregnancies.

In 1918, Stopes married H. V. Roe, a wealthy manufacturer and aviator, an event that made it possible for her to pursue what had become her primary passion in life: the establishment of birth control clinics at which women could be taught methods of contraception and ways of avoiding sexually transmitted infections. She

opened the first of these clinics, the Mother's Clinic for Construc-
tive Birth Control, in Holloway, North London, in 1921, and staffed
the facility with female nurses, believing that they would be less
threatening to patients than would male doctors. The clinic moved
to central London four years later, and remains there today.

Stopes spent the rest of her life working to promote safe contraceptive technology for women. Much of her time was devoted
to writing for and editing her clinic's newsletter, *Birth Control
News.* She also wrote a second book, *Wise Parenthood,* which drew
the wrath of church leaders from most denominations. Later in
life, she devoted much of her time to writing novels and poetry.
She died in Dorking, Surrey, on October 2, 1958, from breast cancer. Today, her name and work are memorialized in the Marie
Stopes International (MSI) organization, which operates more
than 560 family planning clinics in more than 40 nations.

Brandon Teena (1972–1993)

Teena was a biological female who early on in life identified herself as a male and lived as a male for most of her/his life. Teena
was raped and murdered by two male friends on December 31,
1993. Her/his story has been memorialized in the 1999 film *Boys
Don't Cry,* for which Hillary Swank, who played the role of Teena,
received an Academy Award for Best Actress.

Teena was born in Lincoln, Nebraska, on December 12, 1972.
Her parents described her as a "tomboy," and she began thinking
of herself as a "man trapped in a woman's body" early in life. In
high school, she dressed as a boy and dated girls. In 1993, Teena
moved from Lincoln to Falls City, Nebraska, where she lived exclusively as a man. He dated a friend of the family with whom he
was living at the time, Lana Tisdel, and became close friends with
two ex-convicts, John Lotter and Marvin "Tom" Nissen. Tisdel
eventually found out that Teena was a biological female, but the
couple continued dating.

At a New Year's Eve party on December 31, 1993, Lotter and
Nissen forced Teena to expose himself to Tisdel and then took him
to a deserted factory, where they beat and raped Teena. Later in
the evening, they broke into Teena's home and murdered Teena
and two other occupants of the house. Lotter and Nissen were
eventually found guilty of murder and sentenced to death, but
both cases are still on appeal.

The 1999 film about this case brought to public attention an issue with which most Americans are probably unaware, the travails of young men and women who identify as being of the opposite sex. Since the Teena murder, a number of organizations interested in issues of sexuality have made a greater effort to include transgender issues in their work and, in many cases, to include the term *transgender* in their publications and publicity.

Karolina Olivia Widerström (1856–1949)

Widerström was a Swedish doctor who advocated for programs of sex education, especially for young women, as a way of helping people better understand their own anatomy and physiology and to learn how to deal with sexual health issues in their own lives.

Widerström was born in Helsingbord, Sweden, on December 10, 1856, to Otto Fredrik Widerström and Olivia Erika Dillén, a gymnastics teacher and a veterinarian. After completing her secondary education, she studied at the Gymnastic Central Institute in Stockholm from 1873 to 1875. She then served as assistant to professor Lars Gabriel Branting, a pioneer in the field of medical gymnastics. She then completed her undergraduate studies at the Walinska Skolan in Stockholm in 1879 and at the University of Uppsala in 1880 before earning her medical degree at the Karolinska Institute in Stockholm in 1884. In 1888 she received her medical license and established a private practice in Hufvudstaden.

Early on in her practice, Widerström was appalled to learn that her women clients often knew next to nothing about female anatomy and physiology or about sexually transmitted infections, pregnancy, and contraception. She set out to do all she could to change that situation and to provide education for both women and men about issues in sexual health. She gave a number of lectures and wrote a book, *Kvinnohygien* (*Women's Hygiene*), which was first published in 1899 and eventually went through seven editions until 1932. She argued strongly that men should be tested for sexually transmitted infections before marriage at a time when far greater emphasis was being placed on the testing of prostitutes. Widerström was also active politically, elected to the Stockholm city council in 1910, the first year in which public office was available to women. She also held leadership positions in the

Landsföreningen för kvinnans politiska rösträtt (National Union for Women's Political Suffrage), an organization through which she worked to obtain suffrage for women, a goal achieved in 1921. She died in Stockholm on March 4, 1949.

Harald zur Hausen (1936–)

Harald zur Hausen is a German virologist who was awarded the 2008 Nobel Prize in Physiology or Medicine for his discovery of the role of the human papillomavirus (HPV) in cancer of the cervix. His work made possible the eventual development of a vaccine that protects women against HPV and, thus, significantly decreases their risk for both cervical cancer and genital warts.

Harald zur Hausen was born in Gelsenkirchen, Germany, on March 11, 1936. He attended high school in Vechta and then studied medicine at the universities of Bonn, Hamburg, and Düsseldorf, from which he received his M.D. in 1960. After serving for two years as a medical assistant at Düsseldorf, zur Hausen took a position as a laboratory researcher at the Institute for Microbiology at Düsseldorf. In 1966 he emigrated to the United States to work at the Virus Laboratories of the University of Pennsylvania's Children's Hospital with the famous expatriate German virologists, Werner and Gertrude Henle. In 1969, zur Hausen returned to Germany, where he served successively as professor of virology at the University of Würzburg (1969–1972), the University of Erlangen-Nuremberg (1972–1977), and the University of Freiburg (1977–1983). In 1983, he was appointed director of the German Cancer Research Center (Deutsches Krebsforschungszentrum) in Heidelberg and professor of medicine at the University of Heidelberg.

Zur Hausen became interested in the role of viruses in the development of cancer early in his career. At the time, scientists had found that viruses are responsible for cancer in some animals, but their role in any form of cancer in humans was still unclear. In 1983, zur Hausen discovered the presence of one form of the human papillomavirus, called HPV 16, in cervical cancer tumors. A year later, he discovered a second type of HPV, HPV 18, in similar cervical tumors. He became convinced that HPV was the causative agent in at least some types of cervical cancer. Zur Hausen's discovery was greeted with serious doubt by most cancer researchers since the predominant theory at the time was that a different type of virus, the one responsible for herpes simplex, was the causative agent in cervical cancer. Evidence for zur Hausen's hypothesis accumulated over the years, however, and there is now no doubt as to the role of HPV viruses in causing both cervical cancer and genital warts. In addition to his Nobel Prize, zur Hausen has received a number of other important awards, including the Robert Koch Prize, Charles S. Mott Prize, Paul-Ehrlich-und-Ludwig-Darmstaedter-Preis, Virchow Medal, San Marino Prize for Medicine, Great Cross of Merit of the Federal Republic of Germany, William B. Coley Award, and Gairdner Foundation International Award.

References

Bates, Anna. 1995. *Weeder in the Garden of the Lord: Anthony Comstock's Life and Career.* Lanham, MD: University Press of America.

Bates, Stephen. 1993. *Battleground: One Mother's Crusade, the Religious Right, and the Struggle for Control of Our Classrooms.* New York: Simon & Schuster Adult Publishing Group.

6

Data and Documents

Documents

Texas Sex Education Law (1995)

The U.S. Congress has adopted no legislation specifically requiring or recommending the content of sex education programs in U.S. schools. A number of states, however, have struggled with this issue and have considered and/or adopted such legislation. As to be expected, the stance taken in various states differs significantly. At one extreme, a law adopted by the 74th session of the Texas legislature in 1995 emphasized an almost exclusive "abstinence-only" approach to sex education in the state. In light of later studies that suggested that abstinence-only sex education was not particularly effective in reducing teen pregnancies and the spread of sexually transmitted infections, some Texas legislators have called for changing the 1995 act. As of 2009, however, that act remained on the books. Its essential features are contained in section 28.004, "Local School Health Advisory Council and Health Education Instruction," of the state education code. The relevant sections are as follows:

(e) Any course materials and instruction relating to human sexuality, sexually transmitted diseases, or human immunodeficiency virus or acquired immune deficiency syndrome shall be selected by the board of trustees with the advice of the local school health advisory council and must:

(1) present abstinence from sexual activity as the preferred choice of behavior in relationship to all sexual activity for unmarried persons of school age;

153

    (2)   devote more attention to abstinence from sexual activity than to any other behavior;

    (3)   emphasize that abstinence from sexual activity, if used consistently and correctly, is the only method that is 100 percent effective in preventing pregnancy, sexually transmitted diseases, infection with human immunodeficiency virus or acquired immune deficiency syndrome, and the emotional trauma associated with adolescent sexual activity;

    (4)   direct adolescents to a standard of behavior in which abstinence from sexual activity before marriage is the most effective way to prevent pregnancy, sexually transmitted diseases, and infection with human immunodeficiency virus or acquired immune deficiency syndrome; and

    (5)   teach contraception and condom use in terms of human use reality rates instead of theoretical laboratory rates, if instruction on contraception and condoms is included in curriculum content.

(f)   A school district may not distribute condoms in connection with instruction relating to human sexuality.

(g)   A school district that provides human sexuality instruction may separate students according to sex for instructional purposes.

(h)   The board of trustees shall determine the specific content of the district's instruction in human sexuality, in accordance with Subsections (e), (f), and (g).

(i)   A school district shall notify a parent of each student enrolled in the district of:

    (1)   the basic content of the district's human sexuality instruction to be provided to the student; and

    (2)   the parent's right to remove the student from any part of the district's human sexuality instruction.

(j)   A school district shall make all curriculum materials used in the district's human sexuality instruction available for reasonable public inspection.

Source: Education Code. Title 2. Public Education. Subtitle F. Curriculum, Programs, and Services. Chapter 28. Courses of Study; Advancement. Subchapter A. Essential Knowledge and Skills; Curriculum, 9–10. Available at http://www.statutes.legis.state.tx.us/ SOTWDocs/ED/pdf/ED.28.pdf.

Separate Program for Abstinence Education (1996)

On September 8, 1995, Senator Rick Santorum (R-PA) and Senator Lauch Faircloth (R-NC) introduced a provision to the welfare reform bill then being considered by the U.S. Congress to provide funding for sex education programs that taught about abstinence only, with no mention of any other form of contraception or family planning. That provision was included in the final version of the act that was passed by both houses of Congress and signed by President Bill Clinton on August 22, 1996. The program was later reauthorized a number of times, although opponents have constantly tried to demonstrate that it is not effective in the goals it attempts to achieve. The provisions of the original program are included below, now enshrined as section 710 of Title 42 of the U.S. Code.

§ 710. Separate program for abstinence education

    (a) *In general*

For the purpose described in subsection (b) of this section, the Secretary shall, for fiscal year 1998 and each subsequent fiscal year, allot to each State which has transmitted an application for the fiscal year under section 705 (a) of this title an amount equal to the product of—

        (1) the amount appropriated in subsection (d) of this section for the fiscal year; and

        (2) the percentage determined for the State under section 702 (c)(1)(B)(ii) of this title.

    (b) *Purpose of allotment*

        (1) The purpose of an allotment under subsection (a) of this section to a State is to enable the State to provide abstinence education, and at the option of the State, where appropriate, mentoring, counseling, and adult supervision to promote abstinence from sexual activity, with a focus on those groups which are most likely to bear children out-of-wedlock.

        (2) For purposes of this section, the term "abstinence education" means an educational or motivational program which—

            (A) has as its exclusive purpose, teaching the social, psychological, and health gains to be realized by abstaining from sexual activity;

            (B) teaches abstinence from sexual activity outside marriage as the expected standard for all school age children;

            (C) teaches that abstinence from sexual activity is the only certain way to avoid out-of-wedlock pregnancy, sexually transmitted diseases, and other associated health problems;

            (D) teaches that a mutually faithful monogamous relationship in context of marriage is the expected standard of human sexual activity;

(E) teaches that sexual activity outside of the context of marriage is likely to have harmful psychological and physical effects;

(F) teaches that bearing children out-of-wedlock is likely to have harmful consequences for the child, the child's parents, and society;

(G) teaches young people how to reject sexual advances and how alcohol and drug use increases vulnerability to sexual advances; and

(H) teaches the importance of attaining self-sufficiency before engaging in sexual activity.

(c) *Applicability of sections 703, 707, and 708*

(1) Sections 703, 707, and 708 of this title apply to allotments under subsection (a) of this section to the same extent and in the same manner as such sections apply to allotments under section 702 (c) of this title.

(2) Sections 705 and 706 of this title apply to allotments under subsection (a) of this section to the extent determined by the Secretary to be appropriate.

(d) *Appropriations*

For the purpose of allotments under subsection (a) of this section, there is appropriated, out of any money in the Treasury not otherwise appropriated, an additional $50,000,000 for each of the fiscal years 1998 through 2003. The appropriation under the preceding sentence for a fiscal year is made on October 1 of the fiscal year.

Source: U.S. Code. Title 42. Chapter 7. Subchapter V §710.

Memorandum for the Administrator of the United States Agency for International Development (2001)

At the United Nations International Conference on Population held in Mexico City in 1984, the administration of President Ronald Reagan announced a new policy for the funding of family planning programs around the world funded by the U.S. Agency for International Development (USAID). According to that policy, which became known as the Mexico City Policy, any nongovernmental organization receiving USAID funding was required to refrain from offering or promoting abortion services as part of its family planning program. That policy was later revoked by President Bill Clinton on January 22, 1993, and reinstated by President George W. Bush on January 22, 2001. It was revoked once more after the election of President Barack Obama on January 23,

2009 (see below). President Bush's memorandum reinstating the policy in 2001 is given here.

MEMORANDUM FOR THE ADMINISTRATOR OF THE UNITED STATES AGENCY FOR INTERNATIONAL DEVELOPMENT

SUBJECT: Restoration of the Mexico City Policy

The Mexico City Policy announced by President Reagan in 1984 required nongovernmental organizations to agree as a condition of their receipt of Federal funds that such organizations would neither perform nor actively promote abortion as a method of family planning in other nations. This policy was in effect until it was rescinded on January 22, 1993.

It is my conviction that taxpayer funds should not be used to pay for abortions or advocate or actively promote abortion, either here or abroad. It is therefore my belief that the Mexico City Policy should be restored. Accordingly, I hereby rescind the "Memorandum for the Acting Administrator for the Agency for International Development, Subject: AID Family Planning Grants/Mexico City Policy," dated January 22, 1993, and I direct the Administrator of the United States Agency for International Development to reinstate in full all of the requirements of the Mexico City Policy in effect on January 19, 1993.

George W. Bush

Source: USAID. "Memorandum From the White House to USAID." Available at http://www.usaid.gov/whmemo.html.

South Dakota House Bill 1215 (2006)

The U.S. Supreme Court decision in Roe v. Wade (1973) established a national standard for abortion law in the United States that has remained in force for more than three decades. A number of people disagree with that decision, however, and have continued to work for a reversal or reconsideration of the 1973 decision. One of the most forceful efforts in that direction was the passage of a bill in the South Dakota state legislature in 2006 which essentially banned abortions for any and all reasons. The bill was later rejected by a statewide vote in November 2006.

An Act

ENTITLED, An Act to establish certain legislative findings, to reinstate the prohibition against certain acts causing the termination of an unborn human life, to prescribe a penalty therefor, and to provide for the implementation of such provisions under certain circumstances.

Be IT Enacted By The Legislature of The State of South Dakota:

Section 1. The Legislature accepts and concurs with the conclusion of the South Dakota Task Force to Study Abortion, based upon written materials, scientific studies, and testimony of witnesses presented to the task force, that life begins at the time of conception, a conclusion confirmed by scientific advances since the 1973 decision of Roe v. Wade, including the fact that each human being is totally unique immediately at fertilization. Moreover, the Legislature finds, based upon the conclusions of the South Dakota Task Force to Study Abortion, and in recognition of the technological advances and medical experience and body of knowledge about abortions produced and made available since the 1973 decision of Roe v. Wade, that to fully protect the rights, interests, and health of the pregnant mother, the rights, interest, and life of her unborn child, and the mother's fundamental natural intrinsic right to a relationship with her child, abortions in South Dakota should be prohibited. Moreover, the Legislature finds that the guarantee of due process of law under the Constitution of South Dakota applies equally to born and unborn human beings, and that under the Constitution of South Dakota, a pregnant mother and her unborn child, each possess a natural and inalienable right to life.

Section 2. That chapter 22-17 be amended by adding thereto a NEW SECTION to read as follows:

No person may knowingly administer to, prescribe for, or procure for, or sell to any pregnant woman any medicine, drug, or other substance with the specific intent of causing or abetting the termination of the life of an unborn human being. No person may knowingly use or employ any instrument or procedure upon a pregnant woman with the specific intent of causing or abetting the termination of the life of an unborn human being.

Any violation of this section is a Class 5 felony.

Section 3. That chapter 22-17 be amended by adding thereto a NEW SECTION to read as follows:

Nothing in section 2 of this Act may be construed to prohibit the sale, use, prescription, or administration of a contraceptive measure, drug or chemical, if it is administered prior to the time when a pregnancy could be determined through conventional medical testing and if the contraceptive measure is sold, used, prescribed, or administered in accordance with manufacturer instructions.

Section 4. That chapter 22-17 be amended by adding thereto a NEW SECTION to read as follows:

No licensed physician who performs a medical procedure designed or intended to prevent the death of a pregnant mother is guilty of violating section 2 of this Act. However, the physician shall make reasonable medical efforts under the circumstances to preserve both the life of the mother and the life of her unborn child in a manner consistent with conventional medical practice.

Medical treatment provided to the mother by a licensed physician which results in the accidental or unintentional injury or death to the unborn child is not a violation of this statute.

Nothing in this Act may be construed to subject the pregnant mother upon whom any abortion is performed or attempted to any criminal conviction and penalty.

[*The remaining sections of this act deal with definitions and "house-keeping" issues in its implementation.*]

Source: South Dakota Legislature HB 1215. Available at http://legis. state.sd.us/sessions/2006/bills/HB1215enr.htm.

Responsible Education About Life Act (2007)

In recent years, a number of states have considered or adopted legislation that would provide required sex education courses with specific features (see "Texas Sex Education Law" above). The federal government has, however, refrained from adopting specific legislation dealing with the existence or content of sex education classes. Some efforts have been made to change that situation, however. In 2007, for example, Senator Frank Lautenberg (D-NJ) introduced legislation outlining a recommended approach to sex education in American schools. His bill, S. 972, was called the Responsible Education About Life (REAL) Act. The bill was never acted on in committee, as has been the fate for all previous federal legislation in this area. It does outline, however, one philosophy about the type of sex education that might be encouraged in U.S. schools. Footnotes and citations have been omitted from this excerpt.

A Bill

To provide for the reduction of adolescent pregnancy, HIV rates, and other sexually transmitted diseases, and for other purposes.

    Be it enacted by the Senate and House of Representatives of the United States of America in Congress assembled,

Section 1. Short Title.

This Act may be cited as the 'Responsible Education About Life Act.'

Sec. 2. Findings.

[*This section has 15 sub-sections that review research findings and recommendations from professional groups about the status of sexual issues among adolescents in the United States.*]

Sec. 3. Assistance to Reduce Teen Pregnancy, HIV/Aids, and other Sexually Transmitted Diseases and to Support Healthy Adolescent Development.

    (a) In General- Each eligible State shall be entitled to receive from the Secretary of Health and Human Services, for each of the fiscal years 2008 through 2012, a grant to conduct programs of family life education, including education on both abstinence and contraception for the prevention of teenage pregnancy and sexually transmitted diseases, including HIV/AIDS.

(b) Requirements for Family Life Programs- For purposes of this Act, a program of family life education is a program that—

(1) is age-appropriate and medically accurate;

(2) does not teach or promote religion;

(3) teaches that abstinence is the only sure way to avoid pregnancy or sexually transmitted diseases;

(4) stresses the value of abstinence while not ignoring those young people who have had or are having sexual intercourse;

(5) provides information about the health benefits and side effects of all contraceptives and barrier methods as a means to prevent pregnancy;

(6) provides information about the health benefits and side effects of all contraceptives and barrier methods as a means to reduce the risk of contracting sexually transmitted diseases, including HIV/AIDS;

(7) encourages family communication about sexuality between parent and child;

(8) teaches young people the skills to make responsible decisions about sexuality, including how to avoid unwanted verbal, physical, and sexual advances and how not to make unwanted verbal, physical, and sexual advances; and

(9) teaches young people how alcohol and drug use can effect [*sic*] responsible decisionmaking.

(c) Additional Activities- In carrying out a program of family life education, a State may expend a grant under subsection (a) to carry out educational and motivational activities that help young people—

(1) gain knowledge about the physical, emotional, biological, and hormonal changes of adolescence and subsequent stages of human maturation;

(2) develop the knowledge and skills necessary to ensure and protect their sexual and reproductive health from unintended pregnancy and sexually transmitted disease, including HIV/AIDS throughout their lifespan;

(3) gain knowledge about the specific involvement of and male responsibility in sexual decisionmaking;

(4) develop healthy attitudes and values about adolescent growth and development, body image, gender roles, racial and ethnic diversity, sexual orientation, and other subjects;

(5) develop and practice healthy life skills including goal-setting, decisionmaking, negotiation, communication, and stress management;

(6) promote self-esteem and positive interpersonal skills focusing on relationship dynamics, including, but not limited to, friendships, dating, romantic involvement, marriage and family interactions; and

(7) prepare for the adult world by focusing on educational and career success, including developing skills for employment preparation, job seeking, independent living, financial self-sufficiency, and workplace productivity.

Sec. 4. Sense of Congress.
It is the sense of Congress that while States are not required to provide matching funds, they are encouraged to do so.

Sec. 5. Evaluation of Programs.
[*This section requires that an evaluation of all sex education programs receiving federal funding be evaluated on both a national and state level. The criteria to be evaluated at both levels are as follows:*]

(A) the effectiveness of such programs in helping to delay the initiation of sexual intercourse and other high-risk behaviors;

(B) the effectiveness of such programs in preventing adolescent pregnancy;

(C) the effectiveness of such programs in preventing sexually transmitted disease, including HIV/AIDS;

(D) the effectiveness of such programs in increasing contraceptive knowledge and contraceptive behaviors when sexual intercourse occurs; and

(E) a list of best practices based upon essential programmatic components of evaluated programs that have led to success in subparagraphs (A) through (D).

Sec. 6. Definitions.
[*This section defines a number of terms used in the bill.*]

Sec. 7. Appropriations.
[*This section outlines the funding provisions for carrying out this act.*]

Source: "S 972 IS." [Senate bill 972] Available at http://thomas.loc.gov/cgi-bin/query/z?c110:s972:

Mandatory HPV Vaccination (2007)

In June 2006, the Advisory Committee on Immunization Practices of the Centers for Disease Control and Prevention recommended that all girls between the ages of 11 and 12 be vaccinated for the human papillomavirus (HPV), which causes virtually all cases of genital warts and cervical cancer. In response to that recommendation more than 40 states have considered some form of legislation to meet this recommendation, usually to provide funding or education about the vaccine, but in some cases, requiring vaccination for HPV as a condition for attending school. As of 2009, only one state actually adopted a requirement provision, Texas, where Governor Rick Perry issued executive order RP 65 on February 2, 2007, requiring HPV vaccination for admission to the sixth grade. Perry's executive order was overturned by action of the state legislature, but his executive order still outlines the kind of provision that other states have considered in the past and, in some cases, are still considering.

By The Governor of The State of Texas

Executive Department
Austin, Texas
February 2, 2007
WHEREAS, immunization from vaccine-preventable diseases such as Human Papillomavirus (HPV) protects individuals who receive the vaccine; and
WHEREAS, HPV is the most common sexually transmitted infection-causing cancer in females in the United States; and
WHEREAS, the United States Food and Drug Administration estimates there are 9,710 new cases of cervical cancer, many of which are caused by HPV, and 3,700 deaths from cervical cancer each year in the United States; and
WHEREAS, the Texas Cancer Registry estimates there were 1,169 new cases and 391 deaths from cervical cancer in Texas in 2006; and
WHEREAS, research has shown that the HPV vaccine is highly effective in preventing the infections that are the cause of many of the cervical cancers; and
WHEREAS, HPV vaccine is only effective if administered before infection occurs; and
WHEREAS, the newly approved HPV vaccine is a great advance in the protection of women's health; and
WHEREAS, the Advisory Committee on Immunization Practices and Centers for Disease Control and Prevention recommend the HPV vaccine for females who are nine years through 26 years of age;
NOW THEREFORE, I, RICK PERRY, Governor of Texas, by virtue of the power and authority vested in me by the Constitution and laws of the State of Texas as the Chief Executive Officer, do hereby order the following:

Vaccine. The Department of State Health Services shall make the HPV vaccine available through the Texas Vaccines for Children program for eligible young females up to age 18, and the Health and Human Services Commission shall make the vaccine available to Medicaid-eligible young females from age 19 to 21.

Rules. The Health and Human Services Executive Commissioner shall adopt rules that mandate the age appropriate vaccination of all female children for HPV prior to admission to the sixth grade.

Availability. The Department of State Health Services and the Health and Human Services Commission will move expeditiously to make the vaccine available as soon as possible.

Public Information. The Department of State Health Services will implement a public awareness campaign to educate the public of the importance of vaccination, the availability of the vaccine, and the subsequent requirements under the rules that will be adopted.

Parents' Rights. The Department of State Health Services will, in order to protect the right of parents to be the final authority on their children's health care, modify the current process in order to allow parents to submit a request for a conscientious objection affidavit form via the Internet while maintaining privacy safeguards under current law.

This executive order supersedes all previous orders on this matter that are in conflict or inconsistent with its terms and this order shall remain in effect and in full force until modified, amended, rescinded, or superseded by me or by a succeeding governor.

Given under my hand this the 2nd day of February, 2007.
RICK PERRY(Signature)
Governor

Source: Office of the Governor Rick Perry. "RP65—Relating to the Immunization of Young Women from the Cancer-causing Human Papillomavirus." Available at http://governor.state.tx.us/news/executive-order/3455.

Access to Birth Control Act (2007)

In the first decade of the 21st century, a new trend developed among some pharmacists in the United States who defined themselves as "pro-life pharmacists" who operated "pro-life pharmacies." These pharmacists decided that their moral conscience did not allow them to fill prescriptions for birth control and emergency contraceptives, such as the so-called morning-after pill. In many cases, these pharmacists also declined to refer their customers to other establishments where the prescriptions could be filled. In response to this trend, a number of states considered legislation making such actions illegal, requiring that all licensed pharmacists fill legitimately written prescriptions. In 2007, Representative Carolyn B. Maloney (D-NY) filed legislation in the U.S. House of Representatives making the practice of refusing to fill a prescription a federal crime. The earliest version of that bill is as follows. (Line numbering in the bill has been omitted.)

A Bill

To establish certain duties for pharmacies to ensure provision of Food and Drug Administration-approved contraception, and for other purposes.

Be it enacted by the Senate and House of Representatives of the United States of America in Congress assembled,

Section 1. Short Title.

This Act may be cited as the "Access to Birth Control Act".

Sec. 2. Findings.

The Congress finds as follows:

(1) Family planning is basic health care for women. Access to contraception helps women prevent unintended pregnancy and control the timing and spacing of planned births.

(2) Although the Centers for Disease Control and Prevention included family planning in its published list of the Ten Great Public Health Achievements in the 20th Century, the United States still has one of the highest rates of unintended pregnancies among industrialized nations.

(3) Each year, 3,000,000 pregnancies, nearly half of all pregnancies, in the United States are unintended, and nearly half of unintended pregnancies end in abortion.

(4) Women rely on prescription contraceptives for a range of medical purposes in addition to birth control, such as regulation of cycles and endometriosis.

(5) The Food and Drug Administration has declared emergency contraception to be safe and effective in preventing unintended pregnancy and has approved over-the-counter access to the emergency contraceptive Plan B for adults.

(6) If taken soon after unprotected sex or primary contraceptive failure, emergency contraception can significantly reduce a woman's chance of unintended pregnancy and, therefore, the need for abortion.

(7) Emergency contraception works like other hormonal birth control. It does not harm or terminate an already-established pregnancy.

(8) Access to legal contraception is a protected fundamental right in the United States and should not be impeded by an individual's personal beliefs.

(9) Reports of pharmacists refusing to fill prescriptions for contraceptives, including emergency contraceptives, have surfaced in States across the Nation, including Arizona, California, Georgia, Illinois, Louisiana, Massachusetts, Minnesota, Missouri, New Hampshire, New York, North Carolina, Ohio, Oregon, Rhode Island, Tennessee, Texas, Washington, West Virginia, and Wisconsin. Since emergency contraception has become available without a prescription for individuals 18 and over, reports of refusals to provide non-prescription emergency contraception have also been reported.

Sec. 3. Duties of Pharmacies to Ensure Provision of FDA-approved Contraception.

Part B of title II of the Public Health Service Act (42 U.S.C. 238 et seq.) is amended by adding at the end the following:

"Sec. 249. Duties of Pharmacies to Ensure Provision of FDA-approved Contraception.

"(a) IN GENERAL.—Subject to subsection (b), a pharmacy that receives Food and Drug Administration approved drugs or devices in interstate commerce shall maintain compliance with the following:

"(1) If a customer requests a contraceptive that is in stock, the pharmacy shall ensure that the contraceptive is provided to the customer without delay.

"(2) If a customer requests a contraceptive that is not in stock and the pharmacy in the normal course of business stocks contraception, the pharmacy shall immediately inform the customer that the contraceptive is not in stock and without delay offer the customer the following options:

"(A) If the customer prefers to obtain the contraceptive through a referral or transfer, the pharmacy shall—

"(i) locate a pharmacy of the customer's choice or the closest pharmacy confirmed to have the contraceptive in stock; and

"(ii) refer the customer or transfer the prescription to that pharmacy.

"(B) If the customer prefers for the pharmacy to order the contraceptive, the pharmacy shall obtain the contraceptive under the pharmacy's standard procedure for expedited ordering of medication and notify the customer when the contraceptive arrives.

"(3) The pharmacy shall ensure that its employees do not—

"(A) intimidate, threaten, or harass customers in the delivery of services relating to a request for contraception;

"(B) interfere with or obstruct the delivery of services relating to a request for contraception;

"(C) intentionally misrepresent or deceive customers about the availability of contraception or its mechanism of action;

"(D) breach medical confidentiality with respect to a request for contraception or threaten to breach such confidentiality; or

"(E) refuse to return a valid, lawful prescription for contraception upon customer request.

"(b) REFUSALS PURSUANT TO STANDARD PHARMACY PRACTICE.—This section does not prohibit a pharmacy from refusing to provide a contraceptive to a customer in accordance with any of the following:

"(1) If it is unlawful to dispense the contraceptive to the customer without a valid, lawful prescription and no such prescription is presented.

"(2) If the customer is unable to pay for the contraceptive.

"(3) If the employee of the pharmacy refuses to provide the contraceptive on the basis of a professional clinical judgment.

"(c) RULE OF CONSTRUCTION.—Nothing in this section shall be construed to alter any standard under title 18 VII of the Civil Rights Act of 1964.

"(d) PREEMPTION.—This section does not preempt any provision of State law or any professional obligation made applicable by a State board or other entity responsible for licensing or discipline of pharmacies or pharmacists, to the extent that such State law or professional obligation provides protections for customers that are greater than the protections provided by this section.

[*The final two sections of the act deal with enforcement provisions and definitions of terms used in the bill."*]

Source: U.S. House of Representatives. Available at http://maloney. house.gov/documents/reproductivechoice/alpha/041707ABCbill.pdf

Mexico City Policy (2009)

*The so-called Mexico City Policy has determined U.S. policy about
abortion in family planning programs around the world since 1984.
See "Memorandum for the Administrator of the United States
Agency for International Development (2001)" above for details of
that history. The Mexico City Policy has, during its lifetime, been
invoked or not depending on the political party to which the president belongs at the time. In 2009, with the election of Democrat
Barack Obama to the White House, the policy was once again revoked. Obama's reasoning in making this decision is outlined in the
memorandum below.*

MEMORANDUM FOR THE SECRETARY OF STATE;

THE ADMINISTRATOR OF THE UNITED STATES AGENCY FOR
INTERNATIONAL DEVELOPMENT

SUBJECT: Mexico City Policy and Assistance for Voluntary Population Planning

The Foreign Assistance Act of 1961 (22 U.S.C. 2151b(f)(1)), prohibits
nongovernmental organizations (NGOs) that receive Federal funds from
using those funds "to pay for the performance of abortions as a method
of family planning, or to motivate or coerce any person to practice abortions." The August 1984 announcement by President Reagan of what
has become known as the "Mexico City Policy" directed the United
States Agency for International Development (USAID) to expand this
limitation and withhold USAID funds from NGOs that use non-USAID
funds to engage in a wide range of activities, including providing
advice, counseling, or information regarding abortion, or lobbying a
foreign government to legalize or make abortion available. The Mexico
City Policy was in effect from 1985 until 1993, when it was rescinded
by President Clinton. President George W. Bush reinstated the policy in
2001, implementing it through conditions in USAID grant awards, and
subsequently extended the policy to "voluntary population planning"
assistance provided by the Department of State.

These excessively broad conditions on grants and assistance awards
are unwarranted. Moreover, they have undermined efforts to promote
safe and effective voluntary family planning programs in foreign nations. Accordingly, I hereby revoke the Presidential memorandum of
January 22, 2001, for the Administrator of USAID (Restoration of the
Mexico City Policy), the Presidential memorandum of March 28, 2001,
for the Administrator of USAID (Restoration of the Mexico City Policy),
and the Presidential memorandum of August 29, 2003, for the Secretary
of State (Assistance for Voluntary Population Planning). In addition, I
direct the Secretary of State and the Administrator of USAID to take the
following actions with respect to conditions in voluntary population

planning assistance and USAID grants that were imposed pursuant to either the 2001 or 2003 memoranda and that are not required by the Foreign Assistance Act or any other law: (1) immediately waive such conditions in any current grants, and (2) notify current grantees, as soon as possible, that these conditions have been waived. I further direct that the Department of State and USAID immediately cease imposing these conditions in any future grants.

This memorandum is not intended to, and does not, create any right or benefit, substantive or procedural, enforceable at law or in equity by any party against the United States, its departments, agencies, or entities, its officers, employees, or agents, or any other person.

The Secretary of State is authorized and directed to publish this memorandum in the Federal Register.

BARACK OBAMA

THE WHITE HOUSE, January 23, 2009.

Source: The White House. "Memorandum." Available at http://www.whitehouse.gov/the_press_office/MexicoCityPolicy-VoluntaryPopulationPlanning/.

Court Cases

Griswold v. Connecticut (1965)

Most people in the United States probably take the availability of contraceptive materials and techniques for granted today, whether they approve and/or use them or not. Yet, as recently as the mid-1960s, contraceptive use was illegal in the United States. That situation changed in 1965 when the U.S. Supreme Court issued its ruling in the case of Griswold v. Connecticut. The excerpt below briefly reviews the background of the case, the court's decision, and the rationale behind that decision. Although Griswold v. Connecticut applied only to married couples, the court expanded its decision to include nonmarried individuals in Eisenstadt v. Baird in 1972.

Appellant Griswold is Executive Director of the Planned Parenthood League of Connecticut. Appellant Buxton is a licensed physician and a professor at the Yale Medical School who served as Medical Director for the League at its Center in New Haven—a center open and operating from November 1 to November 10, 1961, when appellants were arrested.

They gave information, instruction, and medical advice to married persons as to the means of preventing conception. They examined the wife and prescribed the best contraceptive device or material for her use. Fees were usually charged, although some couples were serviced free.

The statutes whose constitutionality is involved in this appeal are §§ 53-32 and 54-196 of the General Statutes of Connecticut (1958 rev.). The former provides:

"Any person who uses any drug, medicinal article or instrument for the purpose of preventing conception shall be fined not less than fifty dollars or imprisoned not less than sixty days nor more than one year or be both fined and imprisoned."

Section 54-196 provides:

"Any person who assists, abets, counsels, causes, hires or commands another to commit any offense may be prosecuted and punished as if he were the principal offender."

The appellants were found guilty as accessories and fined $100 each, against the claim that the accessory statute, as so applied, violated the Fourteenth Amendment. The Appellate Division of the Circuit Court affirmed. The Supreme Court of Errors affirmed that judgment. 151 Conn. 544, 200 A.2d 479. We noted probable jurisdiction. 379 U.S. 926.

[*The court then considers portions of the Bill of Rights which would appear to guarantee a "right of privacy" and conclude that that "right of privacy" is violated by the Connecticut law. Certain footnotes and references are omitted (as indicated by ellipses) from the following excerpt.*]

The foregoing cases suggest that specific guarantees in the Bill of Rights have penumbras, formed by emanations from those guarantees that help give them life and substance. . . . Various guarantees create zones of privacy. The right of association contained in the penumbra of the First Amendment is one, as we have seen. The Third Amendment, in its prohibition against the quartering of soldiers "in any house" in time of peace without the consent of the owner, is another facet of that privacy. The Fourth Amendment explicitly affirms the "right of the people to be secure in their persons, houses, papers, and effects, against unreasonable searches and seizures." The Fifth Amendment, in its Self-Incrimination Clause, enables the citizen to create a zone of privacy which government may not force him to surrender to his detriment. The Ninth Amendment provides: "The enumeration in the Constitution, of certain rights, shall not be construed to deny or disparage others retained by the people."

The Fourth and Fifth Amendments were described in Boyd v. United States, . . . as protection against all governmental invasions "of the sanctity of a man's home and the privacies of life." . . . to the Fourth Amendment as creating a "right to privacy, no less important than any other right carefully an particularly reserved to the people." . . .

We have had many controversies over these penumbral rights of "privacy and repose." . . . These cases bear witness that the right of privacy which presses for recognition here is a legitimate one.

The present case, then, concerns a relationship lying within the zone of privacy created by several fundamental constitutional guarantees. And it concerns a law which, in forbidding the use of contraceptives, rather than regulating their manufacture or sale, seeks to achieve its goals by means having a maximum destructive impact upon that relationship. Such a law cannot stand in light of the familiar principle, so often applied by this Court, that a "governmental purpose to control or prevent activities constitutionally subject to state regulation may not be achieved by means which sweep unnecessarily broadly and thereby invade the area of protected freedoms."

... Would we allow the police to search the sacred precincts of marital bedrooms for telltale signs of the use of contraceptives? The very idea is repulsive to the notions of privacy surrounding the marriage relationship.

We deal with a right of privacy older than the Bill of Rights—older than our political parties, older than our school system. Marriage is a coming together for better or for worse, hopefully enduring, and intimate to the degree of being sacred. It is an association that promotes a way of life, not causes; a harmony in living, not political faiths; a bilateral loyalty, not commercial or social projects. Yet it is an association for as noble a purpose as any involved in our prior decisions.

Reversed.

Source: Griswold v. Connecticut, 381 U.S. 479 (1965), 480, 484, 486. Available at http://supreme.justia.com/us/381/479/case.html

Roe v. Wade (1973)

One of the most important judicial cases in the last century was argued before the U.S. Supreme Court on December 13, 1971, and again on October 11, 1972. The question at hand was whether a Texas law criminalizing abortion except when a woman's life was at risk was constitutional or not. In announcing its decision on January 22, 1973, the Supreme Court established a national standard for abortion that remains today. The excerpt below from the Court's very long decision provides the essence of the Court's position on the issue.

In view of all this, we do not agree that, by adopting one theory of life, Texas may override the rights of the pregnant woman that are at stake. We repeat, however, that the State does have an important and legitimate interest in preserving and protecting the health of the pregnant woman, whether she be a resident of the State or a nonresident who seeks medical consultation and treatment there, and that it has still another important and legitimate interest in protecting the potentiality of human life. These interests are separate and distinct. Each grows in substantiality as the woman approaches term and, at a point during pregnancy, each becomes "compelling."

With respect to the State's important and legitimate interest in the health of the mother, the "compelling" point, in the light of present medical knowledge, is at approximately the end of the first trimester. This is so because of the now-established medical fact, referred to above at 410 U.S. 149, that, until the end of the first trimester mortality in abortion may be less than mortality in normal childbirth. It follows that, from and after this point, a State may regulate the abortion procedure to the extent that the regulation reasonably relates to the preservation and protection of maternal health. Examples of permissible state regulation in this area are requirements as to the qualifications of the person who is to perform the abortion; as to the licensure of that person; as to the facility in which the procedure is to be performed, that is, whether it must be a hospital or may be a clinic or some other place of less-than-hospital status; as to the licensing of the facility; and the like.

This means, on the other hand, that, for the period of pregnancy prior to this "compelling" point, the attending physician, in consultation with his patient, is free to determine, without regulation by the State, that, in his medical judgment, the patient's pregnancy should be terminated. If that decision is reached, the judgment may be effectuated by an abortion free of interference by the State.

[*The Court summarizes its guidelines for legal abortions twice in its decision, as follows:*]

To summarize and to repeat:
1. A state criminal abortion statute of the current Texas type, that excepts from criminality only a lifesaving procedure on behalf of the mother, without regard to pregnancy stage and without recognition of the other interests involved, is violative of the Due Process Clause of the Fourteenth Amendment.
    (a) For the stage prior to approximately the end of the first trimester, the abortion decision and its effectuation must be left to the medical judgment of the pregnant woman's attending physician.
    (b) For the stage subsequent to approximately the end of the first trimester, the State, in promoting its interest in the health of the mother, may, if it chooses, regulate the abortion procedure in ways that are reasonably related to maternal health.
    (c) For the stage subsequent to viability, the State in promoting its interest in the potentiality of human life may, if it chooses, regulate, and even proscribe, abortion except where it is necessary, in appropriate medical judgment, for the preservation of the life or health of the mother.

Source: U.S. Supreme Court. *Roe v. Wade*, 410 U.S. 113 (1973), 162–65. Available at http://supreme.justia.com/us/410/113/case.html#163.

Curtis v. School Committee of Falmouth (1995)

Many schools in the United States (and other countries) have instituted condom distribution programs for the purposes of reducing teen pregnancies and helping to prevent sexually transmitted infections. Parents sometimes object to such programs on a number of grounds, and schools may respond to these objections by providing for "opt-out" provisions in which parents are notified if their children express a wish to participate in them. A number of court cases have been filed over condom distribution programs, with mixed results. The case below is an example of these cases. The case cited was heard by the Massachusetts Supreme Court in March 1995 on an appeal from a lower court. Citations are omitted from the following excerpt.

[Falmouth High School offered a condom distribution program in which students could receive condoms at no cost from the school nurse, or they could purchase condoms from a vending machine for 75 cents each. Counseling and information materials were also available to all students who requested either or both. A group of 10 parents sued the Falmouth School Committee claiming that the condom distribution program was an unconstitutional intrusion on the right to raise their children as they saw fit. The court responded to each of the plaintiffs' arguments as follows:]

The plaintiffs argue that the condom-availability program violates their substantive due process rights, protected by the Fourteenth Amendment, to direct and control the education and the upbringing of their children. In the same vein, they argue that the program invades the constitutionally protected "zone of privacy" which surrounds the family. Further, they claim the program intrudes on these rights because it allows their minor children unrestricted access to contraceptives without parental input and within the compulsory setting of the public schools. They claim that in these circumstances parents have the right to intervene and prohibit their children from obtaining the condoms (by an opt-out provision in the program), and that they have a right to parental notification if their child requests and obtains a condom.

. . .

We discern no coercive burden on the plaintiffs' parental liberties in this case. No classroom participation is required of students. Condoms are available to students who request them and, in the high school, may be obtained from vending machines. The students are not required to seek out and accept the condoms, read the literature accompanying them, or participate in counseling regarding their use. In other words, the students are free to decline to participate in the program. No penalty or disciplinary action ensues if a student does not participate in the program. For their part, the plaintiff parents are free to instruct their children not to participate. The program does not supplant the parents' role as advisor in the moral and religious development of their children. Although exposure to condom vending machines and to the program itself may offend the moral and religious sensibilities of the plaintiffs, mere exposure to programs offered at school does not amount to unconstitutional interference with parental liberties without the existence of some compulsory aspect to the program.

. . .

The plaintiffs argue that the condom-availability program is coercive because, although participation is voluntary, the program has been implemented in the compulsory setting of the public schools.

. . .

Because we conclude the program lacks any degree of coercion or compulsion in violation of the plaintiffs' parental liberties, or their familial privacy, we conclude also that neither an opt-out provision nor parental notification is required by the Federal Constitution.

. . .

Next, the plaintiffs argue that the condom-availability program violates their Federal constitutional rights to the free exercise of religion. Religious freedom is guaranteed by the free exercise clause of the First Amendment, which provides that "Congress shall make no law respecting an establishment of religion, or prohibiting the free exercise thereof. . . ."

. . .

The preliminary inquiry in a free exercise analysis is whether the challenged governmental action creates a burden on the exercise of a plaintiff's religion. . . . Only if a burden is established must the analysis move to the next step: a consideration of the nature of the burden, the significance of the governmental interest at stake, and the degree to which that interest would be impaired by an accommodation of the religious practice. . . . The degree of interference with free exercise necessary to trigger further analysis of the State's justification for the action in question, must at least rise to the level of a "substantial burden." The Supreme Court has indicated that, just as in the context of a parental liberties claim, a "substantial burden" is one that is coercive or compulsory in nature. . . . The free exercise clause "categorically prohibits government from regulating, prohibiting, or rewarding religious beliefs as such," either directly or indirectly. . . . In our view the plaintiffs are unable to demonstrate sufficient facts to support their argument that the condom policy substantially burdens their rights to freely exercise their religion to any degree approaching constitutional dimensions.

. . .

The plaintiffs argue that the condom-availability program burdens their right freely to exercise their religion by creating a conflict between the religious teaching of parents as to the issue of premarital sexual intercourse, and the view, allegedly endorsed by the school committee, that sexual activity before marriage is not only permissible but also can be made safe. The plaintiffs contend further, as noted in the previous section, that the program is coercive in nature, because it exists in the public schools, to which parents are compelled to send their children, and because it lacks an opt-out provision by which parents could choose to prohibit their children from obtaining condoms at school. The plaintiffs also argue that peer pressure may add to the coercive effect of the program.

    . . .

We conclude that the program in issue which does not violate the plaintiffs' parental liberties or privacy rights also does not violate their rights freely to exercise their religion. There is no requirement that any student participate in the program. The plaintiffs argument that the well-known existence of peer pressure in secondary schools adds to the alleged burden on their free exercise rights simply does not rise to the level of constitutional infringement. . . . The condom-availability program in Falmouth does not penalize students or parents for their religious beliefs or condition the receipt of benefits on a certain belief. Although the program may offend the religious sensibilities of the plaintiffs, mere exposure at public schools to offensive programs does not amount to a violation of free exercise. Parents have no right to tailor public school programs to meet their individual religious or moral preferences.

Source: Elizabeth G. Curtis & others vs. School Committee of Falmouth & Others. 420 Mass. 749. Available at http://masscases.com/cases/ sjc/420/420mass749.html#foot1.

Parker v. Hurley, 474 F. Supp. 2d 261 (2007)

School districts in the United States take a very wide range of positions on the teaching of human sexuality. Some districts are relatively open on the subject, willing to offer instruction in the use of condoms, the validity of homosexual feelings and acts, the importance of instruction about sexually transmitted infections, and related issues. Other districts prefer to limit sex instruction to lessons on abstinence and fidelity and, in some cases, to exclude sex education from classrooms. No matter the choice a school district may make, individual parents may disagree with the implementation of any specific policy. Conservative parents may object to lessons about same-sex marriages, and liberal parents may disagree with a decision to teach about abstinence exclusively in lessons on sexually transmitted infections. Courts at all levels have been asked to arbitrate about these differences of opinion. The case cited below is just one example. In this case, two sets of parents in Lexington, Massachusetts, objected to having their first-grade children (Jacob, Joshua, and Joseph ["Joey"]) exposed to books that discuss same-sex relationships.

They argued that they should have been notified about the use of these materials by school authorities so that they could have withdrawn the children from instruction they found "religiously repugnant" (as cited in the case). When their case was dismissed by the U.S. District Court, the parents appealed to the U.S. Court of Appeals for the First Circuit. On January 31, 2008, that court affirmed the lower court's decision. The decision in this case involves some abstruse legal reasoning, and only the court's final reasoning is cited here. Citations are omitted from this excerpt, as indicated by ellipses.

In the present case, the plaintiffs claim that the exposure of their children, at these young ages and in this setting, to ways of life contrary to the parents' religious beliefs violates their ability to direct the religious upbringing of their children. We try to identify the categories of harms alleged. The parents do not allege coercion in the form of a direct interference with their religious beliefs, nor of compulsion in the form of punishment for their beliefs, as in *Yoder*. [*Yoder is a case concerning a state requirement that Amish children attend public schools.*] Nor do they allege the denial of benefits. Further, plaintiffs do not allege that the mere listening to a book being read violated any religious duty on the part of the child. There is no claim that as a condition of attendance at the public schools, the defendants have forced plaintiffs—either the parents or the children—to violate their religious beliefs. In sum there is no claim of direct coercion.

The heart of the plaintiffs' free exercise claim is a claim of "indoctrination": that the state has put pressure on their children to endorse an affirmative view of gay marriage and has thus undercut the parents' efforts to inculcate their children with their own opposing religious views. The Supreme Court, we believe, has never utilized an indoctrination test under the Free Exercise Clause, much less in the public school context. The closest it has come is *Barnette,* a free speech case that implicated free exercise interests and which *Smith* included in its hybrid case discussion. [*Smith was a case in which two Native Americans claimed that they had a right to ingest peyotte, an illegal drug, because it was part of their religious tradition.*] In *Barnette,* the Court held that the state could not coerce acquiescence through compelled statements of belief, such as the mandatory recital of the pledge of allegiance in public schools. . . . It did not hold that the state could not attempt to inculcate values by instruction, and in fact carefully distinguished the two approaches. . . . We do not address whether or not an indoctrination theory under the Free Exercise Clause is sound. Plaintiffs' pleadings do not establish a viable case of indoctrination, even assuming that extreme indoctrination can be a form of coercion.

First, as to the parents' free exercise rights, the mere fact that a child is exposed on occasion in public school to a concept offensive to a parent's religious belief does not inhibit the parent from instructing the child differently. A parent whose "child is exposed to sensitive topics or information [at school] remains free to discuss these matters and to place them in the family's moral or religious context, or to supplement the information with more appropriate materials." . . . (noting that the school's requirement that Newdow's daughter recite the pledge of allegiance every day did not "impair[] Newdow's right to instruct his daughter in his religious views"). The parents here did in fact have notice, if not prior notice, of the books and of the school's overall intent to promote toleration of same-sex marriage, and they retained their ability to discuss the material and subject matter with their children. Our outcome does not turn, however, on whether the parents had notice.

Turning to the children's free exercise rights, we cannot see how Jacob's free exercise right was burdened at all: two books were made available to him, but he was never required to read them or have them read to him. Further, these books do not endorse gay marriage or homosexuality, or even address these topics explicitly, but merely describe how other children might come from families that look different from one's own. There is no free exercise right to be free from any reference in public elementary schools to the existence of families in which the parents are of different gender combinations.

Joey has a more significant claim, both because he was required to sit through a classroom reading of *King and King* and because that book affirmatively endorses homosexuality and gay marriage. It is a fair inference that the reading of *King and King* was precisely *intended* to influence the listening children toward tolerance of gay marriage. That was the point of why that book was chosen and used. Even assuming there is a continuum along which an intent to influence could become an attempt to indoctrinate, however, this case is firmly on the influence-toward-tolerance end. There is no evidence of systemic indoctrination. There is no allegation that Joey was asked to affirm gay marriage. Requiring a student to read a particular book is generally not coercive of free exercise rights.

Public schools are not obliged to shield individual students from ideas which potentially are religiously offensive, particularly when the school imposes no requirement that the student agree with or affirm those ideas, or even participate in discussions about them. . . . ("[P]ublic schools are not required to delete from the curriculum all materials that may offend any religious sensibility.") The reading of *King and King* was not instruction in religion or religious beliefs. . . . (distinguishing between compelling students to declare a belief through mandatory recital of the pledge of allegiance, which violates free exercise, and "merely . . . acquaint[ing students] with the flag salute so that they may be informed as to what it is or even what it means").

On the facts, there is no viable claim of "indoctrination" here. Without suggesting that such showings would suffice to establish a claim of indoctrination, we note the plaintiffs' children were not forced to read the books on pain of suspension. Nor were they subject to a constant stream of like materials. There is no allegation here of a formalized curriculum requiring students to read many books affirming gay marriage. . . . (concluding that such facts could constitute a burden on free exercise, although such a burden would be constitutionally permissible in the public school context if parents still retained other educational options). The reading by a teacher of one book, or even three, and even if to a young and impressionable child, does not constitute "indoctrination."

Because plaintiffs do not allege facts that give rise to claims of constitutional magnitude, the district court did not err in granting defendants' motion to dismiss the claims under the U.S. Constitution.

III.

Public schools often walk a tightrope between the many competing constitutional demands made by parents, students, teachers, and the schools' other constituents. . . . The balance the school struck here does not offend the Free Exercise or Due Process Clauses of the U.S. Constitution.

We do not suggest that the school's choice of books for young students has not deeply offended the plaintiffs' sincerely held religious beliefs. If the school system has been insufficiently sensitive to such religious beliefs, the plaintiffs may seek recourse to the normal political processes for change in the town and state. . . . They are not entitled to a federal judicial remedy under the U.S. Constitution.

We affirm the district court's dismissal with prejudice of plaintiffs' federal claims and its dismissal without prejudice of the state claims so that they may be reinstated, should plaintiffs choose, in state court.

Source: Parker v. Hurley. 474 F. Supp. 2d 261 (D. Mass 2007), 37–43. Available at http://www.ca1.uscourts.gov/pdf.opinions/07-1528-01A.pdf.

Gonzalez v. School Board of Okeechobee County (2008)

A gay-straight alliance (GSA) is a high school club that brings together gay, lesbian, nongay, and nonlesbian students to discuss issues of mutual interest and concern. As of 2009, more than 1,000 such clubs had been formed in almost every state of the union. In many cases, school administrators are ambivalent about sanctioning such organizations and, in the most extreme cases, have forbidden their presence on school campuses. A number of legal challenges have been filed against efforts to ban gay-straight clubs. One of the most recent and most significant of those cases was argued before the U.S. District Court for the Southern District of Florida in May 2008. In that case, the plaintiff, Yasmin Gonzalez, argued that her high school's refusal to allow a gay-straight club on campus was a violation of the federal Equal Access Act (EAA), which requires schools to provide space for all noncurricular clubs if they provide space for any noncurricular club. The Okeechobee School Board (OSB) responded that banning the club was necessary for four reasons: (1) to maintain the integrity of the school's abstinence only program, (2) to avoid unhealthy premature sexual development of students, (3) to protect GSA members from the risk of contact with potentially dangerous outside adult influences, and (4) to ensure that GSA members do not have access to adult-only materials. Judge K. Michael Moore rejected all four of these arguments in his decision below, and ordered the school to make provisions for hosting the gay-straight alliance on its campus. Certain citations are omitted in this excerpt.

b. Inconsistency of the Abstinence Only Program with the GSA's Mission

SBOC has failed to demonstrate that the GSA's mission to promote tolerance towards individuals of non-heterosexual identity is inherently inconsistent with the abstinence only message SBOC has adopted. SBOC has not clarified how dialogue promoting tolerance towards nonheterosexual individuals is antithetical to principles of abstinence. However, the crux of such a proposition appears to be that because the topic of tolerance relating to sexual identity is a subset of the topic of sexuality generally, the dialogue required to discuss tolerance towards nonheterosexuals is impossible to convey without doing violence to the principle of abstinence. This conclusion, however, relies on the premise that discussing the subject of sexuality undermines the advocation of abstinence. Yet, if such a premise were indeed true, then virtually any topic touching on sexual issues, including those already part of SBOC's curriculum such as pregnancy and sexually transmitted disease, would also undermine an abstinence only policy. SBOC has pointed to no special factor pertaining to tolerance towards non-heterosexuals that distinguishes that topic from other matters concerning sexuality generally. Accordingly, this Court dismisses the unsupported assertion that curriculum based discussions of sexually related topics related to heterosexual activity may occur without violating the abstinence only program but that such a violation would occur in the case of noncurricular based discussions of tolerance towards nonheterosexuals.

. . .

[Judge Moore next cites data about the sexual development of American adolescents before concluding that:]

While the precise accuracy of such figures are [*sic*] uncertain, these statistics merely illustrate the point that premature sexualization of secondary school students is a legitimate concern and a matter of national importance. Nevertheless, this Court is unable to discern how a club whose stated purpose is to promote tolerance towards non-heterosexuals within the student body promotes the premature sexualization of students, either in absolute terms or relative to any other already existing curriculum based instruction which touches on topics of a sexual nature. SBOC's argument that discussions of tolerance towards non-heterosexuals will promote premature sexualization of students is speculative at best and clearly without evidentiary support in the record.

. . .

[*With regard to the school board's third point, Judge Moore observes that:*]
SBOC also contends that recognizing the GSA as a noncurricular student group would place its student members at risk by facilitating access to students by adults who may pose a danger to the students. The simple and obvious solution to this dilemma is to require all noncurricular student groups to seek permission from the principal or a designee in order for any adult who is not a faculty member to attend the meeting of any noncurricular student group or to contribute to its organization or operation. While a host of other measures would be suited to resolve this concern, SBOC may address this concern as it sees fit.

[*With regard to the school board's final point, Judge Moore writes that:*]
As already stated, once a secondary school has established itself as a limited open forum, the EAA provides that "[n]othing in this subchapter shall be construed to limit the authority of the school . . . to maintain order and discipline . . . [or] to protect the well-being of students and faculty." It is self-evident that this language is intended to protect the well-being of all students, heterosexual and non-heterosexual. Accordingly, SBOC is obligated to take into account the well-being of its non-heterosexual students in assessing whether acknowledging the GSA as a noncurricular student group inures to the well-being of students. SBOC has failed to demonstrate that recognition of the GSA, a noncurricular student group promoting tolerance towards nonheterosexual students, would jeopardize the well-being of students. Additionally, SBOC has failed to show that permitting non-heterosexual students to establish a venue promoting unity and collective action is likely to detract from the maintenance of order and discipline.

[*Judge Moore concluded his opinion with the following observation:*]
For the reasons stated above in the analysis pertaining to the EAA, this Court finds that the GSA's tolerance based message would not materially or substantially interfere with discipline in the operation of the school. In order for SBOC to justify its refusals to recognize the GSA as a student organization, "it must be able to show that its action was caused by something more than a mere desire to avoid the discomfort and unpleasantness that always accompany an unpopular viewpoint." This is precisely what SBOC has failed to do. The reasons presented by Defendant for denying the GSA equal access and recognition sound in a desire to avoid the discomfort and unpleasantness of tolerating a minority of

students whose sexual identity is distinct from the majority of students and discordant to SBOC's abstinence only program. Ensuring that this minority of students are afforded meaningful expression secures the precept of freedom from external dominion over thought and expression exalted by the founders and safeguarded by the First Amendment. (citations omitted)

Source: In the United States District Court for the Southern District of Florida. Case No. 06-1 4320-CIV-Moore/Lynch. Available at http://www.aclufl.org/pdfs/GSA_MSJ.pdf.

Reports

The Surgeon General's Call to Action to Promote Sexual Health and Responsible Sexual Behavior (2001)

On July 9, 2001, Surgeon General David Satcher released a report on public health issues related to the sexual health of the nation's citizens. The purpose of the report was to review the current status of a number of sexual issues and to propose a forum by which communities could initiate discussion of and necessary actions on these issues. The report included a section on a Vision for the Future, which summarized information and challenges presented in the study.

VI. Vision for the Future

Strategies that cover three fundamental areas—increasing awareness, implementing and strengthening interventions, and expanding the research base–could help provide a foundation for promoting sexual health and responsible sexual behavior in a manner that is consistent with the best available science.

1. Increasing Public Awareness of Issues Relating to Sexual Health and Responsible Sexual Behavior

- Begin a national dialogue on sexual health and responsible sexual behavior that is honest, mature and respectful, and has the ultimate goal of developing a national strategy that recognizes the need for common ground.
- Encourage opinion leaders to address issues related to sexual health and responsible sexual behavior in ways that are informed by the best available science and that respect diversity.

- Provide access to education about sexual health and responsible sexual behavior that is thorough, wide-ranging, begins early, and continues throughout the lifespan. Such education should:
  - recognize the special place that sexuality has in our lives;
  - stress the value and benefits of remaining abstinent until involved in a committed, enduring, and mutually monogamous relationship; but
  - assure awareness of optimal protection from sexually transmitted diseases and unintended pregnancy, for those who are sexually active, while also stressing that there are no infallible methods of protection, except abstinence, and that condoms cannot protect against some forms of STDs.
- Recognize that sexuality education can be provided in a number of venues–homes, schools, churches, other community settings–but must always be developmentally and culturally appropriate.
- Recognize that parents are the child's first educators and should help guide other sexuality education efforts so that they are consistent with their values and beliefs.
- Recognize, also, that families differ in their level of knowledge, as well as their emotional capability to discuss sexuality issues. In moving toward equity of access to information for promoting sexual health and responsible sexual behavior, school sexuality education is a vital component of community responsibility.

2. Providing the Health and Social Interventions Necessary to Promote and Enhance Sexual Health and Responsible Sexual Behavior

- Eliminate disparities in sexual health status that arise from social and economic disadvantage, diminished access to information and health care services, and stereotyping and discrimination.
- Target interventions to the most socioeconomically vulnerable communities where community members have less access to health education and services and are, thus, likely to suffer most from sexual health problems.
- Improve access to sexual health and reproductive health care services for all persons in all communities.
- Provide adequate training in sexual health to all professionals who deal with sexual issues in their work, encourage them to use this training, and ensure that they are reflective of the populations they serve.

- Encourage the implementation of health and social interventions to improve sexual health that have been adequately evaluated and shown to be effective.
- Ensure the availability of programs that promote both awareness and prevention of sexual abuse and coercion.
- Strengthen families, whatever their structure, by encouraging stable, committed, and enduring adult relationships, particularly marriage. Recognize, though, that there are times when the health interests of adults and children can be hurt within relationships with sexual health problems, and that sexual health problems within a family can be a concern in and of themselves.

3. Investing in Research Related to Sexual Health and Disseminating Findings Widely

- Promote basic research in human sexual development, sexual health, and reproductive health, as well as social and behavioral research on risk and protective factors for sexual health.
- Expand the research base to cover the entire human life span–children, adolescents, young adults, middle age adults, and the elderly.
- Research, develop, disseminate, and evaluate educational materials and guidelines for sexuality education, covering the full continuum of human sexual development, for use by parents, clergy, teachers, and other community leaders.
- Expand evaluation efforts for community, school and clinic based interventions that address sexual health and responsibility.

Source: The Surgeon General's Call to Action to Promote Sexual Health and Responsible Sexual Behavior. [Washington, D.C.: Department of Health and Human Services, 2001], 13–15. Available at http://www.surgeongeneral.gov/library/sexualhealth/call.pdf

The Content of Federally Funded Abstinence-only Education Programs (2004)

Since 1998, the U.S. government has been providing funding for so-called abstinence-only sex education programs, in which abstinence is taught as the only or best acceptable method of birth control and for preventing sexually transmitted infections. For most of that time,

*critics have asked how effective such programs are in providing stu-
dents with information of sexual issues and how effective they are
in achieving their stated objectives. In December 2004, the Special
Investigations Division of the Minority Staff of the Committee on
Government Reform issued a report to Representative Henry Waxman (D-CA) on the first part of this question, with special regard
to the largest federal initiative in this area, the Special Programs of
Regional and National Significance Community-Based Abstinence
Education (SPRANS) program. The major findings of that report are
as follows:*

The report finds that over 80% of the abstinence-only curricula,
used by over two-thirds of SPRANS grantees in 2003, contain false, misleading, or distorted information about reproductive health. Specifically,
the report finds:

- **Abstinence-Only Curricula Contain False Information
  about the Effectiveness of Contraceptives.** Many of the
  curricula misrepresent the effectiveness of condoms in
  preventing sexually transmitted diseases and pregnancy. One
  curriculum says that "the popular claim that 'condoms help
  prevent the spread of STDs,' is not supported by the data";
  another states that "[i]n heterosexual sex, condoms fail to
  prevent HIV approximately 31% of the time"; and another
  teaches that a pregnancy occurs one out of every seven times
  that couples use condoms. These erroneous statements are
  presented as proven scientific facts.
- **Abstinence-Only Curricula Contain False Information about
  the Risks of Abortion.** One curriculum states that 5% to 10%
  of women who have legal abortions will become sterile; that
  "[p]remature birth, a major cause of mental retardation, is
  increased following the abortion of a first pregnancy"; and
  that "[t]ubal and cervical pregnancies are increased following
  abortions." In fact, these risks do not rise after the procedure
  used in most abortions in the United States.
- **Abstinence-Only Curricula Blur Religion and Science.** Many
  of the curricula present as scientific fact the religious view
  that life begins at conception. For example, one lesson states:
  "Conception, also known as fertilization, occurs when one
  sperm unites with one egg in the upper third of the fallopian
  tube. This is when life begins." Another curriculum calls a 43-
  day-old fetus a "thinking person."
- **Abstinence-Only Curricula Treat Stereotypes about Girls and
  Boys as Scientific Fact.** One curriculum teaches that women
  need "financial support," while men need "admiration."
  Another instructs: "Women gauge their happiness and judge

their success on their relationships. Men's happiness and success hinge on their accomplishments."

- **Abstinence-Only Curricula Contain Scientific Errors.** In numerous instances, the abstinence-only curricula teach erroneous scientific information. One curriculum incorrectly lists exposure to sweat and tears as risk factors for HIV transmission. Another curriculum states that "twenty-four chromosomes from the mother and twenty-four chromosomes from the father join to create this new individual"; the correct number is 23.

The report finds numerous examples of these errors. Serious and pervasive problems with the accuracy of abstinence-only curricula may help explain why these programs have not been shown to protect adolescents from sexually transmitted diseases and why youth who pledge abstinence are significantly less likely to make informed choices about precautions when they do have sex.

Source: Special Investigations Division. Minority Staff of the Committee on Government Reform. *The Content of Federally Funded Abstinence-only Education Programs.* [n.p.], December 2004, i–ii.

Data

Cases of Sexually Transmitted Diseases Reported by State Health Departments and Rates per 100,000 Population: United States, 1941–2007

The U.S. Centers for Disease Control and Prevention (CDC) has tracked the incidence of three sexually transmitted infections— syphilis, gonorrhea, and chancroid—for more than 60 years, and the incidence of one other infection, chlamydia, for about 20 years. These data are collected from required reports from state health departments. A summary of these data from 1941 to 2007, the latest year available, is reported in the center's annual surveillance report for STIs, reproduced in Table 6.1.

Estimated Number of Cases of Other Sexually Transmitted Infections in the United States, 1966–2007

In addition to the four "classic" sexually transmitted infections tabulated in Table 6.1, other such infections are also kept under

TABLE 6.1
Cases of Sexually Transmitted Diseases Reported by State Health Departments and Rates per 100,000 Population: United States, 1941–2007

					Syphilis					
	All Stages		Primary & Secondary		Early Latent		Late and Late Latent		Congenital	
Year	Cases	Rate	Cases	Rate	Cases	Rate	Cases	Rate	Cases	Rate
1941	485,560	368.2	68,231	51.7	109,018	82.6	202,984	153.9	17,600	651.1
1942	479.601	363.4	75,312	57.0	116,245	88.0	202,064	153.1	16,918	566.0
1943	575.593	447.0	82,204	63.8	149,390	116.0	251,958	195.7	16,164	520.7
1944	467,755	367.9	78,443	61.6	123,038	96.7	202,848	159.6	13,578	462.0
1945	359,114	282.3	77,007	60.5	101,719	79.9	142,187	111.8	12,339	431.7
1946	363,647	271.7	94,957	70.9	107,924	80.6	125,248	93.6	12,106	354.9
1947	355,592	252.3	93,545	66.4	104,124	73.9	122,089	86.6	12,200	319.6
1948	314,313	218.2	68,174	47.3	90,598	62.9	123,312	85.6	13,931	383.0
1949	256,463	175.3	42,942	28.7	75,045	51.3	116,397	79.5	13,952	382.4
1950	217,558	146.0	23,939	16.7	59,256	39.7	113,569	70.2	13,377	368.3
1951	174,924	116.1	14,485	9.6	43,316	28.7	98,311	65.2	11,094	290.4
1952	167,762	110.2	10,449	6.9	36,454	24.0	105,238	69.1	8,553	218.8
1953	148,573	95.9	8,637	5.6	28,295	18.3	98,870	63.8	6,675	193.0
1954	130,687	82.9	7,147	4.5	23,861	15.2	89,123	56.5	6,676	164.0
1955	122,392	76.2	6,454	4.0	20,054	12.5	86,526	53.8	5,354	130.7
1956	130,201	78.7	6,392	3.9	19,783	12.0	95,096	56.5	5,491	130.4
1957	123,758	73.5	6,576	3.9	17,796	10.6	91,309	54.2	5,288	123.0
1958	113,884	66.4	7,176	4.2	16,556	9.7	83,027	48.4	4,866	114.6
1959	120,824	69.2	9,799	5.6	17,025	9.8	86,740	49.7	5,130	119.7
1960	122,538	68.8	16,145	9.1	18,017	10.1	81,798	45.9	4,416	103.7
1961	124,658	68.8	19,851	11.0	19,486	10.8	79,304	43.8	4,163	97.5
1962	126,245	68.7	21,067	11.5	19,585	10.7	79,533	43.3	4,070	97.7
1963	124,137	66.5	22,251	11.9	18,235	9.8	78,076	41.8	4,031	98.4
1964	114,325	60.4	22,969	12.1	17,781	9.4	68,629	36.3	3,516	87.3
1965	112,842	58.9	23,338	12.2	17,458	9.2	67,317	35.1	3,564	94.8
1966	105,159	54.2	21,414	11.0	15,950	8.2	63,541	32.7	3,170	87.9
1967	102,581	52.2	21,053	10.7	15,554	7.9	61,975	31.5	2,894	82.2
1968	96,271	48.4	19,019	9.6	15,150	7.5	58,564	29.4	2,381	68.0
1969	92,162	45.7	19,130	9.5	15,402	7.6	54,587	27.1	2,074	57.6
1970	91,382	44.8	21,982	10.8	16,311	8.0	50,348	24.7	1,953	52.3
1971	95,997	46.4	23,783	11.5	19,417	9.4	49,993	24.2	2,052	57.7
1972	91,149	43.6	24,429	11.7	20,784	9.9	43,456	20.8	1,758	54.0
1973	87,469	41.4	24,825	11.7	23,548	11.2	37,054	17.5	1,527	48.7
1974	83,771	39.3	25,385	11.9	24,124	11.8	31,854	14.9	1,138	36.0
1975	80,356	37.3	25,561	11.9	26,569	12.3	27,096	12.6	916	29.1
1976	71,761	33.0	23,731	10.9	25,363	11.7	21,905	10.1	625	19.8
1977	64,621	29.4	20,399	9.3	21,329	9.7	22,313	210.2	463	13.9
1978	64,875	29.2	21,656	9.8	19,628	8.8	23,038	10.4	434	13.0
1979	67,049	29.9	24,874	11.1	20,459	9.1	21,031	9.5	332	9.5
1980	68,832	30.3	27,204	12.0	20,297	8.9	20,979	9.2	277	7.7

(*Continued*)

TABLE 6.1
Cases of Sexually Transmitted Diseases Reported by State Health Departments and Rates per 100,000 Population: United States, 1941–2007 (Continued)

	Syphilis								
	All Stages		Primary & Secondary		Early Latent		Late and Late Latent		Congenital	
Year	Cases	Rate	Cases	Rate	Cases	Rate	Cases	Rate	Cases	Rate
1981	72,799	31.7	31,266	13.6	21,033	9.2	20,168	8.8	287	7.9
1982	75,579	32.6	33.613	14.5	21,894	9.5	19,799	8.5	259	7.0
1983	74,637	31.9	32,698	14.0	23,783	10.2	17,896	7.7	239	6.6
1984	69,872	29.6	28,607	12.1	23,131	9.8	17,829	7.6	305	8.3
1985	67,563	28.4	27,131	11.4	21,689	9.1	18,414	7.7	329	8.7
1986	67,779	28.2	27,667	11.5	21,656	9.0	18,046	7.5	410	10.9
1987	87,286	36.0	35,585	14.7	28,233	11.7	22,988	9.5	480	12.6
1988	104,546	42.8	40,474	16.6	35,968	14.7	27,363	11.2	741	19.0
1989	115,089	46.6	45,826	18.4	45,394	18.4	22,032	8.9	1,837	45.5
1990	135,590	54.3	50,578	20.3	55,397	22.2	25,750	10.3	3,865	92.9
1991	128,719	50.9	42,950	17.0	53,855	21.3	27,490	10.9	4,424	107.6
1992	114,730	44.7	34,009	13.3	49,929	19.5	26,725	10.4	4,067	100.0
1993	102,612	39.5	26,527	10.2	41,919	16.1	30,746	11.8	3,420	85.5
1994	82,713	31.4	20,641	7.8	32,017	12.2	27,604	10.5	2,452	62.0
1995	69,359	26.0	16,543	6.2	26,657	10.0	24,296	9.1	1,863	47.8
1996	53,240	19.8	11,405	4.2	20,187	7.5	20,366	7.6	1,282	32.9
1997	46,715	17.1	8,556	3.1	16,631	6.1	20,447	7.5	1,081	27.9
1998	38,289	13.9	7,007	2.5	12,696	4.6	17,743	6.4	843	21.4
1999	35,385	12.7	6,617	2.4	11,534	4.1	16,655	6.0	579	14.6
2000	31,618	11.2	5,979	2.1	9,465	3.4	15,594	5.5	580	14.3
2001	32,284	11.3	6,103	2.1	8,701	3.0	16,976	5.9	504	12.5
2002	32,919	11.4	6,862	2.4	8,429	2.9	17,168	6.0	460	11.4
2003	34,289	11.8	7,177	2.5	8,361	2.9	18,319	6.3	432	10.6
2004	33,423	11.4	7,980	2.7	7,768	2.6	17,300	5.9	375	9.1
2005	33,288	11.2	8,724	2.9	8,176	2.8	16,049	5.4	339	8.2
2006	36,959	12.3	9,756	3.3	9,186	3.1	17,644	5.9	373	9.1
2007	40,920	13.7	11,466	3.8	10,768	3.6	18,256	6.1	430	10.5

	Chlamydia		Gonorrhea		Chancroid	
Year	Cases	Rate	Cases	Rate	Cases	Rate
1941	Data first collected in 1983		193,468	146.7	3,384	2.5
1942			212,403	160.9	5,477	4.1
1943			275,070	213.6	8,354	6.4
1944			300,676	236.5	7,878	6.1
1945			287,181	225.8	5,515	4.3
1946			368,020	275.0	7,091	5.2
1947			380,666	270.0	9,515	6.7

(Continued)

TABLE 6.1

Cases of Sexually Transmitted Diseases Reported by State Health Departments and Rates per 100,000 Population: United States, 1941–2007 (*Continued*)

Year	Chlamydia		Gonorrhea		Chancroid	
	Cases	Rate	Cases	Rate	Cases	Rate
1948			345,501	239.8	7,661	5.3
1949			317,950	217.3	6,707	4.6
1950			286,746	192.5	4,977	3.3
1951			254,470	168.9	4,233	2.8
1952			244,957	160.8	3,738	2.5
1953			238,340	153.9	3,338	2.2
1954			242,050	153.5	3,003	1.9
1955			236,197	147.0	2,649	1.7
1956			224,346	135.7	2,135	1.3
1957			214,496	127.4	1,637	1.0
1958			232,386	135.6	1,595	0.9
1959			240,254	137.6	1,537	0.9
1960			258,933	145.4	1,680	0.9
1961			264,158	145.8	1,438	0.8
1962			263,714	143.6	1,344	0.7
1963			278,289	149.0	1,220	0.7
1964			300,666	158.9	1,247	0.7
1965			324,925	169.5	982	0.5
1966			351,738	181.2	838	0.4
1967			404,836	205.9	784	0.4
1968			464,543	233.4	845	0.4
1969			534,872	265.4	1,104	0.5
1970			600,072	294.2	1,416	0.7
1971			670,268	324.1	1,320	0.6
1972			767,215	366.6	1,414	0.7
1973			842,621	398.7	1,165	0.6
1974			906,121	424.7	945	0.4
1975			999,937	464.1	700	0.3
1976			1,001,994	460.6	628	0.3
1977			1,002,219	456.0	455	0.2
1978			1,013,436	456.3	521	0.2
1979			1,004,058	447.1	840	0.4
1980			1,004,029	442.1	788	0.3
1981			990,864	431.8	850	0.4
1982			960,633	414.7	1,392	0.6
1983			900,435	385.1	847	0.4
1984	7,594	6.5	878,556	372.5	665	0.3
1985	25,848	17.4	911,419	383.0	2,067	0.9
1986	58,001	35.2	892,229	371.5	3,045	1.3
1987	91,913	50.8	787,532	325.0	4,986	2.1
1988	157,854	87.1	738,160	301.9	4,891	2.0
1989	200,904	102.5	733,294	297.1	4,697	1.9

(*Continued*)

TABLE 6.1
Cases of Sexually Transmitted Diseases Reported by State Health Departments and
Rates per 100,000 Population: United States, 1941–2007 *(Continued)*

Year	Chlamydia		Gonorrhea		Chancroid	
	Cases	Rate	Cases	Rate	Cases	Rate
1990	323,663	160.2	690,042	276.4	4,212	1.7
1991	381,228	179.7	621,918	245.8	3,476	1.4
1992	409,694	182.3	502,858	196.0	1,906	0.7
1993	405,332	178.0	444,649	171.1	1,292	0.5
1994	451,785	192.5	419,602	163.9	782	0.3
1995	478,577	187.8	392,651	147.5	607	0.2
1996	492,631	190.6	328,169	121.8	386	0.1
1997	537,904	205.5	327,665	120.2	246	0.1
1998	614,250	231.8	356,492	129.2	189	0.1
1999	662,647	247.2	360,813	129.3	110	0.0
2000	709,452	251.4	363,136	128.7	78	0.0
2001	783,242	274.5	361,705	126.8	38	0.0
2002	834,555	289.4	351,852	122.0	48	0.0
2003	877,478	301.7	335,104	115.2	54	0.0
2004	929,462	316.5	330,132	112.4	30	0.0
2005	976,445	329.4	339,593	114.6	17	0.0
2006	1,030,911	344.3	358,366	119.7	19	0.0
2007	1,108,374	370.2	355,991	118.9	23	0.0

Source: Division of STD Prevention, *Sexually Transmitted Disease Surveillance 2007* (Atlanta, GA: Centers for
Disease Control and Prevention, December 2008), 99–100.

surveillance, although by a less precise method than that used for
syphilis, gonorrhea, chancroid, and chlamydia. Table 6.2 below
provides estimates for some of these other conditions, based on
reported initial visits to physicians' offices for each infection. The
range of possible error for these estimates, unlike that for the diseases listed in Table 6.1, is very large, ranging from 9 to 13 percent
for estimates greater than a million to 20 to 30 percent for estimates between 100,000 and 300,000.

Characteristics of Women Who Obtained Legal
Abortions—United States, 1973–2005

The Centers for Disease Control and Prevention collects data on
the number of legal abortions performed in the United States each
year and the characteristics of women who have those abortions.
Table 6.3 summarizes some of the most recent information on
these characteristics.

TABLE 6.2

**Estimated Number of Cases of Other Sexually Transmitted Infections
in the United States, 1966–2007**

Year	Genital Herpes	Genital Warts	Vaginal Trichomoniasis	Other Vaginitis	Pelvic Inflammatory Disease
1966	19,000	56,000	579,000	1,155,000	Data not available
1967	15,000	72,000	515,000	1,277,000	
1968	16,000	87,000	463,000	1,460,000	
1969	15,000	61,000	421,000	1,390,000	
1970	17,000	119,000	529,000	1,500,000	
1971	49,000	128,000	484,000	1,281,000	
1972	26,000	165,000	574,000	1,810,000	
1973	51,000	198,000	466,000	1,868,000	
1974	75,000	202,000	427,000	1,907,000	
1975	36,000	181,000	500,000	1,919,000	
1976	57,000	217,000	473,000	1,690,000	
1977	116,000	221,000	324,000	1,713,000	
1978	76,000	269,000	329,000	2,149,000	
1979	83,000	200,000	363,000	1,662,000	
1980	57,000	218,000	358,000	1,670,000	423,000
1981	133,000	191,000	369,000	1,742,000	283,000
1982	134,000	256,000	268,000	1,859,000	374,000
1983	106,000	203,000	424,000	1,932,000	424,000
1984	157,000	224,000	381,000	2,450,000	381,000
1985	124,000	263,000	291,000	2,728,000	425,000
1986	136,000	275,000	338,000	3,118,000	457,000
1987	102,000	351,000	293,000	3,087,000	403,000
1988	163,000	290,000	191,000	3,583,000	431,000
1989	148,000	220,000	165,000	3,374,000	413,000
1990	172,000	275,000	213,000	4,474,000	358,000
1991	235,000	282,000	198,000	3,822,000	377,000
1992	139,000	218,000	182,000	3,428,000	335,000
1993	172,000	167,000	207,000	3,755,000	407,000
1994	142,000	239,000	199,000	4,123,000	332,000
1995	160,000	253,000	141,000	3,927,000	262,000
1996	208,000	191,000	245,000	3,472,000	386,000
1997	176,000	145,000	176,000	3,100,000	260,000
1998	188,000	211,000	164,000	3,200,000	233,000
1999	224,000	240,000	171,000	3,077,000	250,000
2000	179,000	220,000	222,000	3,470,000	254,000
2001	157,000	233,000	210,000	3,365,000	244,000
2002	216,000	266,000	150,000	3,315,000	197,000
2003	203,000	264,000	179,000	3,516,000	123,000
2004	269,000	316,000	221,000	3,602,000	132,000
2005	266,000	357,000	165,000	4,071,000	176,000
2006	371,000	422,000	200,000	3,891,000	106,000
2007	317,000	312,000	205,000	3,723,000	146,000

Source: Division of STD Prevention, *Sexually Transmitted Disease Surveillance 2007* (Atlanta, GA: Centers for Disease Control and Prevention, December 2008), 146.

TABLE 6.3

Characteristics of Women Who Obtained Legal Abortions — United States, 1973–2005

Year	Total Number of Legal Abortions
1973	615,831
1974	763,476
1975	854,853
1976	988,267
1977	1,079,430
1978	1,157,776
1979	1,251,92
1980	1,297,606
1981	1,300,760
1982	1,303,980
1983	1,268,987
1984	1,333,521
1985	1,328,570
1986	1,328,112
1987	1,353,671
1988	1,371,285
1989	1,396,658
1990	1,429,247
1991	1,388,037
1992	1,359,146
1993	1,330,414
1994	1,267,415
1995	1,210,883
1996	1,225,937
1997	1,186,039
1998	884,273
1999	861,789
2000	857,475
2001	853,485
2002	854,122
2003	848,163
2004	839,226
2005	820,151

Characteristic	1973	1974	1975	1976	1977	1978	1979	1980	1981	1982
Age										
≤19	32.7	32.6	33.1	32.1	30.8	30.0	30.0	29.2	28.0	27.1
20–24	32.0	31.8	31.9	33.3	34.5	35.0	35.4	35.5	35.3	35.1
≥25	35.3	35.6	35.0	34.6	34.7	35.0	34.6	35.3	36.7	37.8
Race										
White	72.5	69.7	67.8	66.6	66.4	67.0	68.9	69.9	69.9	68.5
Black	27.5	30.3	32.2	33.4	33.6	33.0	31.1	30.1	30.1	31.5
Other	—	—	—	—	—	—	—	—	—	—

(Continued)

TABLE 6.3
Characteristics of Women Who Obtained Legal Abortions — United States, 1973–2005 (*Continued*)

Characteristic	1973	1974	1975	1976	1977	1978	1979	1980	1981	1982
Marital status										
Married	27.4	27.4	26.1	24.6	24.3	26.4	24.7	23.1	22.1	22.0
Unmarried	72.6	72.6	73.9	75.4	75.7	73.6	75.3	76.9	77.9	78.0
Weeks of gestation										
<8	36.1	42.6	44.6	47.0	51.1	52.2	52.1	51.7	51.2	50.6
9–10	29.4	28.7	28.4	28.1	27.2	26.9	26.9	26.2	26.8	26.7
11–12	17.9	15.4	14.9	14.4	13.1	12.3	12.5	12.2	12.1	12.4
>12	16.6	13.3	12.1	10.5	8.6	8.6	8.5	9.9	9.9	10.3

Characteristic	1983	1984	1985	1986	1987	1988	1989	1990	1991	1992
Age										
≤19	27.1	26.4	26.3	25.3	25.8	25.3	24.2	22.4	21.0	20.1
20–24	34.7	35.3	34.7	34.0	33.4	32.8	32.6	33.2	34.4	34.5
≥25	38.2	38.3	39.0	40.7	40.8	41.9	43.2	44.4	44.6	45.4
Race										
White	67.6	67.4	66.7	67.0	66.4	64.4	64.2	64.8	63.9	61.6
Black	32.4	32.6	29.8	28.7	29.3	31.1	31.2	31.9	32.5	33.9
Other	–	–	3.5	4.3	4.3	4.5	4.6	3.3	3.6	4.5
Marital status										
Married	21.4	20.5	19.3	20.2	20.8	20.3	20.1	21.7	21.4	20.8
Unmarried	78.6	19.5	80.7	79.8	79.2	79.7	79.9	78.3	78.6	79.2
Weeks of gestation										
<8	49.7	50.5	50.3	51.0	50.4	48.7	49.8	51.6	52.4	52.1
9–10	26.8	26.4	26.6	25.8	26.0	26.4	25.8	25.3	25.1	24.2
11–12	12.8	12.6	12.5	12.2	12.4	12.7	12.6	11.7	11.5	12.1
>12	10.7	10.5	10.6	11.0	11.2	12.2	11.8	11.4	11.0	11.6

Characteristic	1993	1994	1995	1996	1997	1998	1999	2000	2001	2002
Age										
≤19	20.0	20.2	20.1	20.3	20.1	19.8	19.2	18.8	18.1	17.5
20–24	34.4	33.5	32.5	31.8	31.7	31.8	32.2	32.8	33.4	33.4
≥25	45.6	46.3	47.4	47.9	48.2	48.4	48.6	48.4	48.5	49.1
Race										
White	60.9	60.9	59.6	59.1	58.4	58.7	56.2	56.6	55.4	55.5
Black	34.9	3.47	35.0	35.3	35.9	35.4	37.3	36.3	36.6	36.6
Other	4.2	4.7	5.4	5.6	5.7	5.9	6.5	7.1	8.0	7.9

(*Continued*)

TABLE 6.3
Characteristics of Women Who Obtained Legal Abortions —
United States, 1973–2005 (*Continued*)

Characteristic	1993	1994	1995	1996	1997	1998	1999	2000	2001	2002
Marital status										
Married	20.4	19.9	19.7	19.6	19.0	18.9	19.2	18.7	18.4	18.1
Unmarried	79.6	80.1	80.3	80.4	81.0	81.1	80.8	81.3	81.6	81.9
Weeks of gestation										
<8	52.3	53.7	54.0	54.6	55.4	55.7	57.6	58.1	59.1	60.5
9–10	24.4	23.5	23.1	22.6	22.0	21.5	20.2	19.8	19.0	18.4
11–22	11.6	10.9	10.9	11.0	10.7	10.9	10.2	10.2	10.0	9.6
>12	11.7	11.9	12.0	11.8	11.9	11.9	12.0	11.9	11.9	11.5

Characteristic	2003	2004	2005
Age			
≤19	17.4	17.4	17.1
20–24	33.5	32.8	32.8
≥25	49.1	49.8	50.1
Race			
White	55.0	54.1	55.1
Black	37.1	38.2	36.9
Other	7.9	7.7	8.0
Marital status			
Married	17.9	17.2	16.9
Unmarried	82.1	82.8	83.1
Weeks of gestations			
<8	60.5	61.4	62.1
9–10	18.0	17.6	17.1
11–12	9.7	9.3	9.3
>12	11.8	11.7	11.5

Source: Sonya B. Gamble et al., "Abortion Surveillance — United States, 2005," *Morbidity and Mortality Weekly Report* 57 (SS-13; November 28, 2008): 13–15.

Pregnancy and Live Birthrates for Females 15–19 Years of Age, by Age, Race, and Hispanic Origin: United States, Selected Years, 1980–2000

A number of federal agencies conduct ongoing studies of the sexual behavior of children, adolescents, and adults in the United States. Table 6.4 below summarizes data from some of these surveys on the sexual behavior of adolescent girls with regard to

TABLE 6.4
Pregnancy and Live Birthrates for Females 15–19 Years of Age, by Age, Race, and Hispanic Origin: United States, Selected Years, 1980–2000

	Pregnancies			Live Births		
	15–19	15–17	18–19	15–19	15–17	18–19
All women						
1980	110.0	73.2	162.2	53.0	32.5	82.1
1985	106.9	71.1	158.3	51.0	31.0	79.6
1988	109.9	74.1	158.7	53.0	33.6	79.9
1990	116.3	80.3	162.4	59.9	37.5	88.6
1991	116.0	79.5	166.5	61.8	38.5	94.0
1995	101.1	70.7	148.2	56.0	35.5	87.7
2000	84.5	53.5	129.9	47.7	26.9	78.1
Hispanic						
1990	155.8	101.0	231.4	100.2	65.8	147.6
1995	151.4	103.0	223.3	99.3	68.3	145.4
2000	132.0	83.1	201.7	87.3	55.5	201.7
Non-Hispanic black						
1990	221.3	165.0	295.3	116.2	84.9	157.5
1995	180.1	133.6	253.1	97.2	70.4	139.2
2000	151.0	100.7	224.5	79.2	50.1	121.9
Non-Hispanic white						
1990	87.7	56.5	126.8	42.6	23.3	66.9
1995	71.8	46.8	110.8	39.3	22.0	65.2
2000	56.9	32.5	92.8	32.6	15.8	57.5

Source: J. C. Abma, G. M. Martinez, W. D. Mosher, and B. S. Dawson, "Teenagers in the United States: Sexual Activity, Contraceptive Use, and Childbearing, 2002," National Center for Health Statistics, *Vital Health Statistics* 23 (24; 2004): 3.

pregnancy and childbearing. Although somewhat dated, these are the most recent data available from the federal government on these topics.

Percentage of High School Students Who Were Currently Sexually Active, Who Used a Condom during or Birth Control Pills before Last Sexual Intercourse, by Sex, Race/Ethnicity, and Grade, 2003

The U.S. Centers for Disease Control and Prevention conducts the Youth Risk Behavior Surveillance System (YRBSS), which monitors six categories of health-risk behaviors among adolescents, behaviors

TABLE 6.5
Percentage of High School Students Who Were Currently Sexually Active, Who
Used a Condom During or Birth Control Pills before Last Sexual Intercourse, by Sex,
Race/Ethnicity, and Grade, 2003

Category	Currently Sexually Active			Condom Use			Birth Control Pill Use		
	Female	Male	Total	Female	Male	Total	Female	Male	Total
Race/ethnicity									
White	33.1	28.5	30.8	56.5	69.0	62.5	26.5	17.3	22.3
Black	44.2	54.0	49.0	63.6	81.2	72.8	11.7	4.4	7.9
Hispanic	35.8	38.5	37.1	52.3	62.5	57.4	12.1	10.3	11.2
Grade									
9	18.3	24.0	21.2	66.1	71.2	69.0	11.6	6.6	8.7
10	31.2	30.0	30.6	66.4	71.8	69.0	13.5	11.8	12.7
11	42.9	39.2	41.1	55.5	66.7	60.8	24.1	14.8	19.6
12	51.0	46.5	48.9	48.5	67.0	57.4	27.2	17.5	22.6
Total	34.6	33.8	34.3	57.4	68.8	63.0	20.6	13.1	17.0

Source: Jo Anne Grunbaum et al., "Youth Risk Behavior Surveillance—United States, 2003," *MMWR* 53
(SS02; May 21, 2004): table 44.

that contribute to unintentional injuries and violence. One of these
behaviors is sexual activity. The report on data collected in 2003 provides information on patterns of sexual behavior, condom use, and
birth control use among males and females in grades 9 through 12.
The major findings of that study are shown in Table 6.5.

Worldwide Data on HIV/AIDS, 2008

In 2008, UNAIDS, the United Nations agency responsible for issues related to the HIV/AIDS epidemic published the most recent statistics on the disease in all countries around the world.
Table 6.6 below summarizes a small portion of that data, dealing
with the number of adults and children living with the disease in
various regions and countries of the world.

Estimated Number of Orphans Due to AIDS, 2008

One of the great tragedies of the HIV/AIDS epidemic is the number of children orphaned when both parents die of the disease.
This problem is especially severe in Africa, for which the following data in Table 6.7 are reported. Similar data for other parts of
the world are generally not available because numbers are relatively small compared to this from Africa.

TABLE 6.6
Worldwide Data on HIV/AIDS, 2008

	Estimated Number of People Living with HIV	
Region/country	Adults and Children 2007	Adults and Children 2001
Global	30,000,000–36,700,000	27,000,000–33,700,000
Sub-Saharan Africa	20,500,000–23,600,000	19,200,000–23,200,000
South Africa	4,900,000–6,600,000	4,000,000–5,500,000
Nigeria	2,000,000–3,200,000	1,700,000–4,200,000
Mozambique	1,300,000–1,700,000	880,000–1,200,000
Tanzania	1,300,000–1,500,000	1,300,000–1,500,000
Zimbabwe	1,200,000–1,400,000	1,800,000–2,000,000
Zambia	1,000,000–1,200,000	870,000–1,000,000
East Asia	480,000–1,100,000	330,000–750,000
China	450,000–1,000,000	320,000–730,000
Oceania	66,000–93,000	19,000–41,000
South and Southeast Asia	3,500,000–5,300,000	3,100,000–5,500,000
India	1,800,000–3,200,000	1,700,000–3,800,000
Thailand	410,000–880,000	490,000–850,000
Vietnam	180,000–470,000	97,000–250,000
Eastern Europe and Central Asia	1,100,000–1,900,000	510,000–1,100,000
Russia	630,000–1,300,000	260,000–860,000
Ukraine	340,000–540,000	180,000–260,000
Western and Central Europe	580,000–1,000,000	490,000–810,000
North Africa and Middle East	280,000–510,000	210,000–400,000
North America	760,000–2,000,000	670,000–1,700,000
United States	690,000–1,900,000	620,000–1,600,000
Caribbean	210,000–270,000	180,000–240,000
Latin America	1,500,000–2,100,000	1,200,000–1,900,000
Brazil	600,000–890,000	520,000–810,000
Mexico	150,000–310,000	130,000–260,000
Colombia	110,000–230,000	96,000–190,000
	Children (0–14) 2007	Children (0–14) 2001
Global	1,900,000–2,300,000	1,400,000–2,100,000
Sub–Saharan Africa	1,700,000–2,000,000	1,300,000–1,900,000
South Africa	230,000–320,000	120,000–190,000
Nigeria	170,000–370,000	83,000–580,000
Mozambique	87,000–120,000	41,000–81,000
Tanzania	130,000–150,000	100,000–130,000
Zimbabwe	110,000–140,000	120,000–140,000
Zambia	86,000–110,000	71,000–91,000
East Asia	5,300–11,000	2,500–5,100
Oceania	1,200	<500
South and Southeast Asia	110,000–180,000	50,000–150,000
Thailand	12,000–17,000	7,500–14,000
Eastern Europe and Central Asia	9,100–15,000	2,200–4,800
Western and Central Europe	<1,000–1,800	1,600–3,000

(Continued)

TABLE 6.6

Worldwide data on HIV/AIDS, 2008 (*Continued*)

	Estimated Number of People Living with HIV	
Region/country	Children (0–14) 2007	Children (0–14) 2001
North Africa and Middle East	18,000–34,000	8,800–34,000
North America	2,600–7,300	3,400–8,900
Caribbean	9,400–12,000	6,800–10,000
Latin America	37,000–58,000	29,000–56,000
Honduras	1,000–3,000	<1,000–4,000

Source: 2008 Report on the Global AIDS Epidemic (Geneva: UNAIDS, 2008), Annex 1, 214–233. Available at http://www.unaids.org/en/KnowledgeCentre/HIVData/GlobalReport/2008/2008_Global_report.asp. Used with permission.

TABLE 6.7

Estimated Number of Orphans due to AIDS, 2008

	Number of Orphans, Age 0–17	
Country	2007	2001
South Africa	1,100,000–1,800,000	260,000–590,000
Nigeria	640,000–4,100,000	110,000–3,400,000
Uganda	1,100,000–1,400,000	910,000–1,300,000
Zimbabwe	920,000–1,100,000	610,000–830,000
Tanzania	850,000–1,100,000	500,000–740,000
Ethiopia	540,000–780,000	220,000–430,000
Zambia	530,000–660,000	290,000–490,000
Malawi	470,000–640,000	150,000–340,000
Côte d'Ivoire	320,000–530,000	100,000–370,000
Mozambique	280,000–590,000	53,000–350,000
Sub–Saharan Africa total	10,600,000–15,300,000	5,600,000–10,000,000
Global total	13,000,000–19,000,000	6,900,000–12,000,000

Source: 2008 Report on the Global AIDS Epidemic (Geneva: UNAIDS, 2008), Annex 1, 218. Available at http://www.unaids.org/en/KnowledgeCentre/HIVData/GlobalReport/2008/2008_Global_report.asp. Used with permission.

7

Directory of Organizations, Associations, and Agencies

A number of governmental and nongovernmental organizations are interested in one or another of the issues discussed
in this book: sexually transmitted infections, pregnancy and
contraception, and/or sexual orientation and gender identity. The
organizations listed in this chapter are classified in two general
groups: governmental agencies and nongovernmental agencies.
For each group, a Web site is provided with a brief discussion of
the mission and activities of the group.

Governmental Agencies

Agency for Healthcare Research and Quality (AHRQ)
Web site: http://www.ahrq.gov/

The Agency for Healthcare Research and Quality was created
in December 1989 as the Agency for Health Care Policy and Research, and was renamed the Agency for Healthcare Research and
Quality in December 1999. The purpose of the agency is to support research designed to improve the quality, safety, efficiency,
and effectiveness of health care for all Americans. A subsidiary
of the agency, the U.S. Preventive Services Task Force (USPSTF)
was first convened by the U.S. Public Health Service in 1984 to
conduct assessments of scientific evidence for the effectiveness of
various forms of prevention for medical problems. USPSTF was
incorporated into AHRQ in 1998. In 2008, the task force issued a
recommendation statement on behavioral counseling to prevent
sexually transmitted infections.

Publications: *USPSTF:* Recommendation statements on a number of health issues, including cancer; heart and vascular diseases; infectious diseases; injury and violence; mental health conditions and substance abuse; metabolic, nutritional, and endocrine conditions; musculoskeletal disorders; obstetric and gynecologic conditions; pediatric disorders; vision and hearing disorders.

Centers for Disease Control and Prevention.
See **Division of STD Prevention**

Division of STD Prevention (DSTDP) Centers for Disease Control and Prevention
Web site: http://www.cdc.gov/nchstp/dstd/aboutdiv.htm

The Division of STD Prevention has seven goals: to prevent STD-related infertility, STD-related adverse outcomes of pregnancy, STI-related cancers, and STI-related HIV transmission; to strengthen the capacity and infrastructure elements of STD-prevention programs; to reduce STD health disparities across and within communities and populations; and to address the social and economic effects of STDs among specific populations. On October 1, 2008, the center published a five-year plan outlining its goals and programs for the prevention of sexually transmitted diseases in the United States.

Publications: *Division of STD Prevention Strategic Plan 2008–2013* (strategic plan): many fact sheets on specific diseases; many brochures on specific diseases; "CDCynergy," an interactive CD-ROM program; data and statistics publications; "Sexually Transmitted Diseases Treatment Guidelines 2006" (guidelines).

The Kinsey Institute for Research in Sex, Gender, and Reproduction
Web site: http://www.kinseyinstitute.org/

The origins of the Kinsey Institute can be traced to 1938 when a group of female students at Indiana University asked the university to provide a course on marriage. Alfred Kinsey, then professor of zoology, was hired to teach that course. Over the years, Kinsey expanded his work in the field of human sexuality. Then in 1947, he was appointed director of the newly created Institute for Sex Research at Indiana. A year later, under the auspices of the institute, Kinsey published his now famous book, *Sexual Behavior in the Human Male,* followed five years later by his companion work, *Sexual Behavior in the Human Female.* Today, the institute exists in two parts, a research-oriented division of Indiana University, and a nonprofit Indiana corporation that owns and administers materials from the institute's archives. In addition to having research functions, the institute is an ongoing source of information about a range of issues related to human sexuality, providing a variety of educational events in that area.

Publications: A number of books, including *The Psychophysiology of Sex, Feminine Persuasion: Art and Essays on Sexuality, Sex and Humor: Selections from The Kinsey Institute, Sexual Development in Childhood, Researching Sexual Behavior: Methodological Issues;* monographs, such as *Kinsey Institute Monograph Series, The Kinsey Institute Studies in Sex and Society.*

National Institute of Allergy and Infectious Diseases (NIAID)
Web site: http://www3.niaid.nih.gov/

The National Institute of Allergy and Infectious Diseases began as a single laboratory at the Marine Hospital on Staten Island, New York, in 1887. It achieved its current status in 1948, when the National Institute of Health was redefined as the National Institutes of Health (NIH), and NIAID was established as one of the individual health institutes within NIH. Today, NIAID conducts and supports basic research on the causes, spread, treatment, and cure of infectious, immunologic, and allergic diseases. Over the years, NIAID research programs have led to a number of new diagnostic tests, vaccines, therapies, and other technologies. The agency's research on sexually transmitted infections focuses on basic research, research on diagnostic methodologies and techniques, the development of vaccines and treatment procedures, and additional studies on prevention programs.

Publications: A number of research reports and educational materials, such as *Topical Microbicides—Preventing Sexually Transmitted Diseases* and *Women's Health in the U.S.—Research on Health Issues Affecting Women;* a large number of news releases on topics such as genomic sequencing of causative agents, adult male circumcision in Kenya and Uganda, research on an HIV vaccine, initial trials on a herpes vaccine for women, and new diagnostic tests for specific STIs.

Office of Population Affairs (OPA), Office of Public Health and Science, U.S. Department of Health and Human Services
Web site: http://www.hhs.gov/opa/

The Office of Population Affairs is responsible for two programs established by the U.S. Congress, the family planning program created by Title X of the Public Health Service Act of 1946, as amended (Title 42 of the U.S. Code) and the Adolescent Family Life program authorized by Title XX of the same act. At the present time, OPA is supporting three initiatives in the area of family planning and population affairs: (1) Parents Speak Up National Campaign, which includes television, radio, print, and outdoor advertising, as well as community events encouraging parents to talk to their children about delaying sexual activity until they are married; (2) HIV Prevention and Integration in Family Planning, which provides financial support to clinics for educational, testing, counseling, and other services designed to reduce HIV infection; and (3) Male Services in Family Planning, whose goal is to significantly increase the involvement of males in family planning issues.

Publications: Many free pamphlets and brochures on topics such as "What Is Abstinence?" "Parents, Speak Up!" "Teen Chat," and "The Adoption Option"; many reports such as *Healthy People 2010, Family Planning Annual Report, Youth Development Approaches in Adolescent Family Life Demonstration Projects*, and *Collaborative Evaluation of Strategies to Encourage Couples-Focused Health Service Delivery*.

United Nations Population Fund (UNPF)
Web site: http://www.unfpa.org/public/

The United Nations Population Fund is a subsidiary agency of the United Nations (UN) General Assembly. It was established as a trust fund (the UN Fund for Population Activities) within the UN in 1967 and received its current administrative status in 1972 and its current name in 1987. The work of UNPF is guided by a set of goals established at the 1994 International Conference on Population and Development (ICPD) held in Cairo, Egypt: (1) universal access to reproductive health services by 2015; (2) universal primary education and closing the gender gap in education by 2015; (3) reducing maternal mortality by 75 percent by 2015; (4) reducing infant mortality; (5) increasing life expectancy;

(6) reducing HIV infection rates. In 2007, UNPF spent just over $600 million on hundreds of national and regional projects in every developing nation in the world.

Publications: Many books, booklets, reports, and other print materials on a variety of topics, such as *"Three Ones" in Action: Where We Are and Where We Go From Here*; *2004 Campaign to End Fistula Annual Report*; *24 Tips for Culturally Sensitive Programming: Guide to Working from Within*; *A Holistic Approach to the Abandonment of Female Genital Mutilation/Cutting*; *Financing Healthier Lives: Empowering Women Through Integration of Microfinance and Health Education*; *Contraception: An Investment in Lives, Health and Development*; *Sexual & Reproductive Health and HIV Linkages: Evidence Review & Recommendations*; *Addressing Gender-Based Violence: UNFPA Strategy and Framework for Action*.

U.S. Department of Health and Human Services
See **Office of Population Affairs**

World Health Organization (WHO)
Web site: http://www.who.int/

The World Health Organization is the lead health agency for the United Nations. It is responsible for setting norms and standards for health policies and practices around the world, for providing leadership on global health issues, for fashioning the agenda for research on health problems, for collecting data and statistics and assessing health trends, and for providing technical support to nations on health issues. WHO's primary programmatic focus in the area of sexually transmitted infections is its program for controlling sexually transmitted and reproductive tract infections. Two major emphases of this program are the elimination of congenital syphilis and the general improvement of the reproductive health of men and women around the world. The outlines of this program are set out in a report adopted by the World Health Assembly between 2002 and 2006, *Strategy for the Prevention and Control of Sexually Transmitted Infections*. In addition to providing a host of publications, WHO offers technical information on the prevention of sexually transmitted infections, on the care of STIs, and on other related topics.

Publications: "Sexually Transmitted Infections" (fact sheet); "Effectiveness of Male Latex Condoms" (fact sheet); a number of books, including *Training Modules for the Syndromic Management of*

Sexually Transmitted Infections; Comprehensive Cervical Cancer Control: A Guide to Essential Practice; The Interagency List of Essential Medicines for Reproductive Health; Sexually Transmitted and Other Reproductive Tract Infections—A Guide to Essential Practice; Integrated Management of Adolescent and Adult Illness, and *Sexual and Reproductive Health of Women Living with HIV/AIDS.*

Nongovernmental Agencies

Abortion Access Project (AAP)
Web site: http://www.abortionaccess.org/

The Abortion Access Project was founded in 1992 by a group of physicians and social justice advocates who were concerned about the increasingly violent activities of antiabortion activists attempting to reduce women's access to abortion services. While the organization continues to pursue its traditional goal of ensuring that all women have access to abortion services, it has also expanded its mission to finding common ground among a wide range of organizations and individuals with very different stances on the legitimacy of abortion. The five major initiatives currently supported by AAP are the Rural Abortion Provider Initiative, which attempts to make abortion services more readily available for women in rural settings; the Least Access States Initiative, which focuses on a handful of states in which abortion services are least readily available; the Low Income Access Initiative, which attempts to improve health care services for low-income pregnant women; the Abortion Education and Training Initiative, which attempts to expand the number of professional training programs in which abortion services are taught; and the Advanced Practice Clinicians program, which works to train a group of health care workers known as advanced practice clinicians to perform abortion services.

Publications: Fact sheets; Web site links to a number of articles, reports, news releases, and other publications on abortion topics.

Abstinence the Better Choice (ABC)
Web site: http://www.abstinencebetterchoice.com/

Abstinence the Better Choice is located in Akron, Ohio, where it operates two abstinence programs, Responsible Social Values

Program (RSVP) and Concerned About Teen Sexuality (C.A.T.S.), which are used in the four-county area around Akron. In addition to supplying these two curricula, the organization offers training sessions for teachers who use the programs in their schools.

Publications: *Responsible Social Values Program; Concerned About Teen Sexuality* (both curricula).

Advocates for Youth
Web site: http://www.advocatesforyouth.org/

Advocates for Youth was established in 1980 as the Center for Population Options. Its objective was to help young people make informed and responsible decisions about their reproductive and sexual health. The organization frames its activities within a concept known as the 3Rs, for rights, respect, and responsibilities. In its three-decade history, the organization has achieved a number of successes, including cosponsoring the First Inter-Africa Conference on Adolescent Reproductive Health in 1992; working with the entertainment industry to promote positive and accurate images about adolescent reproductive and sexual health on television programs; establishing the International Clearinghouse on Adolescent Fertility in 1980; creating an innovative sex education program, Life Planning Education, in 1983 that puts sexual issues into a youth development context; and attempting to deal with issues of consistently high rates of teen pregnancy, HIV/AIDS, and other sexually transmitted infections among Latino populations by way of a program called the Spanish Language Media Initiative.

Publications: *Programs That Work* (report); lesson plans for elementary, middle school, and high school students; pamphlets for young people; policy briefs; posters and poster cards; many reports, manuals, and monographs; *The Facts* (a series of more than 60 fact sheets); *From Research to Practice* (27 short essays on a variety of topics); *Issues at a Glance* (39 essays on a variety of topics). Many publications are available in Spanish and French.

American Association of Sex Educators, Counselors and Therapists (AASECT)
Web site: http://www.aasect.org/

The American Association of Sex Educators, Counselors, and Therapists is a professional organization of sex educators, counselors and therapists; physicians and nurses; social workers; psychologists; allied health professionals; clergy members; lawyers; sociologists; marriage and family counselors and therapists; family planning specialists and researchers; and students of these and related professional disciplines. One major focus of the organization's work is providing services to its membership, such as continuing education courses in various topics in human sexuality, as well as online tests for professional credit. AASECT also helps to connect professionals in the field with potential clients, and vice versa. The organization holds an annual conference for all members.

Publications: On its Web site, the organization provides a list of articles and books by members that are available through third-party sources.

American Sexually Transmitted Diseases Association (ASTDA)
Web site: http://depts.washington.edu/astda/

The American Sexually Transmitted Diseases Association is an organization focused on research on sexually transmitted infections with the goal of reducing and eventually eradicating these diseases and disseminating information about STIs. ASTDA also recognizes the work of researchers in the field of STIs with three annual awards: the Thomas A. Parran Award, the Achievement Award, and the Young Investigator Award.

Publications: *Sexually Transmitted Diseases* (journal)

American Social Health Association (ASHA)
Web site: http://www.ashastd.org/

The American Social Health Association was founded in 1914 to provide patients, health care providers, policymakers, and the general public with accurate and reliable information on sexually transmitted diseases. The organization provides two special web sites with information on STDs for teenagers, one in English and one in Spanish. The former is called IwannaKnow.org, at http://www.iwannaknow.org/, and the latter is Quierosaber.org, at http://www.quierosaber.org/. The ASHA Web site also has a special page devoted to information for parents who want to talk with their children about sexually transmitted diseases. Two special sections of the organization's Web page also have information and resources on two specific infections, the Herpes Resource Center and the HPV Resource Center.

Publications: *State of the Nation Report 2005: Challenges Facing STD Prevention in Youth* (report); *"STI Fact Sheets"*; many pamphlets, such as "What You Need to Know about STIs," "Get Tested," "Gonorrhea: Common Disease, Simple Cure," and "Hepatitis: Knowing the Differences Between A, B, and C"; and books such as *Managing Herpes: Living & Loving with HSV* and *Hooking Up: A Girl's All-out Guide to Sex and Sexuality.*

Association of Reproductive Health Professionals (ARHP)
Web site: http://www.arhp.org/

The Association of Reproductive Health Professionals was founded in 1963 as the education arm of the Planned Parenthood Federation of America. It was incorporated as an independent organization in 1972. Its primary goal has always been and still is education, developing information on reproductive health issues that is soundly based in scientific data. The organization carries out its objectives by providing speakers on a variety of topics, such as "Breaking the Contraceptive Barrier: Techniques for Effective Contraceptive Consultations," "A Case-Based Approach for Addressing Hormonal Contraception," "Choosing a Birth Control Method," "A Clinical Update on Intrauterine Contraception," "Environmental Impacts on Reproductive Health," "Evidence-Based Diagnoses and Treatment of Fibromyalgia," and "Managing HPV: A New Era in Patient Care." It also offers ongoing educational programs for the training and updating of professionals in reproductive health care; works to develop and expand curricula in the field of reproductive health care; and conducts an annual convention for professionals in the field.

Publications: *Clinical Proceedings* (monograph series); *Contraception: An International Reproductive Health Journal*; *Quick Reference Guide for Clinicians* (guides on a variety of topics, such as "Managing HPV: A New Era in Patient Care," "Managing Premenstrual Symptoms," "Manual Vacuum Aspiration," and "Non-Hormonal Contraceptive Methods'; clinical fact sheets; *Clinical Practice Tools* (forms, charts, tool kits, etc.); studies and surveys; brochures for patients ("Facts about Emergency Contraception," "Understanding the HPV Vaccine," "How a Woman's Reproductive System Works," etc.)

AVERT
Web site: http://www.avert.org/

AVERT was founded in 1986 in the United Kingdom, where its main offices are still based, as the AIDS Education and Research Trust. Its goal is to reduce the rate of HIV infection and AIDS diseases throughout the world, but especially in nations with very high rates of HIV/AIDS disease. It currently is operating a number of projects in India, Malawi, Mozambique, South Africa, Uganda, and Zambia. The organization is funded by public donations and from an endowment established by Annabel Kanabus, daughter of the founder of the J. Sainsbury supermarket chain. AVERT's Web page has an extensive amount of information on sexual issues, especially with relationship to adolescents.

Publications: None

Bixby Center for Global Reproductive Health
Web site: http://bixbycenter.ucsf.edu/

The Bixby Center for Global Reproductive Health was founded in 1999 to address the health, social, and economic consequences of sex and reproduction through research and training in contraception, family planning, and sexually transmitted infections. Goals of the organization are to increase the range of choices in contraception, abortion, maternal health, and treatment of sexually transmitted infections through the use of new reproductive technologies; improve the understanding of the factors that lead to unwanted adolescent pregnancies and STIs with the objective of improving adolescent reproductive health; develop and evaluate new technologies that will lead to a decrease in maternal mortality associated with childbirth and pregnancy; evaluate national policies to find ways of improving access for men and women to reproductive health care information and technology; train practitioners, researchers, and decision-makers in the United States and other countries of the world on issues of reproductive health care; and provide information and technical assistance to stakeholders on reproductive health care issues. The Bixby Center is a division of the Department of Obstetrics, Gynecology, and Reproductive Sciences at the University of California, San Francisco.

Publications: Briefs, fact sheets, monographs, visual presentations.

BOMA-USA
Web site: http://www.boma-usa.org/

BOMA is an acronym for Billings Ovulation Method Association, an organization formed to promote a method of natural birth control developed by Australian physicians Lyn and John Billings in the 1950s. The method is based on a woman's ability to detect and act on certain natural signs of her reproductive state, allowing her to be sexually active or inactive, depending on whether she wishes to become pregnant or not. The organization offers training sessions in the Billings method and provides access to a list of instructors in all 50 states through its Web site.

Publications: None

Catholics for Choice (CFC)
Web site: http://www.catholicsforchoice.org/

Catholics for Choice was formed in 1973 to provide a voice for members of the Roman Catholic Church who believe that women have the right to follow their own conscience in matters of reproductive health and pregnancy, whether that decision corresponds to the teachings of the church or not. Much of the organization's work is categorized into the fields of abortion, contraception, Catholic health care, sexuality, Catholicism, public policy, and international affairs. The organization currently sponsors four major campaigns: "Condoms4Life," "Catholics in Public Life," "Prevention Not Prohibition," and "The See Change Campaign." An Action Center on the organization's Web site provides a variety of ways in which interested individuals can become active in the work of Catholics for Choice.

Publications: *Conscience* (magazine); *Opinion Polls* (topics covered include sexual behavior and reproductive health, contraception, prevention of HIV and AIDS, and the Catholic vote in 2004); *Conservative Catholic Influence in Europe* series; fact sheets and brochures.

Center for Reproductive Rights (CRC)
Web site: http://reproductiverights.org/

The Center for Reproductive Rights was established in 1992 to use the law to ensure that governments around the world recognize that reproductive freedom is a fundamental human right. The organization's work is currently focused on seven core issues: abortion, the rights of young people, censorship, contraception, safe and healthy pregnancy, HIV/AIDS, and funding for reproductive health care. CRC advances its causes in appearances before various groups affiliated with the United Nations, as advocates in court cases, and in meetings with public policymakers. It also provides training sessions for attorneys in special issues related to reproductive rights. Through its Law School Initiative, the CRC attempts to educate and motivate attorneys to the special issues raised around the topic of reproductive rights.

Publications: Books and reports such as *Maternal Mortality in India: Using International and Constitutional Law to Promote Accountability and Change, Federal Policy Agenda, At Risk: Rights Violations of HIV-Positive Women in Kenyan Health Facilities, Gender-Based Violence Laws in Sub-Saharan Africa, Imposing Misery: The Impact of Manila's Contraception Ban on Women and Families, What If Roe Fell?* and *Beyond the Law: Justice and Gender in Latin America*; briefing papers; fact sheets; shadow letters and reports (letters and reports that follow up on official reports).

Centre for Development and Population Activities (CEDPA)
Web site: http://www.cedpa.org/

The Centre for Development and Population Activities was founded in 1975 for the purpose of improving the lives of women and girls in developing countries around the world. The three major goals of CEDPA are to improve educational opportunities for women and girls; to ensure access to information about reproductive health and the HIV/AIDS epidemic; and to strengthen the role of women in leadership positions in developing nations. Three recent projects designed to meet the second of these goals have been the USAID/Positive Living project, designed to improve the quality of living of people living with AIDS in Nigeria; the Indefinite Quantity Contracts project, which helps provide funding and support for region-specific health-related problems, improving access to neonatal, maternal, and women's health clinics and the development of technical assistance resource centers; and the USAID/Health Policy Initiative, aimed at improving health care services for women across the developing world.

Publications: Research reports such as *Adolescent Girls in India Choose a Better Future: An Impact Assessment* and *Adolescent Sexual and Reproductive Health Behavior in Dodowa, Ghana*; briefs and fact sheets such as "Advocacy for Girls' Education (Egypt)" and "CEDPA in India: Program Highlights"; press releases; CEDPA e-News.

Concerned Women for America (CWA)
Web site: http://cwfa.org/main.asp

Concerned Women for America was founded in 1978 by Beverly LaHaye in response to her concerns about issues raised by spokespersons for the feminist movement, such as Betty Friedan. One of the group's earliest campaigns was in opposition to the Equal Rights Amendment, which would have provided legal protection for the rights of all Americans, regardless of their gender. The organization's mission is to bring biblical principles to bear on all aspects of public policy in the United States. The six core issues that form the focus of CWA activities at the present time are opposition to same-sex marriage, opposition to most forms of contraception and all forms of abortion, returning authority for the education of children to their parents from public schools, bringing about a ban on all pornography and obscenity, removal of any federal restrictions on the practice of religion in public life, and preventing the United Nations or any other international agency from having sovereignty over American citizens and activities. In recent campaigns, CWA has advocated against the extension of hate crimes legislation to individuals on the basis of sexual orientation, the expansion of stem cell research funding, and the Freedom of Choice Act dealing with abortion.

Publications: Books by Beverly LaHaye and Tim LaHaye and coauthors, such as *The New Spirit-Controlled Woman*, *Season of Blessing*, *Seasons under Heaven*, and *Showers in Season*; brochures ("What Your Teacher Didn't Tell You About Abstinence," "How to Lobby From Your Home," "Pro-Life Action Guide," "A Painful Choice: Abortion's Link to Breast Cancer," "High-Tech 'Birth Control': Health Care or Health Risk?" "Why Children Need Fathers: Five Critical Trends," etc.); fact cards ("2009 Issues Alert," "Freedom of Choice Act," "Freedom of Conscience," "'Gays' in the Military," etc.).

Contraceptive Research and Development Program (CONRAD)
Web site: http://www.conrad.org/

The Contraceptive Research and Development Program was established in 1986 at Eastern Virginia Medical School with funding from the U.S. Agency for International Development (USAID). CONRAD also receives funding from the National Institute of

Child Health and Human Development, the Centers for Disease Control and Prevention, the National Institute of Allergy and Infectious Diseases, and private foundations. CONRAD's mission is to develop safe, acceptable, and affordable contraceptive products that also prevent the spread of sexually transmitted infections, such as HIV/AIDS. The agency is engaged at every stage of the development of these products, from initial research to clinical testing to commercial development and distribution of products to training of workers needed to make best use of these products. In 1995, CONRAD established the Consortium for Industrial Collaboration in Contraceptive Research "to help revitalize the pharmaceutical industry's commitment to developing new contraceptives." The consortium focuses on research and development in three priority areas: male methods, monthly methods for women, and vaginal methods that prevent pregnancy and sexually transmitted infections (STIs).

Publications: Biennial reports; *Manual for the Standardization of Colposcopy for the Evaluation of Vaginal Products: Update 2004*; reports on a number of workshops on topics such as "Vaginal Microbicide Formulations"; "Pharmacology, Biology, and Clinical Applications of Androgens: Current Status and Future Prospects"; "Contraceptive Research and Development: Looking to the Future"; "Barrier Contraceptives: Current Status and Future Prospects"; and "Heterosexual Transmission of AIDS."

Couple to Couple League (CCL)
Web site: http://ccli.org/

The Couple to Couple League is an international nonprofit Roman Catholic organization created to promote the use of natural family planning techniques as an alternative to the use of contraceptive technologies and abortion. The organization was founded in 1971 in response to a suggestion by Pope Paul VI that married couples help other married couples to learn about and make use of natural family planning methods. CCL's three objectives are to provide a nationwide and organized method for delivering natural family planning technologies; to provide scientific, technical, moral, and religious instruction in the use of these technologies; and to train volunteer married couples as counselors and teachers of the technologies.

Publications: Press releases, podcasts, reports of past conventions, media kit, *Family Foundations* (magazine).

EngenderHealth
Web site: http://www.engenderhealth.org/

EngenderHealth was founded in 1943 for the purpose of expanding access to sterilization procedures—vasectomies and tubal ligations, primarily—for men and women in the United States. In 1962, the initial voluntary organization was formally constituted as the Association for Voluntary Sterilization. In 1984, it changed its name again to the Association for Voluntary Surgical Contraception, and in 2001, to its present name of EngenderHealth. In 1966, the organization first initiated efforts to expand its services to nations outside the United States, a program that has since become a major focus of its work. Over the past few decades, EngenderHealth has significantly expanded its program to include helping women give birth to healthy babies, preventing the spread of HIV/AIDS and other sexually transmitted infections, and working with stakeholders to expand the variety of reproductive options available to women.

Publications: *EngenderHealth Update* (quarterly newsletter); a variety of training curricula, clinical guidelines, instructional videos, brochures, working papers, and articles on topics such as family planning; HIV/AIDS and sexually transmitted infections; maternal health; counseling, informed choice, and informed consent; improving clinical quality; and promoting gender equity.

Family Health International (FHI)
Web site: http://www.fhi.org/

Family Health International is a research organization whose goal is to increase access to high quality, affordable reproductive health care for people around the world; to prevent sexually transmitted infections, including HIV/AIDS; to stop the spread of malaria, tuberculosis, and similar infectious diseases; and to promote the health and well-being of youth. The organization had its start as a contraceptive research project at the University of North Carolina at Chapel Hill in 1971 and, with a grant from the U.S. Agency for International Development, became an independent nonprofit organization, the International Fertility Research Program (IFRP), in 1975. In 1982, it changed its name to Family Health International. FHI currently operates research program in areas of its interests in 40 countries. Examples of its projects include the Aastha Project, an HIV/AIDS program in Maharashtra, India; The Tomorrow Project, a worldwide project designed to strengthen and improve family life; and TBCTA, an international program for the control of tuberculosis.

Publications: *Family Health Research* (newsletter); *The Guyana HIV/AIDS Reduction and Prevention Project (GHARP) 2004-2009* (report); *Guidance for Nurse Prescription and Management of Antiretroviral Therapy* (booklet); *Network* (quarterly bulletin); many books and reports, such as *Partnering for Care in HIV Prevention Trials—A How-To Manual, Strategy for the Integration of Family Planning and HIV Voluntary Counselling and Testing Services,* and *Health Outcomes Research: How Can It Assist Decision-Making for the Prevention of Cervical Cancer and Other HPV Disease in Asia and the Pacific?*

Family Research Council (FRC)
URL: http://www.frc.org/

The Family Research Council was founded in 1983 to promote the traditional family and traditional marriage. It pursues its work through a number of venues, including books, pamphlets, and other kinds of publications; testimony before a variety of legislative bodies; analysis and review of legal and policy documents with the potential for impacting marriage and the family; and appearances in public debates and discussions. Among the topics that FRC lists as of special concern are "Human Sexuality," with specific emphasis on abstinence and sexual health and homosexuality, and "Human Life," which includes abortion and women's health.

Publications: Press releases, op-eds, and blog available online at Web site.

Focus on the Family
URL: http://www.focusonthefamily.com/

Focus on the Family is a Christian organization that attempts to follow biblical principles in nurturing and defending the (heterosexual) family. It generally tends to oppose any definition of the family other than one consisting of one man, one woman, and one or more children. The guiding principles under which the organization operates is the preeminence of an evangelical interpretation of the Bible, the importance of a permanent marriage between one man and one woman, the value of children to a family, the sanctity of human life, the importance of social responsibility, and the confirmation of clearly defined male and female roles in a family. Among the topics in which the organization is interested are premarital sexual relationships, sex and intimacy, child development, abstinence, and sexual identity. Articles about all of these topics are available on the organization's Web site.

Publications: *Citizen* magazine; the organization's primary news and issue analysis outlet is the Web site CitizenLink at http://www.citizenlink.org/citizenmag/.

Guttmacher Institute (GI)
Web site: http://www.guttmacher.org/

The Guttmacher Institute was founded in 1968 as a semiautonomous division of the Planned Parenthood Federation of America, at least partly in response to a growing national and international concern about the growth of unplanned and unwanted pregnancies in the United States and around the world. The mission of the organization was "to provide a factual basis for the development of sound governmental policies and for public consideration of the sensitive issues involved in the promotion of reproductive health and rights," a mission it retains to this day. The institute provides reports, policy reviews and analyses, and other resources on topics such as abortion, adolescence, pregnancy, sexually transmitted infections, sex and relationships, and technology and bioethics. Much of its work now falls into four major programmatic areas: Protecting the Next Generation: Adolescent Sexual and Reproductive Health; Adding it Up: Sexual and Reproductive Health Services and Financing; Rights and Responsibilities: Healthy Pregnancies, Contraception and Abortion ; and Healthy Sexuality: Relationships.

Publications: *Perspectives on Sexual and Reproductive Health* (periodical); *International Perspectives on Sexual and Reproductive Health* (periodical); *Guttmacher Policy Review* (periodical); media kits; fact sheets; *State Policies in Brief* (reviews of state policies on issues related to sexuality and reproductive rights); *In Brief* (briefing papers); reports; statistical reviews; slide shows.

International Consortium on Emergency Contraception (ICEC)
Web site: http://www.cecinfo.org/

The International Consortium on Emergency Contraception was formed in 1995 as a way of better informing women around the world about postcoital methods of contraception. The original members of the consortium were the Concept Foundation, International Planned Parenthood Federation, Pacific Institute for Women's Health, Pathfinder International, Program for Appropriate Technology in Health, Population Council, and World Health Organization Special Programme of Research, Development, and Research Training in Human Reproduction. Today, a total of 42 nongovernmental organizations are members of the consortium. The five major areas of interest to the organization today are emergency contraception and youth, legal issues related to emergency contraception, products and access, science and technical information, and the use of emergency contraceptives in times of crisis (as in wars and civil unrest). The ICEC Web site provides access to a large number of articles about emergency contraception, to information about the status and availability of emergency contraceptive technologies, and to publications of the organization.

Publications: Policy statements; advocacy materials; *The Emergency Contraception Newsletter* (online newsletter); programmatic resources (e.g., *Medical and Service Delivery Guidelines, Framework for Introducing EC, Adapting Resource Materials for Local Use*).

International Society for Sexually Transmitted Diseases Research (ISSTDR)
Web site: http://www.isstdr.org/
http://www.congrexnetwork.com/dbs/isstdr/cndbz.cfm.

The purpose of the International Society for Sexually Transmitted Diseases Research is to promote research on sexually transmitted infections. The organization's primary activity is a biennial conference on STIs, held alternately in Europe and North America. Among the topics discussed at these meetings are HIV infections and the acquired immunodeficiency syndrome; microbiology; virology; immunobiology; pathogenesis; clinical sciences; social and behavioral sciences; epidemiology; prevention; and research in health services, public health, and prevention policy.

Publications: None

International Union against Sexually Transmitted Infections (IUSTI)
Web site: http://www.iusti.org/

The International Union against Sexually Transmitted Infections is the oldest international organization working to foster international cooperation in controlling the spread of sexually transmitted infections. Membership in IUSTI is open to individuals on a full or associate basis and to organizations and commercial sponsors. The organization sponsors annual international conferences, as well as regional and international conferences and other meetings on specific topics such as HIV/AIDS, the papillomavirus, neisseria vaccines, and clinical microbiology and infectious diseases.

Publications: *International Journal of STD & AIDS*; *Sexual Health—The Official Journal of IUSTI—Asia-Pacific*.

Ipas
Web site: http://www.ipas.org/

Ipas was formed in 1973 as the International Pregnancy Advisory Services to help in establishing family planning and abortion clinics in 11 developing countries. In the early 1980s, the organization expanded its mission to include women's health care issues in general. Today, the organization continues to work to expand the availability of abortion and reproductive health care services for women around the world, but also takes a broader approach to such issues by carrying out and sponsoring research, educating women about healthcare issues and options, advocating for a greater role of women in determining their own health options, working with youth on adolescent and health care issues, and working against sexual violence. The basic principle behind the organization's work is that "no woman should have to risk her life or health because she lacks safe reproductive health choices."

Publications: A large collection of publications, available by language and by region of the world, is listed on the organization's Web site at http://www.ipas.org/Publications/Index.aspx.

Kaiser Family Foundation
Web site: http://www.kff.org/

The Kaiser Family Foundation was established in 1948 by industrialist Henry J. Kaiser and his wife, Bess, with the goal of meeting "the unmet health care needs of the citizenry." The foundation currently has an endowment of about a half billion dollars and an annual operating budget of about $40 million. Its primary programmatic areas are health reform, Medicaid and the Children's

Health Insurance Program, Medicare, medical and insurance costs, insurance coverage and the uninsured, state policies, prescription drugs, HIV/AIDS, U.S. global health policy, minority health issues, women's health policy, and media and health issues.

Publications: Charts and data; fact sheets; issue briefs; news releases; reports and studies (e.g., *2009 National ADAP Monitoring Project Annual Report, Health Care and Medicaid—Weathering the Recession, New, Updated Resources on Community Health Centers, How Is The Primary Care Safety Net Faring in Massachusetts? Community Health Centers In The Midst of Health Reform, The Future of Health Care Journalism, Women and Health Care—A National Profile, Sex on TV: TV Sex is Getting Safer*); surveys; testimonies; video and audio productions.

NARAL—Pro-Choice America
Web site: http://www.prochoiceamerica.org/

NARAL was founded in 1969 as the National Association for the Repeal of Abortion Laws. Four years later it changed its name to the National Abortion Rights Action League, and in 2003, it assumed its present name of NARAL Pro-Choice America. The organization describes itself as "the leading national advocate for personal privacy and a woman's right to choose." NARAL's current efforts are organized around four main issues: abortion, birth control, sex education, and women of color. Under the rubric of abortions, the organization works for access to abortions, an end to abortion bans, and access to the drug RU486. The birth control program focuses on emergency contraception, family planning services, access to prescription birth control materials, and insurance coverage for such materials. The sex education program pushes for greater access to sex education for all children, and the women of color program addresses the special health problems confronting this section of the population.

Publications: *Choice and Change* (electronic newsletter); many press releases, all available online.

National Campaign to Prevent Teen and Unplanned Pregnancy
Web site: http://www.thenationalcampaign.org/

The National Campaign to Prevent Teen and Unplanned Pregnancy was founded in 1996 with the goal of reducing such pregnancies by one-third during the decade from 1996 to 2005.

Having (probably) met that goal, the organization has set its next objective as reducing teen and unwanted pregnancies by an additional third over the next decade, from 2006 to 2015. Among the organization's activities in pursuit of this goal are developing, producing, and disseminating a wide range of educational and informational materials; cooperating with policymakers, members of the news media, governmental officials, and other individuals and organizations to change the way the public thinks about teen and unwanted pregnancies; promoting responsible and healthy relationships among individuals and their attitudes toward family planning; offering personal visits, technical assistance, conference presentations, and other efforts to assist state and community groups working on teen and unwanted pregnancies; working with parents to help them understand their role in reducing teen pregnancies; and partnering with a variety of entertainment media to ensure that prevention messages are included in their work. The organization also works directly with teenagers, more than three million of whom have taken part in the group's online National Day to Prevent Teen Pregnancy.

Publications: Many fact sheets on topics such as abstinence, contraception, effective programs, foster care, males and fatherhood, parents and families, public policy, race and ethnicity, teen birthrates, teen pregnancy rates, teen sexual behavior and activity, and unplanned pregnancy; many reports on topics such as adolescent behavior, the African American community, boys/young men, effective program research, faith and religion, girls/young women, marriage and healthy relationships, sexual abuse, and teen pregnancy costs and connections to other issues.

National Right to Life (NRL)
Web site: http://www.nrlc.org/

The National Right to Life Committee was founded in 1973, a few months after the U.S. Supreme Court's decision in *Roe v. Wade*. Today, the organization has grown to more than 3,000 chapters in all 50 states and the District of Columbia. In addition to its primary campaign in opposition to abortion, NRL is also interested in other issues, such as medical ethics, euthanasia, health care reform, Medicare, and human cloning. An important aspect of NRL's work is an effort to influence federal legislation on abortion and related issues. Its Web page on "Federal Legislation" provides an ongoing record of its work in this field. The organization also sponsors the summer National Right to Life Academy, designed to train young people to continue the battle against the legalization of abortion.

Publications: *National Right to Life News* (newsletter); *Today's News and Views* (daily online news update); *NRL Communications Blog*; *Pro-Life Perspective* (online news and commentary); press releases.

National Women's Health Resource Center (NWHRC)
Web site: http://www.healthywomen.org/

The National Women's Health Resource Center was founded by Dr. Violet Bowen-Hugh in 1986 for the purpose of providing women with up-to-date and accurate information about health issues of interest and concern to them. Its current online library contains information on more than 100 such topics, including bacterial vaginosis, birth control pills, chlamydia, genital herpes, human papillomavirus, infertility, pregnancy, sexual dysfunction, trichomoniasis, and urinary tract infections. The organization's Web site is divided into a number of "health centers" on topics such as diabetes, midlife health, reproductive health, sexual health, pelvic health, heart health, living well and aging well, breast health, and pregnancy and parenting.

Publications: Fast Facts, two-page information sheets on dozens of health topics; Women's Health Updates, short booklets on a variety of topics; Guides, booklet-size publications on a variety of topics; *Healthy Women Take 10* (newsletter); *National Women's Health Report* (irregular newsletter on health topics of current interest); *Questions to Ask* (one-page information sheets on health topics); miscellaneous publications on a variety of health topics.

Pharmacy Access Partnership
Web site: http://www.pharmacyaccess.org/

Pharmacy Access Partnership was founded in California in 1999 to expand consumer access to contraceptive materials and devices and reproductive health services at local pharmacies. It has a four-fold mission in this regard, namely to (1) develop and put into practice new policies; (2) advance new practices in pharmacies and clinics; (3) create more educational opportunities for

consumers in pharmacies; and (4) promote greater public awareness of reproductive health practices and opportunities. Currently,
the organization provides access to emergency contraceptives for
consumers in more than 90 percent of the state's 58 counties and
information about reproductive health practices in 11 languages.
Pharmacy Access Partnership also sponsors the Youth-Friendly
Pharmacy Initiative (YFPI), a program designed to make the information and materials available at local pharmacies more accessible to young women and men.

Publications: *National Survey on Attitudes and Interest for Pharmacy Access for Hormonal Contraception Among Women at Risk for
Unintended Pregnancy* (report); scholarly articles in peer-reviewed
journals; news releases.

Planned Parenthood Federation of America (PPFA)
Web site: http://www.plannedparenthood.org/

Planned Parenthood was founded in 1916 when Margaret Sanger,
her sister, and a friend opened the nation's first birth control
clinic in Brooklyn, New York. Today, the organization provides a
very wide array of services in the fields of abortion, birth control,
emergency contraception, family planning, men's sexual health,
pregnancy, sexual identity and sexual orientation, teenage sexual
health issues, and women's sexual health. Some areas in which
Planned Parenthood is currently working are political activism on
behalf of sexual and women's issues, birth control, abortion, family planning, health care reform, medical privacy, international
health issues, and sex education issues. The organization provides health and educational services and advocates on a number
of issues related to human sexuality. It carries out much of its mission through 97 affiliated organizations in the United States and
around the world.

Publications: A series of podcasts on topics such as "Hanging Out with Herpes," "The Anal Sex Show," "Benefits of Sex,"
and "Tales of Dating"; research reports on topics such as "The
Health Benefits of Sexual Expression," "A History of Birth Control
Methods," and "Masturbation—From Stigma to Sexual Health";
a variety of teaching materials that include curricula, classroom
materials, and evaluation materials.

Population Action International (PAI)
Web site: http://www.populationaction.org/

Population Action International was founded in 1965 as an international nonprofit organization seeking to provide information about and access to sexual and reproductive health with the long-term goal of reducing the number of people in the world who are living in poverty. The three major aspects of PAI's work are research, advocacy, and communication. The six primary issues on which PAI is currently focusing are international advocacy, institutions and partnerships; comparative funding and finances; reproductive health supplies; development and security; population and climate change; and population and the environment.

Publications: Reports; working papers; fact sheets; documentaries; interactive databases, such as "How Do Recent Population Trends Matter to Climate Change?" (working paper); "Condoms and CFLs: Environmental Behavior Change Lessons from Public Health" (commentary); "The Silent Partner: HIV in Marriage" (fact sheet); "Population, Fertility and Family Planning in Pakistan: A Program in Stagnation" (commentary); "A Measure of Survival—Calculating Women's Sexual and Reproductive Risk" (research report).

Population Council (PC)
Web site: http://www.popcouncil.org/

The Population Council was formed in 1952 as the result of a meeting held in Williamsburg, Virginia, sponsored by John D. Rockefeller III and the National Academy of Sciences in response to a growing concern about the rapid pace of increase in the world's population. The guiding principle under which the council has already operated is that it has no desire to impose a single population policy on any nation, but prefers to fund efforts by individual countries to research their own population status and needs and to develop population policies appropriate to that status and those needs. In addition to its programs in more than 60 nations today, PC also supports three research initiatives, the Center for Biomedical Research, which conducts (1) basic research in reproductive biology and immunology and (2) applied research for product development; Frontiers in Reproductive Health, which carries out operational research with individual countries to improve delivery of health services; and (3) Horizons: Global Operation Research on HIV/AIDS/STI Prevention and Care, which conducts operational research to find ways of reducing the spread of HIV/AIDS and sexually transmitted infections.

Publications: *Population and Development Reviews* (journal); *Studies in Family Planning* (journal); *Population Briefs* (newsletter); *Momentum* (biannual newsletter); *Frontiers in Reproductive Health* (journal); *Policy Research Division Working Papers*; *Poverty, Gender, and Youth Working Papers*; many books, articles, and reports indexed by subject on the PC Web site.

Pro-Choice Public Education Project (PEP)
Web site: http://www.protectchoice.org/

The Pro-Choice Public Education Project is affiliated with the Women's Leadership Council, which directs PEP's research and programmatic activities. The organization seeks to bridge the gap between young women as individuals and the organizations that have been created to serve and help them. The organization's activities fall into four major categories: research with young women that can be used for the development of tools and messages for other young women, development and production of those tools and messages, development of leaders who can take a role in bringing about change in their communities, and developing strategic partnerships among organizations with similar goals and objectives. PEP's Technical Assistance Project was launched in the spring of 2007 to help grassroots organizations incorporate the principles of reproductive justice into their own specific policies and programs.

Publications: Online newsletter; *On Our Terms* (report); posters, ads, and campus handouts, available online.

Religious Coalition for Reproductive Choice (RCRC)
Web site: http://www.rcrc.org/

The Religious Coalition for Reproductive Choice was formed in New York City in 1973 in response to an announcement made by the Roman Catholic Church that it planned to work for the overthrow of the U.S. Supreme Court's recent decision in *Roe v. Wade*. Two years later, the organization had grown to include 24 religious organizations in eight states. These groups represent a wide array of religious and theological positions, ranging from conservative, reconstructionist, and reform Judaism to the Episcopal, Presbyterian, and Methodist churches to the American Ethical Union National Service Conference and the Unitarian Universalist Association. In addition to its core issue of abortion, RCRC is concerned with a number of related issues, including contraception, sex education, health care, bioethics, environment and health, and children. RCRC works for its objectives through a number of programs, such as Call to Justice, a response by clergy to efforts by the religious right to overthrow the Supreme Court's *Roe v. Wade* decision; Clergy for Choice, a national registry of clergy of all faiths who support the RCRC position on abortion; Black Church Initiative, a program to assist African American clergy and laity in addressing problems of special concern, including teen pregnancy, sex education, unintended and unwanted pregnancies, and other reproductive health issues; Spiritual Youth for Reproductive Freedom (SYRF), an interfaith, multicultural program by and for young adults ages 16–30; and La Iniciativa Latina, a program to assist Latino communities in addressing issues related to human sexuality from a faith-informed perspective.

Publications: *Between a Woman and Her God: Clergy and Women Tell Their Stories* (booklet); *Hospital Merger Guide*; *Prayerfully Pro-Choice: Resources for Worship* (collection of sermons, prayers, rituals, statements, etc.); *Speak Out for Choice Activist Kit*; *Educational Series Kit*.

Reproductive Health Technologies Project (RHTP)
Web site: http://www.rhtp.org/

The Reproductive Health Technologies Project was founded in 1988 with the specific objective of providing information about the newly developed French abortifacient, RU486. Since its founding RHTP has expanded its agenda to include programs to expand women's access to over-the-counter emergency contraceptives, push for greater integrity in the development of federal reproductive health policy, work for greater cooperation among members of the reproductive health and rights community for the implementation and availability of new genetic technologies, improve communication among reproductive care advocates and pharmaceutical and medical devices companies to increase the availability of reproductive choices for women, and build consensus on the use of the drug misoprostol for reproductive health indications.

Publications: Fact sheets, brochures, and reports on topics such as *Instructions for Use: Misoprostol for Incomplete Pregnancy and Miscarriage*; *Instructions for Use: Misoprostol for Pregnancy Termination*; *Understanding What the Public Thinks About Abortion: Moving*

From Judgment to Empathy. A Report on Findings from Dial Groups; Facts About Fertility; Nonoxynol 9 Facts; The Unfinished Revolution in Contraception: Convenience, Consumer Access, and Choice; The Quinacrine Debate and Beyond.

Sexuality Information and Education Council of the United States (SIECUS)
Web site: http://www.siecus.org/index.cfm

The Sexuality Information and Education Council of the United States was founded in 1964 by Mary S. Calderone, who had previously served as medical director of Planned Parenthood, and her colleagues, Wallace Fulton, William Genne, Lester Kirkendall, Harold Lief, and Clark Vincent. The organization was created to serve as an advocate for sex education, sexual health issues, and sexual rights. Today, SIECUS provides information and services to the general public on a wide variety of topics, including educational programs in human sexuality, abstinence only until marriage programs, adolescent sexuality, teen pregnancy, sexually transmitted diseases, sexual orientation, and sexual and reproductive health. Through a variety of reports and fact sheets, the organization also monitors and disseminates information on a number of topics related to human sexuality and sex education, including Title V "abstinence-only-until-marriage programs," statistics on comprehensive sex education programs, emergency contraception, and the so-called virginity pledges.

Publications: annual reports (available online); position statements on a variety of issues (available online); *Guidelines for Comprehensive Sexuality Education: Kindergarten–12th Grade; Developing Guidelines for Comprehensive Sexuality Education* (handbook); *Filling the Gaps: Hard-to-Teach Topics in Sexuality Education* (teacher's manual); *On the Right Track?* (guide for youth organizations); *Right from the Start: Guidelines for Sexuality Issues, Birth to Five Years* (guidelines); *Talk About Sex?* (booklet).

United States Conference of Bishops
Web site: http://www.usccb.org/index.shtml

The United States Conference of Bishops is an assembly of the hierarchy of the Roman Catholic Church in the United States whose purpose is to "promote the greater good which the Church offers humankind, especially through forms and programs of the apostolate fittingly adapted to the circumstances of time and place." The conference is very interested in and has taken strong stands on a number of issues related to human sexuality, including abortion, contraception, marriage and family, natural family planning, and women's issues. The organization's Web site contains an extensive amount of documents and information on each of these topics, generally arranged under the categories of church documents and teachings, basic information, articles and publications, columns and commentaries, specific aspects of each given issue, testimony and letters, news releases and statements, and additional resources. This Web site is by far the most complete resource available on the official position of the Roman Catholic Church on essentially every issue related to human sexuality.

Publications: Hundreds of books, booklets, pamphlets, prayer cards, prayer books, liturgical documents, posters, and other print materials on every aspect of human sexuality and other social and religious issues.

Young People's Sexual Health (YPSH)
Web site: http://www.ypsh.net/

Young People's Sexual Health is an organization located in Ipswich, England, with a superb Web site containing a host of valuable information on many sexual health issues for young people. It provides information on contraception, sexually transmitted infections, services and clinics, special information for men and boys, and support groups. A special section of the organization's Web site is designed for professionals, who can obtain information and advice on topics in sexual health by joining the service for free online.

Publications: None

Gay and Lesbian Youth Groups

A key resource for gay, lesbian, bisexual, transgender, and questioning (GLBTQ) youth is local groups who provide information and support for young women and men in a specific geographic area. Dozens of such organizations currently exist. The listings below provide a modest sense of the diversity of those organizations. An extensive list of nearly 350 nonprofit organizations that provide services to GLBTQ youth is available at GuideStar (http://www2.guidestar.org/). Also see the Wikipedia Web site at http://en.wikipedia.org/wiki/List_of_LGBT-related_organi zations.

Gay and Lesbian Community Center of the Ozarks (GLCCO)
Web site: http://www.glocenter.org/

The Gay and Lesbian Community Center of the Ozarks was founded in 1996 to provide a safe haven for lesbians, gay men, bisexuals, and transgendered persons in southwest Missouri. The organization provides counseling services, AA meetings, religious services, social nights, and special youth activities.
Publications: None

Gay, Lesbian and Straight Education Network (GLSEN)
Web site: http://www.glsen.org/cgi-bin/iowa/all/home/ index.html

The mission of the Gay, Lesbian and Straight Education Network is to work for safe schools regardless of a person's sexual orientation. The organization was founded by 70 gay and lesbian educators in 1990 as the Gay and Lesbian Independent School Teachers Network (GLSTN). At that point in history, there were two gay-straight alliances in the United States, and only one state with a policy for the protection of lesbian, gay, bisexual, and transgender (LGBT) students. There were also very few opportunities for students to discuss issues of sexual orientation and sexual identity in a formal school setting. The goal of GLSEN has been to change that situation by promoting the creation of gay-straight alliance groups throughout the nation (there are now about 1,300 such clubs) and sponsoring a variety of other activities, such as the promotion of antibullying campaigns and no-name-calling weeks and training of educators in sensitivity issues.
Publications: *The 2007 National School Climate Survey* (report); *The Principal's Perspective* (report); *Involved, Invisible, Ignored: The Experiences of Lesbian, Gay, Bisexual, and Transgender Parents and Their Children in Our Nation's K-12 Schools* (report).

Human Rights Campaign (HRC)
Web Site: http://www.hrc.org/

The Human Rights Campaign was founded in 1980 to work for the civil rights of all gay men and lesbians in the United States. The organization currently claims 700,000 members and calls itself the largest organization of its kind in the country. The organization's Center for the Study of Equality works to improve the general understanding of gay and lesbian issues. HRC has published a number of reports on various aspects of the gay and lesbian rights movement, such as "Transgender Inclusion in the Workplace," "Family Matters," "Equality from State to State: Gay, Lesbian, Bisexual and Transgender Americans and State Legislation," and "Small Business Basics." One of the organization's areas of special concern is Youth and Campus Activism. HRC's Web page for this issue offers articles and news reports, information about state laws on GLBT youth, pending legislation at both federal and state levels, a frequently asked questions section, a place for personal stories from GLBT youth, and a list of HRC resources and publications.

Publications: *GenEQ Newsletter* (for youth); *Resource Guide to Coming Out*; *A Straight Guide to GLBT Americans*; *Coming Out for African Americans*; *Guía de Recursos Para Salir del Clóset*; *Coming Out As Transgender*; *Living Openly in Your Place of Worship*; *Buying for Equality 2008*; *Corporate Equality Index 2008*; *Healthcare Equality Index 2008*.

Matthew Shepard Foundation (MSF)
Web Site: http://www.matthewshepard.org/

The Matthew Shepard Foundation was founded in 1998 by Dennis and Judy Shepard in memory and honor of their son, Matthew, who was murdered by Russell Arthur Henderson and Aaron James McKinney near Laramie, Wyoming. The foundation has three major goals: to eliminate the kind of hate in our society that resulted in Matthew's murder; to work for equal rights for all lesbian, gay, bisexual, and transgendered person (LGBT); and to educate and provide for the needs of young men and women, especially LGBT individuals. In 2007, the foundation launched an online Youth Lounge, providing an opportunity for young people to interact on issues of concern to them.

Publications: Press releases, news announcements, and media resources online.

Parents, Families & Friends of Lesbians & Gays (PFLAG)
Web Site: http://community.pflag.org/

Parents, Families & Friends of Lesbians & Gays is a nonprofit organization of more than 200,000 members and supporters with over 500 chapters in the United States. It operates out of a national office in Washington, D.C., and 13 regional offices. PFLAG has six strategic goals that focus on building an organization strong enough to carry out its objectives; creating a world in which young people can grow up without fear of violence or discrimination; ending the isolation of gay men, lesbians, bisexuals, and transgendered people; working for the inclusion of people of all gender orientations in all religious faiths; eliminating prejudice and discrimination in the workplace; and achieving full civil rights and equality for all gay men, lesbians, bisexuals, and transgendered persons.

Publications: The PFLAG Web site lists a number of press releases, "tools for journalists," "hot topics," and articles about PFLAG in the news.

Sexual Minority Youth Assistance League (SMYAL)
Web site: http://www.smyal.org/

The Sexual Minority Youth Assistance League is a Washington, D.C.-based organization founded in 1984 to provide assistance and information to gay, lesbian, bisexual, transgendered, and questioning (GLBTQ) young men and women. The organization provides a variety of events and activities for GLBTQ youth in the metro D.C. area, including counseling and group support; a youth planning group; youth advocacy internships; HIV testing, counseling, and referrals; discussion meetings and speeches ("Chat It Up!" events); Brotherhood University (HIV/AIDS prevention program); and recreational nights.

Publications: *2006 Annual Report*; *Confronting the Crisis* (report); *SMYAL Literature Review: Risk Factors for LGBTQ Youth* (report).

Utah Pride Center
Web site: http://www.glbtccu.org/

The Utah Pride Center was founded in 1992 as the Utah Stonewall Center to provide a safe space for lesbians, gay men, bisexuals, and transgendered individuals. It was reconstituted in 1997 as the GLBT Community Center of Utah before adopting its current name in 2006 to better express the wider range of its goals and activities. In addition to a very wide range of activities that include support groups, social programs, affinity groups, health and wellness programs, education and training, the center has a very active youth program that includes Tolerant Intelligent Network of Teens (TINT), which provides social and support groups for adolescents of all racial and ethnic backgrounds; Cultural Competency Training for Professionals, for the education and support of teachers, counselors, and other professionals who work with GLBT youth; Resources for Youth, which provides suicide counseling, assistance with housing, and other practical issues for GLBT youth; and Resources for Parents of GLBT Youth, which provides assistance for parents of GLBT youth.

Publications: Annual reports

Youth Guardian Services (YGS)
Web site: http://www.youth-guard.org/

Youth Guardian Services was founded in 1996 by 19-year-old Jason Hungerford, 16-year-old James Miller, and 19-year-old Katherine Lund, some of whom were gay, and others of whom were not, as an online forum through which gay, lesbian, bisexual, transgender, and questioning young women and men could exchange information and questions about their lives and their sexuality. The organization was officially incorporated by the Commonwealth of Virginia on November 5, 1997, as a nonprofit organization. It operates today entirely with private donations. YGS is an entirely online service, providing four major services: the SCHOOLS e-mail list provides a forum aimed at making schools in the United States more GLBTQ friendly; the STR8 email list is aimed at nongay men and nonlesbian women under the age of 25 with interests in and questions about GLBTQ issues; the GLBSO e-mail list provides a means of communication among gay, lesbian, and bisexual student organizations; ELIGHT is an international Web site providing GLBTQ youth with an opportunity to share emotions and feelings about their lives.

Publications: None

Youth Pride
Web site: http://www.youthpride.org/

YouthPride is an Atlanta, Georgia-based 501(c)3 nonprofit organization with the mission of creating positive change in the lives of lesbian, gay, bisexual, transgendered, and questioning youth through education, outreach, support services, community activities, and advocacy. The organization sponsors Safe Zone, a daily after-school program that offers support groups, discussion groups, a print library, Internet resources, HIV testing, movie nights, suicide prevention and counseling, social gatherings, monthly dances, career counseling, job referrals, CITY Academy (a leadership training and empowerment program), and other services for GLBTQ youth.

Publications: None

8

Selected Print and Nonprint Resources

The literature on various aspects of sexual health is extensive, including many books, articles, reports, brochures, fact sheets, Web sites, and other resources. The items listed in this chapter provide a sampling of those resources. The chapter is divided into four major sections: General Resources, Sexually Transmitted Infections, Contraception and Abortion, and Sexual Identity and Sexual Orientation. Each of these sections is divided, in turn, into listings of books, articles, reports, and Web sites. In some cases, there may be overlaps, with a particular item with information on more than one topic. Brief annotations are provided for each item.

General

Books

Basso, Michael J. *The Underground Guide to Teenage Sexuality,* 2nd ed. Minneapolis, MN: Fairview Press, 2003.

This book provides a good, comprehensive discussion of the essential issues that adolescents face with regard to sexuality, with chapters on contraception, abortion, sexually transmitted infections, sexual orientation, date rape, and inappropriate sexual behavior with adults.

Bekaert, Sarah. *Adolescents And Sex: The Handbook for Professionals Working with Young People.* Abingdon, UK: Radcliffe Publishing, 2004.

The author provides a comprehensive review of major sexual health issues with which adolescents have to deal, the role of professionals in educating and assisting them in dealing with these issues, and legal and ethical issues that arise within this practice. The book is written from a British perspective, but provides excellent background information for adolescents and workers of any national background.

Danoff, Dudley Seth. *The Hard Facts: What Every Man (and Woman!) Should Know About Male Sexual Health.* **Los Angeles: Volt Press, 2009.**

The author discusses a wide variety of information about male sexual health which, he suggests, many men avoid discussing with health care professionals, but about which they should be well informed.

Francoeur, Robert T., and Raymond J. Noonan, eds. *The Continuum Complete International Encyclopedia of Sexuality.* **New York and London: The Continuum International Publishing Group, 2004.**

An enormously valuable resource that deals with issues of human sexuality in 63 nations around the world. Although somewhat out-of-date in some respects, the publication has attempted to stay current with special "update" sections on some topics for some countries.

French, Kathy, ed. *Sexual Health.* **New York: Wiley-Blackwell, 2009.**

This book considers a variety of sexual health issues especially for nurses, with chapters on not only the most common sexually transmitted infections, but also clinical issues such as consent and confidentiality and sexual assault and abuse.

Henderson, Elisabeth, and Nancy Armstrong. *100 Questions You'd Never Ask Your Parents.* **Richmond, VA: Uppman Publishing, 2007.**

The authors provide a selection of specific and down-to-earth questions about sexuality, such as whether virgins can contract sexually transmitted infections, how to use a condom, and what a morning-after pill is. The answers are as direct and straightforward as the questions.

Levine, Judith. *Harmful to Minors: The Perils of Protecting Children from Sex.* Minneapolis, MN: University of Minnesota Press, 2002.

The author takes a somewhat difficult position in arguing that sexual relationships between young adults should be viewed as positive experiences that should be treated rationally and without fearmongering. She reviews some approaches to adolescent sexuality that she views as harmful and counterproductive, such as the "panic" over pedophilia, the problem of "no-sex" sex education (abstinence), "compulsory motherhood" (because of the lack of abortion services), and the "expurgation of pleasure." The second part of the book is devoted to the argument that sexual relationships can have enriching and satisfying benefits for young adults.

Murray, Thomas R. *Sex and the American Teenager: Seeing Through the Myths and Confronting the Issues.* Lanham, MD: Rowman and Littlefield, 2009.

The author provides a general overview of the development of adolescent sexuality with special attention to some specific issues with which teenagers have to deal, including sexual abuse, pregnancy, sexually transmitted infections, and gender confusion. He also reviews the status of sex education programs and their effects on adolescent sexual behaviors.

Tepper, Mitchell, and Annette Fuglsang Owens, eds. *Sexual Health.* Westport, CT: Praeger, 2007.

This four-volume collection of essays covers a very broad range of topics in the area of sexual health, ranging from health problems to emotional difficulties to positive aspects of sexuality.

Articles

Bleakley, Amy, Michael Hennessy, and Martin Fishbein. "Public Opinion on Sex Education in US Schools." *Archives of Pediatric and Adolescent Medicine* 160 (11; November 2006): 1151–56.

The authors summarize some of the best information currently available on how the American public views the legitimacy of various topics in sexual health for public school instruction.

Blum, R. W. et al. "The Effects of Race/Ethnicity, Income, and Family Structure on Adolescent Risk Behaviors." *American Journal of Public Health* 90 (12; 2004): 1879–84.

This article is based on the results of the National Longitudinal Study of Adolescent Health (AddHealth), the largest and most comprehensive survey of adolescent health characteristics and trends in the United States. It was initiated in 1994 and continues to the present day as researchers follow up on original participants, who are now in their twenties. This study reviews a number of adolescent risk-behavior characteristics, including cigarette smoking, alcohol use, involvement with violence, suicidal thoughts or attempts, and sexual intercourse.

Chandrasekhar, Cahru A. "Rx for Drugstore Discrimination: Challenging Pharmacy Refusals to Dispense Prescription Contraceptives under State Public Accommodations Laws." *Albany Law Review* 70 (1; Winter 2006): 55–115.

This article considers in great depth one of the most serious issues involving the distribution of contraceptive devices in the United States, namely the reluctance or unwillingness of some pharmacists to fill prescriptions for such materials because they offend their religious or ethical beliefs.

International Journal of Sexual Health. ISSN: 1931-7611 (paper); 1931-762X (electronic).

This publication is the official journal of the World Association for Sexual Health. It is intended primarily for specialists in the field of human sexuality and carries articles on a wide range of issues within the field.

Jones, Rachel K., Jacqueline E. Darroch, and Susheela Singh. "Religious Differentials in the Sexual and Reproductive Behaviors of Young Women in the United States." *Journal of Adolescent Health* 36 (4; 2005): 279–88.

The authors used data from the 1995 National Survey of Family Growth to determine the effects of religious background on the levels of sexual risk to which young women are exposed. Their primary finding was that strong religious affiliations tend to delay the age at which young women begin to engage in sexual behavior, but it has little or no further effects once sexual intercourse has been initiated.

Kennedy, Kristy. "Frankly Speaking: How to Talk to Teens about Sexuality, Abstinence, Appropriate Contraceptive Use and Protection from Sexually Transmitted Infections." *AAP News* 28 (11; November 2007): 1–9.

The author discusses a wide range of issues related to sexual health faced by adolescents, with special attention to a recent policy statement released by the American Academy of Pediatrics in November 2007.

"Sexual and Reproductive Health of Adolescents." *Progress in Reproductive Health Research* 58 (2002): 1–8.

This article reviews some basic issues in adolescent sexual health care around the world, with special features on adolescent boys and unsafe sex in Kenya, sexual coercion among young Nigerians, and sexual behavior and contraceptive use among female migrant workers in China.

Tolman, Deborah L. et al. "Sowing the Seeds of Violence in Heterosexual Relationships: Early Adolescent Narrate Compulsory Heterosexuality." *Journal of Social Issues* 59 (1; January 2003): 159–78.

The authors describe how elements of violence become a part of their earliest romantic relationships because of certain, often unstated but clearly understood, societal expectations, including the role of males as sexual predators.

Tripp, John, and Russell Viner. "Sexual Health, Contraception, and Teenage Pregnancy." *BMJ* 330 (7499; March 12, 2005): 590–93.

The authors provide a very general introduction to important aspects of adolescent sexual health with long-term data on pregnancies, births, and sexually transmitted infections in the United Kingdom.

Tucker, Carolyn et al. "Smart Teens Don't Have Sex (or Kiss Much Either)." *Journal of Adolescent Health* 26 (3; March 2000): 213–25.

The authors make use of data from the National Longitudinal Study of Adolescent Health from approximately 12,000 adolescents enrolled in the 7th to 12th grades to determine the relationship, if any, between intelligence and sexual activity. They find that, when other factors are controlled, adolescents who score higher on intelligence measures tend to be less sexually active than those who score lower on such tests. They conclude that intelligence acts as a "protective factor" against early sexual activity.

Reports

Albert, Bill, Sarah Brown, and Christine M. Flanigan, eds. *14 and Under: The Sexual Behavior of Young Adolescents.* **Washington, DC: The National Campaign to Prevent Teen Pregnancy, 2003.**

This report contains seven papers presented on the subject of sexual activity among young adolescents, specifically, those under the age of 14. A number of interesting trends are noted, such as that nearly one in five adolescents has had sex before her or his 15th birthday; the use of contraceptive devices among young adolescents is low, partly explaining the fact that one in seven sexually active 14-year old girls becomes pregnant; and young adolescents who engage in sexual behavior tend also to be engaged in other forms of risky behavior. A summary of this report is available at http://www.thenationalcampaign.org/resources/pdf/pubs/14summary.pdf, while the full report is available at http://www.eric.ed.gov/ERICDocs/data/ericdocs2sql/content_storage_01/0000019b/80/1b/29/51.pdf.

[Alford, Sue et al.]. *Science And Success: Sex Education and Other Programs That Work to Prevent Teen Pregnancy, HIV & Sexually Transmitted Infections,* **2nd ed. Washington, DC: Advocates for Youth, 2008.**

This report reviews a number of sex education programs across the United States that it deems to have been a success in dealing with teen pregnancy and/or sexually transmitted infections based on their having been published in peer-review journals, using a well-recognized method of evaluation, and having included at least 100 participants. The successful programs are classified in the report as school-based, community-based, or clinic-based programs. The publication contains an impressive amount of very practical information for anyone working with the sexual issues of adolescents.

Grunbaum, Jo Anne et al. "Youth Risk Behavior Surveillance—
United States, 2003." *MMWR* [*Morbidity and Mortality Weekly
Report*] 53 (SS02; May 21, 2004): 1–96.

This report reviews data collected in the Youth Risk Behavior Surveillance System (YRBSS), which monitors six categories of health-
risk behaviors among adolescents, behaviors that contribute to
unintentional injuries and violence. These behaviors include tobacco use; alcohol and other drug use; sexual behaviors that contribute to unintended pregnancy and sexually transmitted diseases
(STDs), including human immunodeficiency virus (HIV) infection;
unhealthy dietary behaviors; and physical inactivity and over-
weight. Examples of data collected on sexual behaviors include the
rate of sexual intercourse before the age of 13, the number of cases
of four or more sexual partners, the use of condoms during intercourse, the use of birth control devices, and rate of pregnancy.

Kaiser Family Foundation. *Sexual Health of Adolescents and
Young Adults in the United States.* Washington, DC: Kaiser
Family Foundation, September 2008.

This publication summarizes the latest statistics on the sexual behavior of adolescents and young adults in a number of areas, including sexually transmitted infections, abortion, pregnancy, use
of contraceptives, and sexual activity.

National Guidelines Task Force. *Guidelines for Comprehensive
Sexuality Education,* 3rd ed. New York: Sexuality Information
and Education Council of the United States.

The Sexuality Information and Education Council of the United
States has produced a set of guidelines that can be used in the
development of sex education programs at any age in primary
and secondary schools. The report is accompanied by a Web site
that lists more than a hundred lesson plans for implementing the
general principles expressed in these guidelines. That Web site is
at http://www.sexedlibrary.org/.

NBC/People Topline Report. *National Survey of Young Teens
Sexual Attitudes and Behaviors.* Princeton, NJ: Princeton Research Associates, January 2005.

This survey consists of a number of similar questions asked of
both parents and their children about patterns of teen sexual

behavior for NBC News and *People* magazine. One of the interesting findings in the survey is that teenagers tend to talk most often (62%) with friends and parents (41%) about sexual matters, and least often with teachers or the school nurse or with religious leaders (12% in both cases).

NPR/Kaiser/Kennedy School Poll. *Sex Education in America: General Public/Parents Survey.* **http://www.kff.org/newsmedia/ upload/Sex-Education-in-America-General-Public-Parents-Survey-Toplines.pdf.**

This poll, completed in 2004, provides probably the most comprehensive review of the attitudes of the American public on the teaching of sex education in American schools, with questions ranging over virtually every aspect of human sexuality.

The Surgeon General's Call to Action to Promote Sexual Health and Responsible Sexual Behavior. **[Washington, DC: U.S. Department of Health and Human Services], July 9, 2001.**

This report was prepared by the office of the U.S. Surgeon General as a device for encouraging a discussion of the present status of sexual health in the United States, some important problems faced by the nation, and some possible solutions for those problems.

Wellings, Kay, and Rachel Parker. *Sexuality Education in Europe: A Reference Guide to Policies and Practices.* **Brussels: IPPF European Network, 2006.**

An excellent overview of the status of policies and practices about sex education in member nations of the European Union.

World Health Organization. *Defining Sexual Health: Report of a Technical Consultation on Sexual Health 28–31 January 2002, Geneva.* **Geneva: World Health Organization, 2006.**

In January 2002, the World Health Organization (WHO) and the World Association of Sexology held a joint conference in Geneva to discuss the state of sexual health in various countries around the world and to determine ways in which WHO could provide guidance to national health managers, policymakers, and care providers to improve the status of sexual health in their countries. This volume summarizes the results of that conference and lists a number of conclusions (recommendations) for future action.

Web Sites

Advocates for Youth. "Adolescent Sexual Behavior." Available at http://www.advocatesforyouth.org/index.php?option=com_content&task=view&id=30&Itemid=59.

This Web site provides one of the most complete and most clearly presented discussions of a host of issues related to adolescent sexual health. It offers dozens of essays on specific topics under three general categories: General Facts about Adolescent Sexual Behavior; Adolescent Sexual Behavior and Youth in Low- and Middle-Income Countries; and Redressing Reproductive and Sexual Health Disparities Among Young People. Examples of specific topics within these categories include Adolescent Pregnancy and Protective Behaviors, Adolescent Protective Behaviors: Abstinence and Contraceptive Use, Adolescent Sexual Behavior: Demographics and Sociopsychological Factors, Facts by State, Facts by Global Region, the Sexual and Reproductive Health of Youth: a Global Snapshot, Giving Up Harmful Practices, Not Culture (Renunciar a Las Prácticas Nocivas, No a La Cultura; Abandonner Les Pratiques Nuisibles et non La Culture), Youth and the Global HIV/AIDS Pandemic (Los Jóvenes Y La Pandemia Global De VIH/SIDA), Youth of Color—at Disproportionate Risk of Negative Sexual Health Outcomes, and GLBTQ Youth.

Centers for Disease Control and Prevention. "Sexual Health." Available at http://www.cdc.gov/sexualhealth/.

This Web site provides extensive and reliable information on a number of topics in sexual health, including sexually transmitted infections, HIV/AIDS prevention and testing, pregnancy and sexual health issues, sexual violence prevention, reproductive health, and preconception health care.

Coalition for Positive Sexuality. "Positive.org." Available at http://www.positive.org/Home/index.html.

This Web site is based on the premise that sexuality is a positive characteristic, but that young people need the best available information to make good judgments about their own sexual behaviors. It contains answers to or thoughts about a number of fundamental questions, such as "Should I have sex?" "What's safe sex and condoms?" "What about birth control?" "What if I'm gay?" "Could I be pregnant?" "What about abortion?" and

"Could I have a disease ("STDs")?" The Web site also provides an interactive section through which individuals can talk with each other online.

Columbia University. Health Promotion Programs. "Go Ask Alice!" Available at http://www.goaskalice.columbia.edu/Cat7. html.

This interactive Web site allows readers to review or pose questions on any aspect of sexual health, including topics such as safer sex, reproduction, contraception, pregnancy options, sexually transmitted infections, men's sexual health, and women's sexual health.

Country Papers. "Youth Sex Education in a Multicultural Europe." http://english.forschung.sexualaufklaerung.de/filead min/fileadmin-forschung/pdf/country_papers_XXX.pdf.

In preparation for a conference on Youth Sex Education in a Multicultural Europe, 16 nations presented reports about the status of various topics in the sex education programs offered in their countries. The Web address above provides access to all these papers, where "XXX" is the name of the country.

Music Television. "It's Your Sex Life." Available at http://www. itsyoursexlife.com/iysl.

This Web site offers four videos dealing with being in control of one's own sexual choices, talking with one's partners about sexual choices, protecting oneself from sexually transmitted infections and unwanted pregnancy, and getting tested for STIs.

Pardini, Priscilla. "The History of Sexuality Education." Available at http://www.rethinkingschools.org/sex/sexhisto.shtml.

The author provides a brief review of the history of sex education in the United States within a broader context of articles dealing with the history of and controversy about abstinence education.

Scarleteen. "Sex Ed for the Real World." Available at http:// www.scarleteen.com/.

This Web site is a very down-to-earth resource with information about sexual issues for teenagers. Some topics included are

"Boyfriend," "Sexual Politics," "Gaydar," "Sexpert Advice," "Skin Deep," and "Crisis Hotline."

"Sexual Health InfoCenter." Available at http://www.sexhealth. org/main.shtml.

The Sexual Health InfoCenter was created in June 1997 by two students at McGill University in Montreál as a way of providing accurate information about sexual topics to users of the Internet. The Web site contains a number of articles on topics such as safer sex, birth control, sexually transmitted infections, sexual problems, and sex and aging.

Teens Health. "Sexual Health." Available at http://kidshealth. org/teen/sexual_health/.

An excellent page from the Web site of the Nemours company that provides information on a range of issues related to sexual health, including "Your Changing Body," "For Girls," "For Boys," "STDs and Other Infections," and "Birth Control." A free weekly newsletter is also available through the Web site.

World Health Organization. "RHL The WHO Reproductive Health Library." Available at http://apps.who.int/rhl/en/.

This Web site contains an extensive array of technical articles reviewing scientific evidence on the safety and efficacy of products for adolescent sexual and reproductive health; fertility regulation; gynecology, infertility, and related cancers; HIV / AIDS; newborn health; pregnancy and childbirth; and sexually transmitted infections.

Sexually Transmitted Infections

Books

Adler, Michael W. *ABC of Sexually Transmitted Infections*, **5th ed. New York: BMJ Books, 2004.**

This book provides a collection of articles on all sexually transmitted infections for professionals in the field, along with additional chapters on procedural and technical issues.

Clutterbuck, Dan. *Specialist Training in Sexually Transmitted Infections and HIV.* Edinburgh and New York: Elsevier Mosby, 2004.

This book is written at a level above that for the general public, but at less than that of a medical professional, especially designed for specialists working in the field of sexually transmitted infections. It includes a number of full-color photographs and useful charts and tables, with a list of references.

Holmes, King et al. *Sexually Transmitted Diseases,* 4th ed. New York: McGraw-Hill Professional, 2007.

This textbook on sexually transmitted infections has been described by one reviewer as "the ultimate reference in this area."

Marr, Lisa. *Sexually Transmitted Diseases: A Physician Tells You What You Need to Know.* Baltimore, MD: Johns Hopkins Press, 2007.

Part 1 of this book includes chapters on some general topics, such as genital anatomy, keys to symptoms, and what to expect from an STI examination. Part 2 is an encyclopedic presentation of the major sexually transmitted infections. The book also contains a glossary and a list of useful references.

World Health Organization. *Guidelines for the Management of Sexually Transmitted Infections.* Geneva: World Health Organization, 2003.

This book may be the most complete resource for all aspects of the medical treatment for sexually transmitted infections. Individual chapters deal with topics such as Treatment of STI-Associated Syndromes; Treatment of Specific Infections; Key Considerations Underlying Treatments; Practical Considerations in STI Case Management; and Children, Adolescents, and Sexually Transmitted Infections. The information in the book evolved out of two meetings sponsored by the World Health Organization on sexually transmitted infections in 1999 and 2001.

World Health Organization. *Sexually Transmitted Infections: Briefing Kit for Teachers.* Manila: World Health Organization, Regional Office for the Western Pacific, 2001.

This publication is a superb guide to educating young people about sexually transmitted infections. Individual sections deal with topics such as Understanding Sexually Transmitted Infections, STI Education, Understanding Young People's Behavior, and Teaching STI Prevention. The annex to the publication contains references to a number of other educational resources from WHO and other sources.

Yancey, Diane. *STDs: What You Don't Know Can Hurt You.* **Minneapolis, MN: Twenty-First Century Books, 2002.**

This book provides a straightforward presentation of factual information about the major sexually transmitted infections for adolescents.

Articles

Bearman, Peter S., James Moody, and Katherine Stovel. "Chains of Affection: The Structure of Adolescent Romantic and Sexual Networks." *American Journal of Sociology* **110 (1; 2004): 44–91.**

This very interesting paper traces the structure of sexual networks among 800 adolescents in a mid-size city in the Midwest United States in an effort to better understand how sexually transmitted infections are spread within such a network.

Brückner, Hannah, and Peter Bearman. "After the Promise: The STD Consequences of Adolescent Virginity Pledges." *Journal of Adolescent Health* **36 (2005): 271–78.**

The authors discover that young adults who take virginity pledges as teenagers tend to marry later, have fewer sex partners, and start having sex later, but have about the same rate of infections from sexually transmitted diseases as do their counterparts who have not taken the pledge. The authors attempt to explain this unexpected phenomenon. This article later became the focus of a number of attacks by pro-abstinence groups and individuals who found a number of methodological problems with the Brückner-Bearman research. See, for example, Robert Rector and Kirk A. Johnson, "Adolescent Virginity Pledges and Risky Sexual Behaviors," online at http://www.heritage.org/research/abstinence/whitepaper06142005-2.cfm.

Halpern, Carolyn Tucker et al. "Implications of Racial and Gender Differences in Patterns of Adolescent Risk Behavior for HIV and Other Sexually Transmitted Diseases." *Perspectives on Sexual and Reproductive Health* 36 (6; 2004): 239–47.

The authors of this study use data from the National Longitudinal Study of Adolescent Health to group 13,998 non-Hispanic black and white participants into categories with the highest degree of risk for sexually transmitted infections. They found that 47 percent of their sample was classified in the lowest risk group, consisting of those who were abstinent and did not use illegal drugs. One interesting finding was that black females tended to be in the lowest risk groups, but reported the highest rate of sexually transmitted infections.

Low, Nicola et al. "Global Control of Sexually Transmitted Infections." *Lancet* 368 (9551; December 2, 2006): 2001–06.

The authors note that sexually transmitted infections are a serious global health problem, but that they tend to receive relatively little attention from public health officials. They explore the reasons for this failing and suggest a number of steps that can be taken to make prevention of and treatment for STIs more readily available to a much wider range of the world's population.

Rothschild, Bruce M. "History of Syphilis." *Clinical Infectious Diseases* 40 (10; May 2005): 1454–63.

Until the rise of the AIDS pandemic in the 1980s, syphilis was probably the most feared of all sexually transmitted infections. This paper provides an excellent review of the history of the disease in Western civilization.

Sexually Transmitted Diseases, **journal of the American Sexually Transmitted Diseases Association. http://www.stdjournal. com/pt/re/std/home.htm;jsessionid=J7JQFGL3h0mTpZxsGhXJ JyLbh3tGyQvR1xNT2j12wgn7hN7wC9rn!928310026!181195629 !8091!-1.**

Sinding, Steven W. "Does 'CNN' (Condoms, Needles and Negotiation) Work Better than 'ABC' (Abstinence, Being Faithful and Condom Use) in Attacking the AIDS Epidemic?" *International Family Planning Perspectives* 31 (1; March 2005): 38–40.

The author assesses the relative merits of two approaches to dealing with the HIV/AIDS epidemic in Africa, and concludes that both approaches have their values and should probably be used in conjunction with each other.

U.S. Preventive Services Task Force. "Behavioral Counseling to Prevent Sexually Transmitted Infections: U.S. Preventive Services Task Force Recommendation Statement." *Annals of Internal Medicine* 149 (7; October 7, 2008): 491–96, W95.

The U.S. Preventive Services Task Force is an agency of the Agency for Healthcare Research and Quality of the U.S. Department of Health and Human Services, whose purpose is to assess the scientific information available on a variety of health care issues. This report discusses the need for and effectiveness of counseling for adolescents and adults about the risks posed by sexual behaviors that lead to sexually transmitted infections. The main recommendation made by the task force is that programs of counseling for such purposes should be readily available to the public in general and, in particular, to adolescents.

Reports

Dehne, Karl L., and Gabriele Riedner. *Sexually Transmitted Infections among Adolescents: The Need for Adequate Health Services.* **Geneva: Department of Child and Adolescent Health Development. World Health Organization, 2005.**

This report examined the status of sexually transmitted infection services for adolescents around the world. It discusses barriers to providing young adults with the information and services needed for dealing with STIs, some programs that have been developed to deal with these problems, and some ways of measuring the success of such programs. The specific questions addressed in the review were: "What characterizes adolescent sexuality and risk for STIs?" "What data exist on the risk and prevalence of STIs in adolescents?" "What kinds of adolescent sexual and reproductive health services are available generally and, in particular, for treatment of STIs?" "What evidence is there that current programmes and programme approaches for delivering STI services are successful in reaching adolescents who need those services?" and "To what extent is an adolescent-specific approach to STI services warranted, and to what extent is an STI-specific approach to adolescent health services warranted?" The authors make a number of recommendations for improving the accessibility of STI services for young adults throughout the world.

Division of STD Prevention. *Sexually Transmitted Disease Surveillance 2007.* **Atlanta, GA: Department of Health And Human Services. Centers for Disease Control and Prevention. National Center for HIV/AIDS, Viral Hepatitis, STD, and TB Prevention. Division of STD Prevention, December 2008.**

This annual publication provides probably the most exhaustive and detailed selection of statistics dealing with sexually transmitted infections in the United States. It focuses on the three traditional STIs of interest, chlamydia, syphilis, and gonorrhea, as well as a number of other infections, such as herpes, hepatitis, and pelvic inflammatory disease.

[Hawkes, Sarah]. *Prevention and Treatment of HIV and Other Sexually Transmitted Infections among Men Who Have Sex with Men and Transgender Populations.* **Geneva: World Health Organization, 2009.**

This report summarizes the findings of a technical consultation held in Geneva on September 15–17, 2008, on the role that health agencies can play in dealing with the growing public health problem of the transmission of HIV among men who have sex with other men and transgendered individuals, with special attention to means by which such transmissions can be prevented.

Kirby, Douglas, B. A. Laris, and Lori Rolleri. *Impact of Sex and HIV Education Programs on Sexual Behaviors of Youth in Developing and Developed Countries.* **Youth Research Working Paper No. 2. Research Triangle Park, NC: Family Health International, 2005.**

This report provides a superb overview of the effectiveness of various types of sex education programs on behaviors of students who have been enrolled in those programs.

Sexually Transmitted Diseases and Substance Use. **Washington, DC: Office of Applied Studies. Substance Abuse and Mental Health Services Administration. U.S. Department of Health & Human Services, March 30, 2007.**

This report summarizes the most recent information collected in the National Survey on Drug Use and Health, with special attention to the relationship of STDs and drug use. The study found that STDs are more common among adolescents who use alcohol or illegal drugs.

Sexually Transmitted Infection—The Silent Menace. **New York: Datamonitor, November 2005.**

This publication offers a general overview to the status of sexually transmitted infections and then devotes a separate chapter each to gonorrhea, syphilis, chlamydia, genital herpes, and genital warts. In each case, the presentation includes information about the etiology and epidemiology of the disease, diagnosis, disease management, and new methods available for treatment.

2008 Report on the Global AIDS Epidemic. **Geneva: UNAIDS, 2008.**

This report provides the most recent data available on the status of the worldwide HIV/AIDS epidemic with charts and tables on almost every conceivable aspect of the disease.

UNAIDS. "Country Progress Indicators." *2008 Report on the Global AIDS Epidemic.* **http://data.unaids.org/pub/GlobalReport/2008/jc1510_2008_global_report_pp235_324_en.pdf.**

The United Nations agency primarily responsible for issues related to the HIV/AIDS pandemic, UNAIDS, provides in this report updated information on the status of the disease in almost every nation of the world.

Workowski, Kimberly A., and Stuart M. Berman. "Sexually Transmitted Diseases Treatment Guidelines, 2006." *MMWR* **[***Morbidity and Mortality Weekly Report***] 51 (RR06; May 10, 2006): 1–80.**

This article summarizes the best information currently available on the treatment of all common sexually transmitted infections, with recommendations for prevention, follow-up and treatment of partners, and management of each condition. This publication is generally considered to be the authoritative resource in the United States for current procedures in the treatment and management of STIs.

Web Sites

About.com. "Sexually Transmitted Diseases STDs." Available at http://parentingteens.about.com/cs/stds/a/stdsfact.htm.

A very comprehensive Web site that contains detailed information on most common sexually transmitted infections. Also included are articles on teenage sexuality, statistics on STIs, body image, parenting classes on building self-esteem, and screening quizzes for parents.

American Social Health Association. "STD/STI Statistics > Fast Facts." Available at http://www.ashastd.org/learn/learn_statistics.cfm.

An excellent summary of some fundamental factual information about sexually transmitted infections, with a number of valuable resources from which the data are taken.

Centers for Disease Control. "National Prevention Information Network." Available at http://www.cdcnpin.org/.

This Web site is the Centers for Disease Control's central source of information on all aspects of sexually transmitted infections, tuberculosis, and related conditions and issues. The Web site contains information on organizations, materials, news, conferences, funding, HIV testing sites, statistics, campaigns and initiatives, electronic mailing lists, and links to related sites.

Condyloma.org. "Complete Disease Information Site." Available at http://www.condyloma.org/main.html.

Condyloma is a wart-like growth in the genital area caused by the human papillomavirus (HPV). This Web site provides an extensive array of information on all aspects of genital and venereal warts caused by the HPV. It provides images of various manifestations of the condition, news of recent developments, and information on research and treatments for the condition.

eMedTV. "About STD." Available at http://std.emedtv.com/.

This Web site provides basic scientific information on common sexually transmitted infections, including chlamydia, gonorrhea, syphilis, HIV/AIDS, and HPV infections. It also reviews a number of medications used in the treatment of these conditions. Other portions of the Web site discuss a host of other issues related to sexual health, including contraception and general sexual health.

FamilyDoctor.org. "STIs: Common Symptoms & Tips on Prevention." Available at http://familydoctor.org/online/famdocen/ home/common/sexinfections/sti/165.html.

This Web site provides a good general introduction to the subject of sexually transmitted infections, with sections on signs and symptoms, risk factors, diagnosis, prevention, and additional resources on STIs.

Guttmacher Institute. "State Policies in Brief as of June 1, 2009: Sex and STI/HIV Education." Available at http://www.gutt macher.org/statecenter/spibs/spib_SE.pdf.

The Guttmacher Institute provides a thorough review of state policies on educational programs for sexually transmitted infections, current as of June 1, 2009.

Patient UK. "Sexually Transmitted Disease (STD)." Available at http://www.patient.co.uk/showdoc/40000397/.

This Web page is intended for physicians and other health care professionals involved in the treatment of sexually transmitted infections, but its language is clear and understandable for the layperson. The information is exhaustive and complete with an excellent and extensive list of links and other resources on the topic.

Teens Health. "About Sexually Transmitted Diseases (STDs)." Available at http://kidshealth.org/teen/sexual_health/stds/std. html#.

In addition to a general overview of the subject of sexually transmitted diseases, this Web site provides detailed and easily understandable information on specific conditions: chlamydia, genital herpes, genital warts, gonorrhea, hepatitis B, HIV and AIDS, pelvic inflammatory disease, pubic lice (crabs), syphilis, and trichomoniasis, The Web site is also available in Spanish.

womenshealth.gov. "Sexually Transmitted Diseases. Overview." Available at http://www.womenshealth.gov/FAQ/sexually-transmitted-infections.cfm.

This Web site is maintained by the National Women's Health Information Center of the U.S. Department of Health and Human Services to provide health information of special interest to women. In addition to providing information about 10 sexually transmitted infections, the Web site contains sections on statistics, means of transmission, symptoms, testing, health problems related to STDs, treatment, pregnancy and STDs, breastfeeding and STDs, and further information on the topic.

Contraception and Abortion

Books

Connell, Elizabeth B. *The Contraception Sourcebook*. Chicago, IL: Contemporary Books, 2002.

This book provides an exhaustive review of the topic of contraception, with sections on the history of contraceptive technologies, oral contraceptives, contraceptive implants, injectable contraceptives, intrauterine devices, female barrier devices, periodic abstinence, lactational amenorrhea, male contraception, the current status of contraception, and future prospects in contraceptive technology. A superb overview of the topic.

Gordon, Linda. *The Moral Property of Women: A History of Birth Control Politics in America*, 3rd ed. Urbana and Chicago, IL: University of Illinois Press, 2002.

The author points out that, while birth control technology has a very long history, it has become an issue of women's rights only in the recent past. She discusses the role of contraception in the development of the women's movement in the United States.

Guillebaud, John. *Contraception: Your Questions Answered*. Edinburgh and New York: Churchill Livingstone, 2008.

This book makes use of an interesting format, with questions posed by general practitioners and answered by specialists in the field of contraception. In spite of this specialist approach, the text should be understandable to most readers with some scientific background.

Hatcher, Robert A. et al. *Contraceptive Technology,* 19th ed. Montvale, NJ: Thomson Reuters, 2008.

This book, designed for specialists in the field, has long been a standard work and is now in its 19th edition. The authors cover almost every conceivable issue related to contraceptive technology, providing the most up-to-date information available on each topic.

Jütte, Robert. *Contraception: A History.* Cambridge, UK, and Malden, MA: Polity Press, 2008.

The author provides a very interesting and very readable account of the use of contraceptives from the earliest days of human civilization, along with a brief consideration of the future of contraceptive technology.

Kubba, Ali. *Contraception.* London: Mosby, 2005.

This book is part of Elsevier's Rapid Reference series that makes general information about a topic readily available to practitioners or anyone else interested in a topic. It includes basic information about epidemiology, management, and therapy, along with useful ancillary information, such as drug listings, clinical trials, possible future developments, patient organizations, and Web site listing. A list of frequently asked questions is also available.

Senanayake, I. Pramilla, and Malcolm Potts. *Atlas of Contraception,* 2nd ed. London: Informa Healthcare, 2008.

This book makes use of about 150 full-color photographs and sketches to illustrate a number of topics related to contraception, including contraceptive methods, family planning and practice methods, contraceptive counseling, reproductive health issues, and preventative medicines.

United States Agency for International Development. Office of Population and Reproductive Health; World Health Organization. Reproductive Health and Research; INFO Project. *Family Planning: A Global Handbook for Providers.* Baltimore, MD: Johns Hopkins University. Bloomberg School of Public Health. Center for Communication Programs. INFO Project; [Geneva]: World Health Organization. Department of Reproductive Health and Research, 2007.

This book is the definitive guideline for clinic-based health care providers around the world who are responsible for dispensing contraceptive information and materials.

Articles

Contraception is an international journal that carries technical articles on the topic and is published monthly. Its ISSN is 0010-7824. *Population Reports* is a group of journals published by the Population Information Program at Johns Hopkins University. The 10 journals in the series deal with oral contraceptives (Series A; ISSN: 0097-9074), intrauterine devices (Series B; ISSN: 0092-9344), female sterilization (Series C; ISSN: 0891-0030), pregnancy termination (Series D; ISSN: 0091-9284), barrier methods (Series H; ISSN: 0093-4496), maximizing access and quality (Series Q: ISSN: 0887-0241), family planning programs (Series J; ISSN: 0091-925X), injectables and implants (Series K; ISSN: 0097-9104), issues in world health (Series L; ISSN: 0887-0241), and special topics (Series M; ISSN: 0733-9135).

Blythe, Margaret J., and Angela Diaz. "Contraception and Adolescents." *Pediatrics* 120 (5; November 2007): 1135–48.

This article presents the position of the American Academy of Pediatrics Committee on Adolescence with regard to the use of contraceptives by adolescents. The authors note that abstinence is always the first choice in dealing with sexual behavior, but that, realistically, the vast majority of adolescents do not remain abstinent until they become adults or are married. As a consequence, the committee recommends that pediatricians and other professional health care workers become familiar with the best information on contraceptive technology and the counseling methods available for making this information accessible to adolescents.

Espey, Eve, and William F. Rayburn, eds. "Contraception." *Obstetrics and Gynecology Clinics of North America* 34 (1; 2007): 1–172.

The whole issue of this journal is devoted to a discussion of a variety of contraceptive devices that have been developed in recent years, such as the contraceptive patch and ring, hormonal implants, and hormonal intrauterine systems. Nonmedical issues, such as current legislation, regulations, and funding options related to the use of contraceptives are also discussed.

Ramos, Pilar S. "The Condom Controversy in the Public Schools: Respecting a Minor's Right of Privacy." *University of Pennsylvania Law Review* 145 (1; November): 149–92.

This law article examines in great detail the legal and ethical issues involved in school programs for the distribution of condoms.

Reddy, Diane M., Raymond Fleming, and Carolyne Swain. "Effect of Mandatory Parental Notification on Adolescent Girls' Use of Sexual Health Care Services" *JAMA* 288 (6; August 14, 2002): 710–14.

The authors report on a survey of 950 teenage girls at 33 Planned Parenthood clinics in Wisconsin to determine the possible effects of a law requiring parents to be notified that their daughters sought sexual health services. Fifty-nine percent of respondents said that they would not make use of at least one or more of such services, and an additional 11 percent indicated that they would delay or discontinue testing for sexually transmitted infections. The authors conclude that "mandatory parental notification for prescribed contraceptives would impede girls' use of sexual health care services, potentially increasing teen pregnancies and the spread of STDs."

Santelli, John et al. "Abstinence and Abstinence-only Education: a Review of U.S. Policies and Programs." *Journal of Adolescent Health* 38 (2006): 72–81.

The authors agree that abstinence is a desirable behavioral objective for adolescents, but that few people remain abstinent until they are married. The recent emphasis by the U.S. government on abstinence programs has undermined more comprehensive sex education programs and, for that reason, threatens "fundamental human rights to health, information, and life."

Society for Adolescent Medicine. "Position Paper on Abstinence-only Education Policies and Programs: A Position Paper of the Society of Adolescent Medicine." *Journal of Adolescent Health* 38 (2006): 83–87.

The Society of Adolescent Medicine commends the intent of abstinence-only education, but points out that a well-rounded program in sex education should also provide information on other forms of contraception.

Reports

Abma, J. C., G. M. Martinez, W. D. Mosher, and B. S. Dawson. *Teenagers in the United States: Sexual Activity, Contraceptive Use, and Childbearing, 2002.* National Center for Health Statistics. *Vital Health Statistics* 23 (24; 2004).

This report summarizes and discusses national data on sexual activity, contraceptive use, and births among males and females 15–19 years of age in the United States in 2002 collected in the National Survey of Family Growth (NSFG). Data are also presented from the 1988 and 1995 NSFGs, and from the 1988 and 1995 National Survey of Adolescent Males (NSAM). The report contains a vast amount of information on nearly every aspect of these issues and is an invaluable resource on the subject.

Guttmacher Institute. *U.S. Teenage Pregnancy Statistics National and State Trends and Trends by Race and Ethnicity.* New York: Guttmacher Institute, 2006.

This report provides some of the best, most complete information on nearly every aspect of teenage pregnancy, including national and state trends for teenage abortions, births, and pregnancies by age, race, and ethnicity.

Nass, Sharyl J., and Jerome F. Strauss III, eds. *New Frontiers in Contraceptive Research: A Blueprint for Action.* Washington, DC: National Academies Press, 2004.

This report reviews recent events in research on and development of contraceptive technologies. The four major chapters deal with target discovery and validation, product identification and development, improving accessibility to and use of contraceptives, and capitalizing on recent scientific achievements. Of particular interest is Appendix A, which discusses progress and impediments in research and development of new contraceptive technologies.

Pro-Choice Public Education Project. *She Speaks: African American and Latino Young Women on Reproductive Health and Rights: Focus Group Research Commissioned by the Pro-Choice*

Public Education Project. **New York: Pro-Choice Public Education Project, 2004.**

Between January and June 2004, researchers for Pro-Choice Public Education Project met with eight focus groups of African American and Latino women ages 16–25 in New Orleans, Louisiana; Los Angeles, California; West Palm Beach, Florida; and New York, New York, to listen to their "thoughts, opinions, feelings, struggles, and experiences" about issues of their reproductive health. This report summarizes the results of those interviews and is available online at http://www.protectchoice.org/downloads/She%20Speaks%20Report%20Full.pdf.

Ross, David A., Bruce Dick, and Jane Ferguson. *Preventing HIV/AIDS in Young People. A Systematic Review of the Evidence from Developing Countries.* **UNAIDS Inter-agency Task Team on Young People. Geneva, Switzerland: World Health Organization. WHO Technical Report Series No. 938, 2006.**

This report summarizes research on methods that have been developed to reduce the rate of HIV/AIDS infection among young people in a number of countries around the world and the effectiveness of those programs.

Special Investigations Division. Minority Staff of the Committee on Government Reform. *The Content of Federally Funded Abstinence-only Education Programs.* **[n.p.], December 2004.**

At the request of Representative Henry Waxman (D-CA), the Special Investigations Division of the Minority Staff of the U.S. House of Representatives Committee on Government Reform assessed the accuracy of information of sexual health provided by a number of abstinence-only sex education programs funded by the U.S. government.

World Health Organization. *Selected Practice Recommendations for Contraceptive Use,* **2nd ed. Geneva: World Health Organization, 2005.**

The recommendations in this reported were developed at a meeting of experts on contraceptive technology held in Geneva on April 13–16, 2004. It covers a variety of issues, including family planning methods: combined oral contraceptives, combined injectable contraceptives, progestogen-only pills, depot medroxyprogesterone acetate, norethisterone enanthate, levonorgestrel implants, emergency contraceptive pills, copper-bearing intrauterine devices, levonorgestrel-releasing intrauterine devices, fertility awareness-based methods, and sterilization. The report is intended for use by policymakers, program managers, and the scientific community for the purpose of preparing service delivery guidelines for women in specific countries.

Web Sites

AVERT. "Birth Control and Contraception for Teenagers." Available at http://www.avert.org/birth-control-contraception.htm.

AVERT is an international organization working to reduce rates of HIV infection and AIDS cases worldwide. Its Web site provides information on a variety of issues related to sexual health, including this page on pregnancy and contraception. The information provided here is up-to-date and clearly written, easily understandable by the target audience of sexually active or curious teenagers.

Barnack, Jessica L. "Improving Access to Emergency Contraception for Female Adolescents." Available at http://www.prochoiceforum.org.uk/psy_research8.asp.

This article appears on the "Psychological Issues" section of the Pro-Choice Forum Web site of Psychology and Reproductive Choice. The author reviews the scientific evidence about the safety and efficacy of emergency contraception and finds that it does not lead to increased sexual activity by minor females nor does it affect the use of conventional contraceptives by members of that group. She also discusses the current legal and regulatory status of emergency contraceptives in the United States.

Bovo, Mary Jane. "Contraceptive Guide." Available at http://www.mjbovo.com/Contracept/.

This Web site provides a very exhaustive review of many types of contraceptive devices and methods, including topics such as abstinence, the cervical cap, condoms, the diaphragm, emergency contraception, implants, injections, intrauterine devices, The Pill, natural family planning, safer sex, sexually transmitted infections, spermicides, the sponge, sterilization, and what doesn't work.

The topics are very well illustrated with helpful line drawings and written at a level readily accessible to most adolescents.

Center for Reproductive Rights. "Adolescents' Access to Reproductive Health Services and Information." Available at http://reproductiverights.org/en/project/adolescents-access-to-reproductive-health-services-and-information.

The Center for Reproductive Rights provides information on obstacles faced by adolescent boys and girls in obtaining information about and services in the area of reproduction. The primary focus in this article is on legislation and laws requiring parental notification before a female minor can have an abortion. Links to two important court cases on this issue are available from the main Web site.

Centers for Disease Control and Prevention. "Unintended Pregnancy Prevention: Contraception." Available at http://www.cdc.gov/ReproductiveHealth/UnintendedPregnancy/Contraception.htm.

The Centers for Disease Control and Prevention provides here one of the most complete and dependable sources of information about all forms of contraception.

The Emergency Contraception Web site. "Plan B and the Bush Administration." http://ec.princeton.edu/pills/planbhistory.html.

This Web site provides a good review of the history of the development and certification of Plan B emergency contraceptive by the U.S. Food and Drug Administration, and the issues raised by the decision of the Bush administration to become involved in this decision.

Helium. "Should Schools Give Teens Birth Control?" http://www.helium.com/debates/161091-should-schools-give-teens-birth-control.

This blog provides an opportunity for teenagers and adults to express their views about the distribution of contraceptive devices by schools. The statements are generally well thought out and expressed.

Mayo Clinic Staff. "Birth Control Guide." Available at http://www.mayoclinic.com/health/birth-control/BI99999.

This very useful and complete review of birth control techniques is divided into sections dealing with condoms and other barrier methods, The Pill and other hormonal contraceptives, intrauterine devices, natural family planning, sterilization, withdrawal, emergency contraceptive techniques, and emergency methods. This Web site also has links to more than 50 related sexual health issues on the Mayo site, including birth control pill FAQs, benefits, risks and choices; women's sexual health: how to reach sexual fulfillment; emergency birth control; Viagra for women: why doesn't it exist?; sex after years of abstinence: OK to resume?; vaginal ring; withdrawal birth control method; essure; standard days birth control method; lactational amenorrhea birth control method; emerging birth control methods; and skin patch for birth control.

National Women's Health Resource Center. "Contraception." Available at http://www.healthywomen.org/healthtopics/con traception.

This Web site provides one of the most exhaustive discussions of a variety of contraceptive technologies on the Internet, with detailed discussions of benefits, risks, possible side effects, and additional information on the most widely used methods of birth control. A valuable chart of the rate of effectiveness for each technique is also supplied.

nelsmiley. "Abstinence Only Sex Education." Available at http:// nelsmiley.deviantart.com/art/Abstinence-Only-Sex-Education-71481378.

An excellent overview and review of the legislative and administrative history for federal funding of abstinence-only sex education in the United States.

New York Times. **"Birth Control and Family Planning." Available at http://health.nytimes.com/health/guides/specialtopic/ birth-control-and-family-planning/in-depth-report.html.**

This Web page is part of the *New York Times* Health Guide, which provides detailed, reliable information on dozens of health topics. This site discusses a number of contraceptive options, including implant contraception, injected contraception, intrauterine devices, fertility awareness methods, spermicidal and barrier contraception, emergency contraception, and female sterilization. A number of up-to-date print references are also provided.

"No Room for Contraception." Available at http://www.noroom-forcontraception.com/.

The purpose of this Web site is "to expose the potential harms that contraception, birth control and sterilization bring to marriage and society." It provides information from its point of view about pregnancy, abstinence, abortion, and contraception, with special commentaries on the role of religion and issues faced by adolescents with regard to these topics. The Web site is updated on a regular basis with new information, testimonies, and news reports. A brochure, *Pregnancy, Contraception, and Abortion: Frequently Asked Questions*, is available online.

Office of Population Research. Princeton University. "The Emergency Contraception Website." Available at http://ec.princeton. edu/.

The purpose of the Emergency Contraception Website is to provide women with accurate scientific information about emergency contraception, to provide a database of service providers for individuals seeking access to emergency contraceptive materials, to provide a database of existing emergency contraceptive materials, and to serve as a resource for clinicians, pharmacists, researchers, members of the media, policymakers, and others seeking up-to-date scientifically based information about emergency contraception.

Samra-Latif, Omnia M., and Ellen Wood. "Contraception." Available at http://emedicine.medscape.com/article/258507-over view.

This page is part of the WebMD Web site emedicine, which provides detailed, expert information on a very large number of medical topics. This article deals with a number of topics, ranging from coitus interruptus and mechanical barriers to sterilization and emergency postcoital contraception. For each topic, the authors discuss the efficacy, advantages, and disadvantages of each technique.

"Should Schools Give Teens Birth Control?" Available at http:// www.helium.com/debates/161091-should-schools-give-teens-birth-control/side_by_side?page=4.

This blog does an unusually good job of presenting pro and con arguments with respect to the distribution of birth control information and devices in schools. Each argument in favor or opposed to the practice is matched with a contrary view. Most of the opinions are well reasoned and well written.

U.S. Food and Drug Administration. "Birth Control Guide." Available at http://www.fda.gov/Fdac/features/1997/babytabl. html.

This Web site was originally published in *FDA Consumer* magazine in April 1997, but it has been revised and updated since that time, most recently in December 2003. The page lists all methods of birth control that have been approved by the FDA, their failure rate, associated risks, convenience, availability with or without prescription, and their effectiveness against sexually transmitted infections.

Sexual Identity and Sexual Orientation

Books

Girshick, Lori B. *Transgender Voices: Beyond Women and Men.* Lebanon, NH: UPNE, 2009.

This book draws on interviews with more than 150 sex- and gender-variant individuals in the United States. Those interviews provide some of the greatest dramatic and emotional impact for the book. With the information gained from these interviews, the author attempts a reconsideration of gender theory and suggests that new approaches be developed for working with youth who are experiencing nontraditional sexual awakenings.

Huegel, Kelly. *GLBTQ: The Survival Guide for Queer and Questioning Teens.* Minneapolis, MN: Free Spirit Publishing, 2003.

This book begins with a review of some basic issues, such as the meaning of terms like *gay, lesbian, queer,* and *questioning,* and stereotypes about GLBTQ youth; homophobia, the process of coming out; life at school; dating and relationships; sex, sexuality, and sexual health; religion and culture; and transgender teens. The author attempts to answer questions about these topics both for GLBTQ themselves as well as for young adults who classify themselves as heterosexual.

Jennings, Kevin, and Pat Shapiro. *Always My Child: A Parent's Guide to Understanding Your Gay, Lesbian, Bisexual,*

Transgendered or Questioning Son or Daughter. New York: Simon & Schuster, 2003.

This book provides a comprehensive and valuable resource for parents with gay, lesbian, bisexual, transgender, or questioning teenagers. It provides fundamental information about the development of sexual orientation, the social and family issues with which adolescents have to deal, and the ways in which parents can support their children. Later chapters deal with transgendered and questioning teens, and with teens of color who may be GLBTQ.

Just the Facts Coalition. *Just the Facts about Sexual Orientation and Youth: A Primer for Principals, Educators, and School Personnel.* **Washington, DC: American Psychological Association, 2008.**

This publication is endorsed by 12 groups, the American Academy of Pediatrics, American Association of School Administrators, American Counseling Association, American Federation of Teachers, American Psychological Association, American School Counselor Association, American School Health Association, Interfaith Alliance Foundation, National Association of School Psychologists, National Association of Secondary School Principals, National Association of Social Workers, National Education Association, and School Social Work Association of America. It deals with the development of sexual orientation, efforts to change sexual orientation through therapy and religious ministries, and legal principles relevant to the subject. The book concludes with a description of the 12 members of the Just the Facts Coalition, along with the resources they have to offer in dealing with this topic.

Levithan, David, and Billy Merrell. *The Full Spectrum: A New Generation of Writing About Gay, Lesbian, Bisexual, Transgender, Questioning, and Other Identities.* **New York: Knopf Books for Young Readers, 2006.**

This book consists of 40 selections written by young women and men under the age of 23 in conjunction with the Gay, Lesbian, and Straight Network describing their own experiences growing up as nonstraight youth. The selections include autobiographical sketches, poems, and written and photographic essays.

Marcus, Eric. *Is It a Choice? Answers to the Most Frequently Asked Questions about Gay & Lesbian People,* 3rd rev. ed. San Francisco: HarperOne Publishing, 2005.

In spite of what the title may suggest, the development of sexual orientation is only one of many questions answered by the author in this book. Other questions deal with families, dating and relationships, sexual behaviors, religion, work and the military, education, sports, the media, politics and activism, and aging.

Ryan, Caitlin, and Donna Futterman. *Lesbian & Gay Youth : Care & Counseling.* New York: Columbia University Press, 1998.

This book grew out of a conference on the primary health care and prevention needs of lesbian, gay, and bisexual youth sponsored by the Health Resources and Services Administration of the U.S. Department of Health and Human Services. It deals with the special physical and mental health challenges faced by lesbian, gay, and bisexual youth; the HIV/AIDS epidemic and its effects on young people; transgendered youth and other special populations; and the development of gender identity.

Savin-Williams, Ritch C. *The New Gay Teenager.* Cambridge, MA: Harvard University Press, 2006.

Based on interviews with numerous adolescents, the author concludes that young people today have a very different view about same-sex relationships than do their parents or grandparents. They tend to be much more at ease with a variety of sexual issues, sexual orientation among them. The author devotes considerable attention to methodological problems that were developed more than a generation ago in studying gay and lesbian adolescents and recommends some changes in the way professionals view these individuals.

Articles

Barber, Heather, and Vikki Krane. "Creating a Positive Climate for Lesbian, Gay, Bisexual, and Transgender Youths." *JOPERD: Journal of Physical Education, Recreation & Dance* 78 (7; September 2007): 6–8.

The authors point out that a number of athletes notable in their own fields of sports have recently come out to the general public.

They argue that adult teachers, leaders, and others responsible for sports activities for adolescents need to be more open and more welcoming to young men and women who classify themselves as nontraditionally sexually oriented.

Graham, Chad. "Milwaukee's Finest: One Lesbian Teacher's Vision of a Safe Place for LGBT High School Students Is a Reality for 107 Kids in Wisconsin—for Now at Least." *The Advocate* 965 (June 20, 2006): 62.

In response to the harassment experienced by GLBT students in many schools, some efforts have been made to establish schools intended solely for this population. This article describes the development of such a school in Milwaukee, Wisconsin, and some of the problems it has experienced in trying to stay in business.

Lehoczky, Etelka. "Young, Gay, and OK: Cultural Shifts and Supportive Parents Are Leading Gay Youths to Come out Earlier, Some Before Their Teens." *The Advocate* 931 (February 1, 2005): 24–31.

The author points out that young people who consider themselves to be gay, lesbian, bisexual, or transgender are now coming out at an earlier age than ever before, largely but not entirely because of a more welcoming and positive attitude by parents, teachers, other gay men and lesbians, and the society at large.

Rienzo, Barbara A. "The Politics of Sexual Orientation Issues in American Schools." *Journal of School Health* 76 (3; March 2006): 93–97.

The authors point out that schools in the United States are under greater pressure at a local level to recognize and meet the special needs of lesbian, gay, bisexual, and transgender youth, but the national mood in the first years of the 21st century has made programs with this objective politically sensitive. They report on a study of public school districts across the United States to see how well they are managing these conflicting demands and make recommendations as to how this issue can be handled in the future.

Rosario, Vernon A. "Transgenderism Comes of Age." *Gay & Lesbian Review Worldwide* 7 (4): 31–33.

The author briefly discusses the rise of what is perhaps the most extreme form of nonheterosexual identification among some school-age youth, transgenderism, and attempts to provide a theoretical introduction to the topic.

Stone, Carolyn B. "Counselors as Advocates for Gay, Lesbian, and Bisexual Youth: A Call for Equity and Action." *Journal of Multicultural Counseling and Development* 31 (2; April 2003): 143–55.

The author points out that the U.S. Supreme Court has validated the role of school counselors in advocating for gay, lesbian, and bisexual youth in public schools and suggests a number of ways in which school counselors can carry out this aspect of their jobs.

Van Wormer, Katherine, and Robin McKinney. "What Schools Can Do to Help Gay/lesbian/bisexual Youth: a Harm Reduction Approach." *Adolescence* 38 (151; Fall 2003): 409–20.

The authors point out the very strong heterosexist atmosphere that prevails in U.S. schools and argue that, if not countered by the actions of school officials, can lead to a host of emotional and psychological problems for lesbian, gay, and bisexual youth. They offer some suggestions as to policies and actions that can support nonheterosexual young people in schools.

Reports

Cianciotto, Jason, and Sean Cahill. *Youth in the Crosshairs: The Third Wave of Ex-Gay Activism*. Washington, DC: National Gay and Lesbian Task Force, 2006.

This report explores the status of religious-based programs that purport to be able to convert young men and women with same-sex feelings to a "normal" heterosexual lifestyle. It found that not only is so-called conversion therapy largely unsuccessful, but it also has a tendency to result in social, psychological, and interpersonal harm to those who experience the treatment. The report also considers a number of ethical issues involved in the use of conversion therapy to change sexual attitudes and behaviors.

Greytak, Emily A., Joseph G. Kosciw, and Elizabeth M. Diaz. *The Experiences of Transgender Youth in Our Nation's Schools*. New York: GLSEN, 2009.

This report provides the findings of a study of the school experiences of 295 students between the ages of 13 and 20 who identified themselves as transgender. Researchers found that these students experienced a significantly higher amount of bullying and harassment than did students self-identified or perceived as gay, lesbian, and bisexual, resulting in poorer school attendance, lower grades, and decreased educational aspirations.

Kosciw, Joseph G., Elizabeth M. Diaz, and Emily A. Greytak. *The 2007 National School Climate Survey: The Experiences of Lesbian, Gay, Bisexual and Transgender Youth in Our Nation's Schools.* **New York: GLSEN, 2008.**

In 2007, researchers for the Gay, Lesbian and Straight Education Network conducted a survey of 6,209 LGBT students from all 50 states and the District of Columbia, between the ages of 13 and 21 in grades K through 12. About two-thirds of the sample (64.4%) was white, over half (57.7%) was female, and over half identified as gay or lesbian (53.6%). The survey collected information on a wide variety of topics and issues, including biased language, overall safety in schools, verbal and physical harassment and assault, racial and ethnic factors in GLBT issues, and availability and utility of school resources and support systems. The report includes more than 90 tables and figures summarizing its findings.

Markow, Dana, and Jill Dancewicz. *Perspective: School Safety, Bullying And Harassment: A Survey of Public School Principals.* **New York: Harris Interactive, 2008.**

From June 15 through August 3, 2007, Harris Interactive conducted a survey for the Gay, Lesbian and Straight Education Network and the National Association of Secondary School Principals on the attitudes of 1,580 K–12 principals about the school climate in their institution for gay, lesbian, bisexual, and transgender students. About half of all respondents said that bullying and harassment based on perceived or actual sexual identity and/or sexual orientation was a serious problem in their schools. About a third said that gay, lesbian, and bisexual students would feel safe in their institutions, and about a quarter said that transgender students would feel safe. In general, principals appear to feel that they would receive the greatest support for improving the environment for GLBT students from other administrators, somewhat less support from teachers, and significantly less support from parents and members of the community at large.

Markow, Dana, and Jordan Fein. *From Teasing to Torment: School Climate in America: A Survey of Students and Teachers.* **New York: Harris Interactive, 2005.**

This study was commission by the Gay, Lesbian and Straight Education Network (GLSEN) to better understand the nature of bullying and harassment of gay, lesbian, bisexual, and other non-traditional sexually identified youth in a wide variety of schools in the United States. Findings suggest that perceived or actual sexual orientation and/or sexual identification are the second most common cause of bullying and harassment after physical characteristics, such as skin color. The study also found that most teachers and counselors are supportive of efforts to deal with this issue and believe that stronger school policies, regulations, and activities would help reduce the problem for youth affected by bullying and harassment.

Ottosson, Daniel. *State-sponsored Homophobia: A World Survey of Laws Prohibiting Same Sex Activity Between Consenting Adults.* **[Brussels]: International Lesbian, Gay. Bisexual, Trans, and Intersex Association, 2009.**

This report is a remarkable piece of research that provides up-to-date information on the legal status of same-sex relationships in every country in the world with an extensive bibliography that contains links to legal documents in almost every country.

Ray, Nicholas. *Lesbian, Gay, Bisexual And Transgender Youth: an Epidemic of Homelessness.* **Washington, DC: National Gay and Lesbian Task Force, 2006.**

The research leading to this report was inspired by evidence that 20 to 40 percent of all homeless youth identify as gay, lesbian, bisexual, or transgender, compared to an estimated 3 to 5 percent of the general population. Researchers reviewed professional literature, academic research, government programs, and other available evidence to determine reasons for this disturbing statistic. The report also contains five detailed descriptions of local programs that have been developed to deal with the problem of GLBT homelessness and concludes with a number of recommendations for action at the federal, state, local, and practitioner levels.

Web Sites

Advocates for Youth. "ambienteJoven.org." Available at http:// www.ambientejoven.org/.

This Spanish-language Web site is aimed at young Spanish-speaking men and women, with information about issues in sexual health and other topics of concern to adolescents.

Advocates for Youth. "YouthResource." Available at http://www. youthresource.com/.

This Web site is designed for gay, lesbian, bisexual, transgendered, and young people who are questioning their own sexual identity and/or sexual orientation (GLBTQ). It provides information on sexual issues of special interests to such individuals, suggests ways of becoming involved in community activities, provides news updates on topics of interest to GLBTQ individuals, and provides online contacts with other GLBTQ individuals.

American Academy of Pediatrics. "Gay, Lesbian, and Bisexual Teens: Facts for Teens and Their Parents." Available at http:// www.pomonapeds.com/download/gay_teen.pdf?PHPSESSID= 500c54f8a4ed98c83f791f66ba60bb27.

This brochure, developed by the American Academy of Pediatrics, presents fundamental information about sexual orientation and provides guidance for parents and health care professionals about working with lesbian, gay, and bisexual youth.

American Psychological Association. "Answers to Your Questions: For a Better Understanding of Sexual Orientation & Homosexuality." Available at http://www.apa.org/topics/sorientation.pdf.

This six-page brochure provides answers to many common questions about sexual orientation, such as "What is sexual orientation?" "How do people know if they are gay, lesbian, or bisexual?" "What causes a person to have a particular sexual orientation?" "Is homosexuality a mental disorder?" "At what age should lesbian, gay, or bisexual youths come out?" and "Can lesbians and gay men be good parents?"

The Body. "Fact Sheet: Lesbian, Gay, Bisexual and Transgender Youth Issues." Available at http://www.thebody.com/content/ whatis/art2449.html.

This Web site provides an excellent summary of some important issues faced by gay, lesbian, bisexual, and transgender youth, along with a short discussion of each issue.

Mental Health America. "What Does Gay Mean?" Available at http://www.mentalhealthamerica.net/go/what-does-gay-mean.

This booklet was prepared to help parents, teachers, counselors, and other interested professionals in helping young people to better understand the nature of sexual orientation and issues that surround the topic. Sections of the booklet are designed specifically for children and young adults of varying age groups.

OutProud.org. "I Think I Might Be Gay . . . Now What Do I Do? A Brochure for Young Men." Available at http://www.outproud. org/brochure_think_gay.html.

Outproud.org. "I Think I Might Be a Lesbian . . . Now What Do I Do? A Brochure for Young Women." Available at http://www. outproud.org/brochure_think_lesbian.html.

These two comparable brochures discuss the ways in which young men and young women may experience and learn how to deal with homosexual feelings. They discuss questions such as how does one know that he/she is gay/lesbian? who should one tell about these feelings? how does one meet other gay men/lesbians? and what unique health problems might one have to think about?

PFLAG. "Be Yourself: Questions and Answers for Gay, Lesbian and Bisexual Youth." Available at http://www.pflag.org/filead min/user_upload/Publications/Be_Yourself.pdf.

This booklet has been prepared by Parents and Friends of Lesbians and Gays (Pflag) to answer most of the basic questions that young people have about sexual orientation in general, and their own sexual orientation in particular.

Sanders, Douglas. "Human Rights and Sexual Orientation in International Law." http://www.ilga.org/news_results.asp?Lang uageID=1&FileCategory=44&FileID=577, 2005.

The author provides an excellent review of the history of efforts to expand tolerance of same-sex relationships in a variety of regional and international law reports and pronouncements.

Glossary

This chapter contains definitions for a number of terms commonly used in the fields of sexually transmitted infections, contraception, sexual orientation and sexual identity, and related fields of sexual health.

abstinence   In general, the practice of abstaining from particular behavior, such as eating certain types of food. In the field of sexual health, abstinence means abstaining from (usually) sexual intercourse, although it may also refer to abstaining from all forms of sexual behavior.

acquired immunodeficiency syndrome (AIDS)   The late stage of an infection, often but not necessarily transmitted by sexual contact, caused by the human immunodeficiency virus (HIV).

acute   In describing a medical condition, symptoms or diseases that last for relatively short periods of time before becoming better or developing into long-term conditions, known as chronic conditions.

AIDS   *See* acquired immunodeficiency syndrome.

antiretroviral   Any drug that is effective in stopping the action of a virus.

asymptomatic   Not displaying any symptoms.

bacterial vaginosis   A bacterial infection of the vagina that occurs commonly among women of childbearing age, characterized by a watery discharge and a fishy-smelling odor. Previously called nonspecific vaginitis.

basal body temperature method   A method of birth control in which a woman monitors her body temperature to determine the times at which she is fecund, and when she is not.

benign   Not cancerous.

bisexual   A term that refers to acts, fantasies, or feelings that involve individuals of either sex. People who call themselves bisexual experience

269

an erotic interest in both men and women, although not necessarily to an equal extent.

candida   A genus of yeast-like fungi responsible for the infection known as candidiasis.

candidiasis   A fungal infection caused by any one of the members of the Candida family of fungi. Such infections occur most commonly in the mucous membranes of the throat and lungs, esophagus, and vagina.

cervical cap   A contraceptive device consisting of a small thimble-shaped cup that is placed over the cervix to prevent sperm from entering the uterus.

chancroid   A highly contagious sexually transmitted infection caused by the *Hemophilus ducreyi* bacterium.

chlamydia   A very common sexually transmitted infection caused by any one of a number of bacteria belonging to the genus of the same name.

chronic   In referring to medical conditions, symptoms or diseases that persist for long periods of time, usually many years. *Also see* acute.

coitus interruptus   A birth control method that involves a male withdrawing his penis before ejaculating.

colposcopy   A medical procedure by which the surface of the vagina and cervix are examined with a special type of microscope called a colposcope.

combination oral contraceptive   A form of "The Pill" that contains two hormones, forms of progesterone and estrogen.

condom   A flexible sleeve made of latex rubber or some other material placed over a man's penis during intercourse to prevent release of sperm into a woman's uterus and to help protect against sexually transmitted infections. *Also see* female condom.

consensual sexual act   Any sexual act to which both (or all) parties agree.

contraceptive patch   A piece of material containing progesterone and estrogen placed on the skin which releases these hormones through the skin into the bloodstream over a period of time.

contraceptive sponge   A small sponge containing a spermicide that is inserted into the vagina prior to sexual intercourse.

cryosurgery   A medical procedure by which a section of tissue is frozen, usually with liquid nitrogen, and then removed.

D and C   *See* dilation and curettage.

Depo provera   A progesterone-like hormone (medroxyprogesterone acetate [DMPA]) contraceptive administered by injection, usually over three-month periods.

diaphragm   A flexible, dome-shape cup covered with a spermicide and fitted over the uterine cervix to prevent entry of sperm.

dilation and curettage (D and C)   A medical procedure in which the cervix is dilated, allowing the surface of the uterus and cervical canal to be scraped.

douching   Cleaning of the cervix and vagina with water or an aqueous solution.

dyspareunia   Painful or difficult sexual intercourse, most commonly experienced by women.

dysuria   Painful or difficult urination, often associated with a sexually transmitted infection.

emergency contraceptive   Any type of contraceptive method that can be administered within a few days of sexual intercourse.

Essure   A sterilization procedure developed by the Conceptus corporation that involves the insertion of a spiral device into a woman's fallopian tubes to prevent implantation of an embryo.

fecund   Capable of producing offspring.

female condom   A tubular pouch that fits into a woman's vagina to prevent sperm from entering the uterus during sexual intercourse.

fertility awareness   Any birth control method used that depends on a woman's being aware of the times each month during which she is and is not fecund.

gay   A term that has come to be associated with individuals, organizations, acts, events, or other phenomena involving two individuals of the same gender, most commonly, two men.

gay bashing   Any activity in which individuals—most commonly, young men—beat up gay men, lesbians, or other individuals whom they judge to be of a sexual orientation to which they object, usually without any apparent rational basis, often "just for the fun of it."

gender   A term that refers to a person's social identity as a man or a woman. The concept of gender includes not only one's biological sex (male or female), but also the social constructs created by a culture that tend to be associated with one or the other sex.

gender identity   The perception that a person has as to whether he or she is a man or a woman. Gender identity and gender or gender identity and sex are not always the same. Some individuals who are biologically male and who may assume all the characteristics of a man may feel that he is actually "a woman trapped in a man's body."

granuloma inguinale   A sexually transmitted infection caused by the *Calymmatobacterium granulomatis* bacterium.

hate crime Any criminal act that is based solely or primarily on prejudice against some group of individuals, such as women, blacks, Hispanics, or gay men and lesbians.

hepatitis An inflammation of the liver caused by microorganisms or chemicals. About a half dozen forms of the disease are known, the most common of which are characterized as hepatitis A, hepatitis B, and hepatitis C.

herpes The name given to a group of diseases and the viruses that cause them, characterized by painful blisters on the skin or mucous membranes.

HIV *See* human immunodeficiency virus.

homosexual A term that should probably best be used as an adjective, referring to any feeling, fantasy, or act that involves two people of the same sex. Historically, the word has also been used to refer to an individual or group of individuals. It is less successful in that context because it tends to define individuals and groups of individuals solely on the basis of their erotic interests.

HPV *See* human papillomavirus.

human immunodeficiency virus The virus that causes acquired immunodeficiency syndrome (AIDS).

human papillomavirus (HPV) Any one of a large number of viruses that cause infections of the skin and mucous membrane, the best known of which are genital warts, which are associated with the onset of cervical cancer.

informed consent A legal principle that means a person understands and agrees to participate in some type of research or treatment.

intrauterine device (IUD) A thin piece of plastic or metal inserted through the vagina into the uterus to prevent a pregnancy from developing.

in vitro From the Latin meaning "in glass," referring to any procedure carried out in laboratory equipment, and not in a living organism.

in vivo From the Latin meaning "in life," referring to any procedure carried out in connection with a living organism.

IUD *See* intrauterine device.

lactational amenorrhea method A method of birth control that makes use of a woman's natural tendency to stop ovulating while she is breastfeeding. In the absence of any synthetic form of contraception, lactational amenorrhea can be considered a form of natural birth control.

latency In medicine, that period of time that elapses after a person has been infected with a disease before signs or symptoms of that disease develop.

menarche   The time in a young woman's life when her menstrual periods first begin.

morning after pill   A form of emergency contraception that can be taken any time up to about five days after sexual intercourse to prevent a pregnancy from developing.

natural family planning   Any method of birth control that does not make use of synthetic chemicals or devices to prevent pregnancy. *Also see* fertility awareness.

nongonococcal urethritis (NGU)   Inflammation of the urethra that is not caused by a gonococcal bacterium.

nonspecific vaginitis   *See* bacterial vaginitis.

Norplant   A form of birth control developed by the Population Council in which small capsules containing hormones are inserted beneath the skin of the upper arm.

off-label   Use of a drug for a purpose other than that for which it has been approved by the U.S. Food and Drug Administration (FDA).

opportunistic infection   An infection that develops as a consequence of a person's having a weakened immune system.

oral contraceptive   Any contraceptive formulation that is designed to be taken by mouth.

over-the-counter contraceptive   Any substance or device that prevents pregnancy that can be purchased without a prescription.

pap smear   *See* pap test.

pap test   A test in which cells are collected from the lining of the cervix and vagina to determine the presence or absence of an inflammation in those tissues.

patch   *See* contraceptive patch.

pedophilia   The condition of being erotically attracted to children. Although pedophilia is sometimes associated with homosexuality, most studies suggest that the vast majority of pedophiliacs are heterosexual men, or men with a troubled heterosexual orientation who are attracted to young girls or to all young children of either sex.

pelvic inflammatory disease (PID)   An infection, usually transmitted by sexual activity, which spreads upward from the vagina to the upper parts of the reproductive tract.

permanent birth control   Any procedure that causes a man or woman to become permanently infertile. *Also see* sterilization; vasectomy.

PID *See* pelvic inflammatory disease.

The Pill A common name given to any contraceptive taken orally, usually, but not necessarily, containing a combination of progesterone- and estrogen-like hormones.

Plan B A form of oral contraceptive that contains a form of the hormone progestin and can be used to prevent a pregnancy from developing for up to 72 hours after sexual intercourse.

postcoital contraception *See* emergency contraception.

prenatal transmission The transmission of an infection from mother to child during the birth process.

prodrome A sign or symptom or set of signs or symptoms taken as a warning sign of a disease that will develop later.

prognosis A prediction of the likely course or outcome of a disease.

prophylactic *See* condom.

prophylaxis Any treatment intended to prevent the onset of a disease.

queer A once-derogatory word used to describe gay men and lesbians. The term has now been adopted by many gay men and lesbians as an act of defiance against those who would use the term in a disparaging manner.

recurrence The return of signs, symptoms, or a disease itself after a period of apparent recovery.

remission The disappearance of the signs and symptoms of a disease, which may indicate that the disease has disappeared permanently or temporarily.

risk factor Any substance or situation increasing a person's chance of contracting a disease.

seroconversion The process by which the status of a person's blood tests changes from negative to positive for some particular disease, such as AIDS.

sexual orientation The tendency of a person to be erotically attracted to someone of the same gender, the opposite gender, or both genders. The term *orientation* usually suggests that this tendency is not consciously chosen by a person, but is determined by some genetic or biological factor.

spermicide Any substance that kills sperm.

sponge *See* contraceptive sponge.

sterilization Any method for making a male or female infertile. *Also see* tubal ligation; vasectomy.

systemic Any condition that affects the body as a whole rather than some specific part of the body.

toxoplasmosis A disease caused by the protozoan *Toxoplasma gondii.*

transgendered person A person who has undergone one or more steps in the process of changing one's sex, from male to female or from female to male.

transsexual A person who identifies as belonging to a gender other than the one to which he or she was assigned at birth.

transvestite A person (almost always a man) who enjoys dressing in the clothing of someone of the opposite sex and, often, takes on the social characteristics of that sex. A man who enjoys dressing as a woman and then going shopping in that attire is a transvestite. The great majority of transvestites are heterosexual males.

trichomoniasis An infection caused by the protozoan *Trichomonas vaginalis,* responsible for vaginitis in women and urethritis in men.

tubal ligation Any procedure that involves the blocking of a woman's fallopian tubes (by cutting and/or tying them off) to prevent sperm from reaching an egg.

vasectomy A surgical procedure in which the vas deferens are cut, preventing sperm from traveling from the testes to the prostate gland.

withdrawal A natural method of birth control in which a man withdraws his penis from a woman's vagina before he ejaculates.

Index

Abortion Access Project (AAP),
202–203
Abortion in the United States
(Calderone), 128
Abortion issues
Abortion Access Project,
202–203
characteristics of women
obtaining, 188–192
Freedom of Choice Act, 209
Roe v. Wade, 157–159, 170–171
sex education, 50–52
Abstinence/fertility awareness,
19–20
Abstinence-only education, 36–42.
See also Content of Federally
Funded Abstinence-only
Education Programs; *Gonzales
v. School Board of Okeechobee
County*; Separate Program
for Abstinence Education;
SPRANS-CBAE
arguments in favor of, 38–39
books out of favor, 47
future of, 41–42
Guttmacher Institute study,
50, 51
historical background, 36–38
Obama's funding withdrawal,
41
research on, 39–41
Abstinence the Better Choice
(ABC), 202

Access to Birth Control Act (2007),
61, 62, 163–166
The Act of Marriage (LaHaye), 137
Adolescence Education Program
(AEP) (India), 82
Adolescent Family Life Act
(AFLA), 37
Adolescents
GLBT groups, 23
GLBTQ youth, 24–26
Plan B age controversy, 58–59
sexual activity, NYC, 43
sexual behavior patterns, 34
sexual identity issues, 21–28
suicides/suicide attempts, 25,
228
virginity pledge taken by, 39
Advisory Committee on
Immunization Practices of the
Centers for Disease Control,
161–163
Advocates for Youth, 27, 203
Africa
HIV/AIDS epidemic, 88
HIV/AIDS programs, 91
sex education in, 87
African Medical and Research
Foundation (AMREF), 91
Agency for Healthcare Research
and Quality (AHRQ),
197–198
AIDS Education and Research
Trust, 206

Alcohol use, by GLBTQ students, 26
American Association of Sex Educators, Counselors, and Therapists (AASECT), 203–204
American Birth Control League, 145, 146
American Ethical Union National Service Conference, 221
American Medical Association (AMA), 60
American Pharmaceutical Association (APhA), 60
American Sexually Transmitted Diseases Association (ASTDA), 204
American Social Health Association (ASHA), 4, 204–205
Anal cancer, 63, 64
Antibiotic treatments, 6, 8
Antiharassment (in schools) protection, 50
Argentina
HIV/AIDS programs, 92
sex education in, 85–86
Association of Reproductive Health Professionals (ARHP), 205
Athar, Shahid, 84
Australia, sex education in, 83–84
AVERT program, 205–206

Barnes, Melody, 41
Barrier methods of contraception, 15–17
Bataclan, Bren, 139
Berrill v. Houde, 48
Bill of Rights (U.S. Constitution), 168–169
Billings, Lyn and John, 207
Birth control. *See also* Contraceptive devices; Contraceptive issues; Knowlton, Charles

abstinence method, 19–20, 182–184
Access to Birth Control Act, 61, 62, 163–166
barrier methods, 15–17
devices, 54, 140–141
hormonal control, 19
opposition to, 61–62
oral contraceptives, 14, 17–18, 39, 54, 141
Pope Paul VI position on, 140–141
Rock's Harvard discussions of, 142–143
Sanger's activism for, 145–146
school dispensing issues, 54–57
Stopes' Great Britain clinics, 148–149
use by sexually active high school students, by sex, race, ethnicity, 193–194
Birth Control News (Stopes), 149
Bisexual individuals, 23
Bixby Center for Global Reproductive Health, 206
Black Church Initiative, 222
Blagojevich, Rod, 61
BOMA-USA (Billings Ovulation Method Association), 206–207
Bowen-Hugh, Violet, 218
Boyd v. United States, 169
Boys Don't Cry movie, 149
Brazil, sex education in, 85–86
Broadhead, George, 80
Brotherhood University (SMYAL), 227
Brown v. Hot, Sexy, and Safer Productions, 48
Bucharest World Population Conference, 96–97
Bush, George W., 36, 98, 156–157

Calderone, Frank, 128
Calderone, Mary Steichen, 127–129, 223
Calvert, Simon, 80

Cambodia, HIV/AIDS programs, 91–92
Cameroon, syphilis data, 95
Caribbean, sex education in, 86
The Case for Birth Control (Sanger), 146
Catholic Church, 78, 86
Catholics for Choice (CFC), 207
Catholics in Public Life campaign, 207
Center for Development and Population Activities (CEDPA), 208
Center for Population Options, 203
Center for Reproductive Rights (CRC), 207–208
Center for the Study of Equality, 226
Centers for Disease Control and Prevention (CDC)(U.S.), 9, 34, 44
  Advisory Committee on the Immunization Practices, 161–163
  characteristics of women obtaining legal abortions, 188–192
  chlamydia data (U.S.), 4, 6
  Division of STD Prevention, 198
  gonorrhea recommendations, 9
  hepatitis recommendations, 11
  HIV/AIDS data, 12, 13
  Youth Risk Behavior Surveillance System, 193–194
Cervical cancer, 63, 64
Cervical caps, 17
Chang, Min-Chueh, 129–130
Chat It Up! events (SMYAL), 227
Chicago Experiment, 31–33
Chicken pox (human herpesvirus 4), 9
China
  HIV/AIDS epidemic, 90
  sex education in, 81–82

China Family Planning Association, 82
Chlamydia, 5–6
Christian Institute, 80
Christian Legal Society's Center for Law and Religions Freedom, 60
Christian viewpoint on sex education, 35
Christmas, David, 80
Clinton, Bill, 98, 155, 156
Coitus interruptus, 15
Collaborative Evaluation of Strategies to Encourage Couples-Focused Health Service Delivery, 200
Colombia, sex education in, 85–86
Committee on Petitions (India), 82
Comprehensive Adolescent Care program (Cuba), 86
Comstock, Anthony, 130–131
Concerned About Teen Sexuality (C.A.T.S.) program, 203
Concerned Women for America (CWA), 62, 136, 209
Condoms, 15, 39
  opposition to distribution, 43, 171–174
  usage instruction, 42–44
Condoms4Life campaign (CFC), 207
Consortium for Industrial Collaboration in Contraceptive Research, 210
Content of Federally Funded Abstinence-only Education Programs, 182–184
The Continuum Complete International Encyclopedia of Sexuality, 76, 85–86
Contraceptive devices. *See also* Birth control
  access to, 53–57
  Internet access to, 58
  Ipsos Public Affairs poll, 54
  male vs. female access, 57

Contraceptive issues
  access outside of schools, 53–57
  Curtis v. School Committee of Falmouth, 171–174
  Griswold v. Connecticut, 168–170
  school provisions controversy, 53–57
  SPRANS-CBAE report, 183
  worldwide perspective, 96–98
Contraceptive Research and Development Program (CONRAD), 209–210
Copper T IUD, 19
Costa Rica, sex education in, 85–86
Côte d'Ivoire, women's counseling services, 97
Couple to Couple League (CCL), 210
Course of Study sex education (Japan), 81
Court cases, 168–180
  Berrill v. Houde, 48
  Boyd v. United States, 169
  Brown v. Hot, Sexy, and Safer Productions, 48
  Curtis v. School Committee of Falmouth, 171–174
  Godkin v. San Leandro School District, 48
  Gonzales v. School Board of Okeechobee County, 177–180
  Griswold v. Connecticut, 168–170
  Parker v. Hurley, 174–177
  Roe v. Wade, 157–158, 170–171, 217
Cuba, sex education in, 86
Cultural Competency Training for Professionals, 228
Curtis v. School Committee of Falmouth (1995), 171–174

Danish Family Planning Association, 77
Denmark, mandatory sex education in, 77

Department of Health and Human Services (U.S.), 200
Diaphragms, 17
Discovering Roads program (Cuba), 86
Division of STD Prevention (DSTDP)(CDC), 198
Division of STD Prevention Strategic Plan 2008–2013, 198
Dominican Republic, HIV/AIDS programs, 91
Due Process Clause (Fourteenth Amendment, U.S. Constitution), 171, 177

Ectopic pregnancy, 9
Education. *See* Abstinence-only education; Gay, Lesbian, and Straight Education Network (GLSEN); Sex education
Education for Family Life (EFL) program (Poland), 78
Ehrlich, Paul, 8, 131–132
ELIGHT Web site (for GLBTQ youth), 228
Emergency contraception (EC). *See* Plan B (emergency contraception)
EngenderHealth, 211
Enovid (oral contraceptive), 17
Equal Rights Amendment, 209
Estrogen derived oral contraceptives, 17–18
Europe, sex education perspective, 76–80

Faircloth, Lauch, 36, 38, 154–156
The Family, a Place for Human Development program (Cuba), 86
The Family Book about Sexuality (Calderone and Johnson), 128
Family Education Trust (UK), 80
Family Health International (FHI), 211–212

Family Limitations (Sanger), 146
Family planning, worldwide
   perspective, 96–98
Family Planning Annual Report,
   200
Family Research Council (FRC),
   212
Female condoms, 15
Fertility awareness and
   abstinence, 19–20
Fifth Amendment (U.S. Constitu-
   tion), 169
First Amendment (U.S. Constitu-
   tion), 169, 173, 180
First Inter-Africa Conference on
   Adolescent Reproductive
   Health (1992), 203
Flagg, Ella, 31–33
Focus on the Family (Christian
   organization), 43–44,
   212–213
Food and Drug Administration
   (U.S. FDA), 17, 58–59
Fourteenth Amendment (U.S.
   Constitution), 169, 171, 172
Fourth Amendment (U.S.
   Constitution), 169
Free Exercise Clause (First
   Amendment, U.S. Constitu-
   tion), 173, 175
Freedom of Choice Act, 209
Friedan, Betty, 136, 209
Frontiers in Reproductive Health,
   220
The Fruits of Philosophy, or the
   Private Companion of Young
   Married People by a Physician
   (Knowlton), 135–136
Fulton, Wallace, 223

Gabon (country)
   education campaigns, 97
   gonorrhea data, 96
Gallup Poll on homosexuality,
   24–25
Gardasil HPV vaccine, 63

Gay, Lesbian, and Straight
   Education Network (GLSEN),
   27, 132–133, 139, 225. *See*
   also Jennings, Kevin; Parlin,
   Robert
Gay, lesbian, bisexual, and
   transgendered (GLBT)
   groups, 23
Gay, lesbian, bisexual, transgender
   and questioning (GLBTQ)
   youth, 24–28
Gay and Lesbian Community
   Center of the Ozarks
   (GLCCO), 225
Gay and Lesbian Humanist
   Association (UK), 80
Gay and Lesbian School Teacher
   Network (GLSTN), 139
Gay marriage, 49, 174–177. *See also*
   Parker v. Hurley
Gay-straight alliance (GSA) high
   school club, 177–178
Gender identity, 21–28
Gender Public Advocacy Coalition
   (GenderPAC), 50
Genital herpes, 9–10
GENIUS Index (2008)(Gender
   Equality National Index for
   Universities and Schools), 50
Genne, William, 223
Ghana, sex education in, 87
GLBSO e-mail list, 228
Global Strategy for the Prevention
   and Control of Sexually
   Transmitted Infections:
   2006–2015 (WHO RHR
   Department), 95
Godkin v. San Leandro School
   District, 48
Gonorrhea, 8–9, 94–95
Gonzales v. School Board of Okeechobee
   County (2008), 177–180
Griswold v. Connecticut (1965),
   168–170
Growing During Adolescence
   program (Cuba), 86

Guidelines for Comprehensive Sexuality Education (SIECUS), 52–53
Guttmacher Institute (GI), 50, 51, 213

Harkin, Tom, 38
Harvard University, 35
Health Policy Initiative (CEDPA), 208
Helium poll on STDs, 57
Helium Web site
  STD poll, 57
  teenage sexuality blog, 55–57
Henry J. Kaiser Family Foundation, 35–36, 215. *See also* NPR/KFF/JFK poll on sex education
Hepatitis (A/B), 10–12
Herpes infections, 9–10
Herpes Resource Center, 204
Heterosexually oriented (sexual orientation), 22
Hispanic females, 15–19 years of age, pregnancy/live birth-rates (1980–2000), 192–193
HIV/AIDS, 12–14
  Aastha Project (India), 211
  abstinence-only programs and, 40
  Advocates for Youth program, 203
  African epidemic, 87
  AIDS Education and Research Trust, 206
  Brotherhood University prevention programs, 227
  CDC data estimates, 12
  curricular educational inclusion, 47
  dismissal/denial, 88–90
  evaluation, 93–94
  Focus on the Family claims, 43–44
  in Indian sex ed, 82

infection description, 12–13
in Japanese sex ed, 81
orphans due to (2008), 194, 198
REAL Act, 159
treatment/prevention programs, 13–14, 90–92
worldwide data (2008), 194–196
Homosexuality (in sex education), 44–50
  bias studies on, 45
  lawsuits about, 48–49
  NPR/KFF/JFK poll on, 44–45
Homosexually oriented (sexual orientation), 22
Horizons: Global Operation Research on HIV/AIDS/STI Prevention and Care, 220
Hormonal methods (of pregnancy/birth control), 17–19
  implants, 18–19
  injections, 18
  oral contraceptives, 14, 17–18, 39, 54, 143
  patches, 18
  Plan B (emergency contraception), 19
  vaginal rings, 18
HPV Resource Center, 204
Human papillomavirus (HPV), 62–65
  description/varieties, 62
  immigrants to U.S./ vaccinations, 64
  Mandatory HPV Vaccination executive order, 161–163
  treatment modalities, 63
  vaccination for, 63–65
Human Rights Campaign (HRC), 225–226
Human sexuality, issues of concern, 87–101
  contraception/family planning, 96–101
  evaluations, 93–94

HIV/AIDS pandemic, 88–94
Parker v. Hurley (2007), 48, 174–177
sexual orientation/gender identity, 98–101
sexually transmitted infections, 94–95

Implants, hormonal, 18–19
Indefinite Quantity Contracts project (CEDPA), 208
India
  Aastha Project, 211
  HIV/AIDS programs, 82, 92
  sex education in, 82–83
La Iniciativa Latina program, 222
Injections, of hormones, 18
Institute for Media Education, 46
International Clearinghouse on Adolescent Fertility, 203
International Conference on Population and Development (ICPD), 200
International Consortium on Emergency Contraception (ICEC), 213–214
International Fertility Research Program (IFRP), 211
International Planned Parenthood Federation, 214
International Pregnancy Advisory Services, 215
International Society for Sexually Transmitted Diseases Research (ISSTDR), 214
International Union against Sexually Transmitted Infections (IUSTI), 214–215
Intrauterine devices (IUDs), 19
Ipsos Public Affairs poll, 54
IwannaKnow.org, 204

Japan, sex education in, 81
Jennings, Kevin, 132–133
Jensen, Albert, 138

John F. Kennedy School of Government (Harvard University), 35–36. *See also* NPR/KFF/JFK poll on sex education
John XXIII (Pope), 140
Johns Hopkins University School of Public Health, 39
Johnson, Eric, 128

Kaiser Family Foundation, 35–36, 215–216
Kanabus, Annabel, 206
Kaposi's sarcoma (human herpesvirus 8), 9
Kinsey, Alfred, 133–135, 198
Kinsey Institute for Research in Sex, Gender, and Reproduction, 198–199
Kirkendall, Lester, 223
Knowlton, Charles, 135–136
Koch, Robert, 131–132
Korman, Edward R., 59

La Iniciativa Latina program, 222
LaHaye, Beverly, 136–137, 209
The Laramie Project, 147
Latin America
  HIV/AIDS programs, 91–92
  sex education in, 85–86
Lautenberg, Frank, 61, 159
Lawsuits about teaching of homosexuality, 48–49
Left Behind novels (LaHaye), 136
Lesbians, 23
Lesotho, women's counseling services, 97
Lief, Harold, 223
Life Planning Education, 203
Lotter, John, 149

"Making Schools Safe for Gay & Lesbian Youth" (Jennings), 133
Mali, women's status promotion, 97

Maloney, Carolyn B., 61, 164–166
Mama's Boy (Jennings), 133
Mandatory HPV Vaccination
  (2007), 161–163
Manford, Jeanne, 27
*Manual of Family Planning and
  Contraceptive Practices*
  (Calderone), 128
*Married Love: A New Contribution
  to the Solution of the Sex
  Difficulties* (Stopes), 148
Marshal, Michael P., 26
Martin, Lon, 128
Martinez, Mel, 98
Massachusetts
  *Curtis v. School Committee of
    Falmouth*, 171–174
  Department of Public Health, 25
  free condom programs, 42
Maternal deaths during childbirth,
  14
Mathematica Policy Research,
  Inc., 39
Matthew Shepard Foundation
  (MSF), 226
Mbeki, Thabo, 88–89
McCormick, Katherine, 129–130,
  142
Memorandum for the
  Administrator of the
  United States Agency for
  International Development
  (2001), 156–157
Men
  chlamydia-specific symptoms, 6
  gonorrhea symptoms, 8–9
Mexico, sex education in, 85–86
Mexico City Policy (2009), 157,
  167–168. *See also* Memoran-
  dum for the Administrator of
  the United States Agency for
  International Development
Mirena intrauterine system (IUS),
  19
Modern Materialism (Knowlton),
  135

Mononucleosis, infectious (human
  herpesvirus 5), 9
Morning-after pill (Plan B), 19
Morocco, sexually transmitted
  diseases, 95
Mujeres en Desarrollo
  Dominciano (MUDE)
  organization (Dominican
  Republic), 91
Muslim World, sex education in,
  84–85
My Fight for Birth Control (Sanger),
  146
Myanmar, absence of HIV/AIDS
  in, 90

NARAL Pro Choice America, 216
National Abstinence Education
  Association, 38, 41
National Campaign to Prevent
  Teen and Unplanned
  Pregnancy, 216–217
National Center of Sexual
  Education (CENESEX)
  (Cuba), 86
National Committee on Federal
  Legislation for Birth Control,
  146
National Day to Prevent Teen and
  Unplanned Pregnancy, 217
National Institute of Allergy and
  Infectious Diseases (NIAID),
  199–200
National Institute of Child Health
  and Human Development,
  209–210
National Network of Adolescents
  for Sexual and Reproductive
  Health (Argentina), 92
National Organization for Women
  (NOW), 64
National Public Radio (NPR),
  35–36. *See also* NPR/KFF/JFK
  poll on sex education
National Right to Life (NRL),
  217–218

National Survey of Family Growth, 34
National Union for Women's Political Suffrage, 151
National Women's Health Resource Center (NWHRC), 218
National Youth Advocacy Coalition, 27
Natural family planning (NFP) methods, 20
Neisseria gonorrhoeae, 8–9
Netherlands
  pregnancy rate data, 77
  sex education in, 77–78
The New Spirit Controlled Woman (LaHaye), 137
New York Society for the Suppression of Vice (NYSSV), 130–131
Nigeria, education campaigns, 97
Ninth Amendment (U.S. Constitution), 169
Nissen, Marvin "Tom," 149
Nixon, Richard M., 145
Noguchi, Hideyo, 137–138
Nonoxynol-9 spermicide, 16
NPR/KFF/JFK poll on sex education, 35–36, 49–50, 90

Obama, Barack, 38, 41
  family funding policy reversals, 98
  Mexico City Policy revocation, 157, 167–168
Office of Population Affairs (OPA), 200
Office of Public Health and Science, 200
Oral contraception, 14, 17–18, 39, 54, 143
Orphans due to AIDS (estimates), 194, 198
Ottesen-Jensen, Elise, 138–139

Pacific institute for Women's Health, 214

Parents, Families and Friends of Lesbians and Gays (PFLAG), 27–28, 226–227
Parker v. Hurley (2007), 48, 174–178
Parlin, Robert, 139
Patches, of hormones, 18
Pathfinder International, 214
Paul VI (Pope), 140
Pediculosis capitis (head louse), 4
Pediculosis pubis infections, 3–4
Pelvic inflammatory disease (PID)
  from chlamydia, 6
  from gonorrhea, 9
Penile cancer, 63
Perry, Rick, 64–65, 125, 162–163. *See also* Mandatory HPV Vaccination
Personal, Social, Health, and Economic Education (PSHE) rubric (United Kingdom), 79
Pharmacists and Plan B controversy, 59–62
  AMA position, 60
  APhA position, 60
  Christian group position, 60
  Concerned Women for America action, 62
  federal/state regulation attempts, 61
  Walgreen pharmacy example, 59
Pharmacy Access Partnership, 218–219
The Pill. *See* Oral contraception
Pincus, Gregory Goodwin, 129, 141–142
Pink Triangle Trust, 80
The Pivot of Civilization (Sanger), 146
Plan B (emergency contraception), 19
  age/availability controversy, 58–59
  pharmacist dispensing controversy, 59–62
  prescription vs. over-the-counter, 58

Planned Parenthood Federation of America (PPFA), 128, 219
Poland, sex education in, 78
Population Action International (PAI), 219–220
Population Council (PC), 144, 220–221
Positive Living Project (USAID), 208
Preacher's Son (Jennings), 133
Pregnancy and contraception, 14–21
  abstinence/fertility awareness, 19–20
  barrier methods, 15–17
  historical background, 14–15
  hormonal methods, 15, 17–19
  intrauterine devices, 19
  sterilization, 20–21
Pregnancy/live birthrates for females 15–19 years of age, by age, race. Hispanic origin (1980–2000), 192–193
Premarital pregnancy, 33
Preparing Young People for Adult Life: Personal, Social, Health, and Economic Education (PSHE) (UK), 79
Prevention Not Prohibition campaign (CFC), 207
Prevention programs, for HIV/AIDS, 13–14, 90–92
  in Argentina, 92
  in Cambodia, 91–92
  in the Dominican Republic, 91
  in India, 92
  in Tanzania, 91
Pro-Choice Public Education Project (PEP), 221
Program for Appropriate Technology in Health, 214
Programme of Action (World Population Plan of Action), 96–97
PROJECT 10 teachers, 46

PSHE rubric. See Personal, Social, Health, and Economic Education (PSHE) rubric
Public Health Service Act (1981) (Title XX), 37, 200
Public opinion polls
  on homosexuality, 24–25
  on sex education, 34–36
Public sexual health issues, 180–182

Questions and Answers about Love and Sex (Calderone), 128
Quierosaber.org, 204

Reagan, Ronald, 98, 156. *See also* Mexico City Policy
Reisman, Judith A., 46
Release from Sexual Tensions (Calderone), 128
Religious Coalition for Reproductive Choice (RCRC), 221–222
Religious freedom rights (First Amendment, U.S. Constitution), 173
Report of the Fourth Meeting of the Follow-Up Committee on the Implementation of the Dakar/Ngor Declaration (DND) and the Programme of Action of the International Conference on Population and Development (ICPD-PA), 97
Reproductive Health and Research (RHR) Department (WHO), 95
Reproductive Health Technologies (RHTP), 222–223
Research on abstinence-only education, 39–41
Resources for Parents of GLBT Youth, 228
Resources for Youth suicide counseling, 228

Responsible Education About Life (REAL) Act (2007), 159–161
Responsible Social Values Programs (RSVP), 203
Riksförbundet för Sexuell Upplysning (Swedish Association for Sexuality Education), 138
Rock, John, 142–143
Rockefeller, John D., III, 143–145
Roe v. Wade (1973), 157–158, 170–171, 217
Roman Catholic Church, 78, 85
Romania World Population Conference, 96–97
Rosenbaum, Janet E., 39
Rusk, Dean, 134

Safe Schools Program for Gay and Lesbian Students (Massachusetts), 139
Sainsbury, J., 206
Sanger, Margaret, 129, 142, 145–146, 219. See also Planned Parenthood Federation of America
Santorum, Rick, 36, 38, 154–156
Satcher, David, 180–182
School programs, issues transcending, 31, 33, 53–65
contraceptive access, 57–58
contraceptive devices access, 53–57
contraceptives, pharmacist prescriptions, 59–62
human papillomavirus, 62–65
Plan B controversy, 58–59
Search and Seizure (Fourth) Amendment (U.S. Constitution), 169
The See Change Campaign (CFC), 207
Self-Incrimination Clause (Fifth Amendment, U.S. Constitution), 169

Separate Program for Abstinence Education (1996), 154–156
Sex education, 33–53. See also Abstinence-only education
abortion, 50–52
in Africa, 87
in Australia, 83–84
Chicago Experiment, 31–33
in China, 81–82
condom instruction, 42–44
course content, 36–42
decisions about teaching, 52–53
in Denmark, 77
homosexuality, 44–50
in India, 82–83
in Japan, 81
in Latin America, 85–86
in the Muslim World, 84–85
in the Netherlands, 77–78
NPR/KFF/JFK poll on, 35–36, 49–50
opposition to, 33
Parker v. Hurley, 48, 174–177
in Poland, 78
public opinion on, 34–36
school-based, 31, 33
in Spain, 78–79
in the United Kingdom, 79–80
Vision for the Future, 180–182
Sex Education: An Islamic Perspective (Athar), 84
Sex Education Guidelines (Japan), 81
Sexual Behavior in the Human Female (Kinsey), 133, 134, 199
Sexual Behavior in the Human Male (Kinsey), 133, 199
Sexual Health and Family Planning (Calderone), 128
Sexual Minority Youth Assistance League (SMYAL), 227
Sexual orientation and gender identity, 21–28
GLBTQ youth issues, 24–28
hormonal basis, 21–22
public opinion polls, 24–25

terminology, 22–24
worldwide perspectives, 98–101
Sexuality and Human Values
(Calderone), 128
Sexuality Information and
Education Council (SIEC)
(U.S.), 223
Sexually active high school
students using condoms or
birth control pills by sex, race,
ethnicity (2003), 193–194
Sexually Information and
Education Council (SIECUS),
51, 128
Sexually transmitted diseases
(STDs), 38–39, 44, 94–95
American Social Health
Association, 4, 204–205
cases, in U.S. (2007), 5
Helium poll, 56–57
historical background, 2–3
symptoms, prognosis,
treatment, 5–14
types of, 3–5
Vision for the Future, 180
WHO focus on, 95, 201–202
Sexually transmitted infections
(STIs). *See* Sexually
transmitted diseases
Sexually transmitted infections
(U.S., 1966–2007), 184–188
Sheldon, Louis, 45
Shepard, Matthew, 146–147, 226
Shingles (human herpesvirus 4), 9
Social Security Act, Title VI, 36, 38
Soranus of Ephesus (Greek
physician), 15
South Africa
education campaigns, 97
gonorrhea data, 96
HIV/AIDS epidemic, 88–89
South Dakota House Bill 1215
(2006), 157–159
South Dakota Task Force to Study
Abortion, 157
Spain, sex education in, 78–79

Spanish Language Media
Initiative, 203
Special Investigations Division
(SID) of the House Committee
on Government Reform, 51
Special Programme of Research,
Development, and Research
Training in Human
Reproduction (WHO), 214
Special Programs of Regional
and National Significance-
Community-Based
Abstinence Education
(SPRANS-CBAE), 37–38, 40,
183
Specter, Arlen, 38
Spermicides, 15–16
Spiritual Power for the Family
(LaHaye), 137
Spiritual Youth for Reproductive
Freedom (SYRF), 222
SPRANS-CBAE. See Special
Programs of Regional and
National Significance-
Community-Based
Abstinence Education
Steichen, Edward, 127
Sterilization, 20–21
Stonehill College, 42
Stopes, Marie, 148–149
Sudan, syphilis data, 95
Suicides/suicide attempts, 25, 229
*A Supplementary Brief and
Statement of Facts* (Sanger),
146
Surgeon General's Call to Action
to Promote Sexual Health and
Responsible Sexual Behavior,
180–182
Swank, Hillary, 149
Swaziland, HIV/AIDS epidemic,
89
Symptoms, prognosis, treatment
of STIs, 5–14
chlamydia, 5–6
gonorrhea, 8–9

hepatitis, 10–12
herpes, 9–10
HIV/AIDS, 12–14
syphilis, 6–8, 94–95
Syphilis, 6–8, 94–95

Talking with Your Child about Sex
  (Calderone), 128–129
Tanzania
  education campaigns, 97
  HIV/AIDS programs, 91
TBCTA tuberculosis control
  program, 212
Teena, Brandon, 149–150
Telling Tales Out of School
  (Jennings), 133
Texas
  Mandatory HVP Vaccination,
  161–163
  Roe v. Wade, 157–158, 170–171,
  217
  Sex Education law, 153–154
Tisdel, Lana, 149
Tolerant Intelligent Network of
  Teens (TINT), 228
Tomorrow Project, 211
Traditional Values Coalition, 45
Transgendered individuals, 23
Treatment/prevention programs,
  for HIV/AIDS, 13–14, 90–92
  in Argentina, 92
  in Cambodia, 91–92
  in the Dominican Republic, 91
  in India, 92
  in Tanzania, 91
Treponema pallidum, 6–7
Tubal ligation, 20–21

Unitarian Universalist
  Association, 221
United Kingdom
  Family Education Trust, 80
  Gay and Lesbian Humanist
  Association, 80
  gay/lesbian organizations, 80
  Pink Triangle Trust, 80

PSHE rubric, 79
  sex education in, 79–80
United Nations Economic
  Commission for Africa, 97
United Nations International
  Conference on Population
  (Mexico), 97–98, 156–157
United Nations Population Fund
  (UNFPA), 97, 200–201
United States Conference of
  Bishops, 223–224
U.S. Agency for International
  Development (USAID),
  156–157, 167–168, 208
U.S. Department of Health and
  Human Services, 200
U.S. Preventive Services Task
  Force (USPSTF), 197
Utah Pride Center, 227–228

Vaccinations
  for hepatitis A, 11
  for hepatitis B, 12
  for human papillomavirus,
  63–65
Vaginal film (barrier method), 16
Vaginal rings, 16, 18
Values and Sexuality program
  (Cuba), 86
Vasectomies, 20–21
Vincent, Clark, 223
Virginity pledge, 39
Vision for the Future section (from
  Surgeon General's report),
  180–182
Vulvar cancer, 63

Walters, Barbara, 136
Wells, Norman, 80
What Every Girl Should Know
  (Sanger), 146
What Every Mother Should Know
  (Sanger), 146
Widerström, Karolina Olivia,
  150–151
Wise Parenthood (Stopes), 149

Woman and the New Race (Sanger), 146

A Woman's Path to True Significance (LaHaye), 137

Women
chlamydia cases/consequences, 4
gonorrhea symptoms, 8
obtaining legal abortions, characteristics of, 188–192

Women's counseling services, 97

Worcester Foundation for Experimental Biology, 129

World Health Assembly, 95

World Health Organization (WHO), 201–202
on maternal deaths during childbirth, 14
on sexually transmitted infections, 95, 201–202
Special Programme of Research, Development, and Research Training in Human Reproduction, 214

World Population Conference, 96, 144

World Population Plan of Action (WWPA), 96

Young Communist Union (UJC) (Cuba), 86

Young People's Sexual Health (YPSH), 224

Youth and Campus Activism program, 226

Youth Development Approaches in Adolescent Family Life Demonstration Projects, 200

Youth Guardian Services (YGS), 228

Youth Lounge (online), 226

Youth Pride, 228–229

Youth Resource (Advocates for Youth), 27

Youth Risk Behavior Surveillance System (YRBSS), 193–194

Zur Hausen, Harald, 151–152

About the Author

David E. Newton holds an associate's degree in science from Grand Rapids (Michigan) Junior College, a B.A. in chemistry (with high distinction) and an M.A. in education from the University of Michigan, and an Ed.D. in science education from Harvard University. He is the author of more than 400 textbooks, encyclopedias, resource books, research manuals, laboratory manuals, trade books, and other educational materials. He taught mathematics, chemistry, and physical science in Grand Rapids, Michigan, for 13 years; was professor of chemistry and physics at Salem State College in Massachusetts for 15 years; and was adjunct professor in the College of Professional Studies at the University of San Francisco for 10 years. Previous books for ABC-CLIO include *Global Warming: A Reference Handbook* (1993), *Gay and Lesbian Rights: A Reference Handbook* (1994, 2010), *The Ozone Dilemma: A Reference Handbook* (1995), *Violence and the Mass Media: A Reference Handbook* (1996), *Encyclopedia of Cryptology* (1997), and *Social Issues in Science and Technology: An Encyclopedia* (1999), and *DNA Technology* (2010).